New Frontiers in Pharmacognosy
and Phytotherapy

New Frontiers in Pharmacognosy and Phytotherapy

Edited by Kendall Jefferson

hayle
medical

New York

Hayle Medical,
750 Third Avenue, 9th Floor,
New York, NY 10017, USA

Visit us on the World Wide Web at:
www.haylemedical.com

ISBN: 978-1-63241-793-0

Cataloging-in-Publication Data

New frontiers in pharmacognosy and phytotherapy / edited by Kendall Jefferson.
    p. cm.
Includes bibliographical references and index.
ISBN 978-1-63241-793-0
1. Pharmacognosy. 2. Materia medica, Vegetable. 3. Drugs. 4. Pharmacy.
5. Herbs--Therapeutic use. 6. Medicinal plants. I. Jefferson, Kendall.
RS160 .N49 2019
615.321--dc23

Table of Contents

Preface

The branch of pharmacy which studies the medicinal drugs derived from plants and other natural sources is known as pharmacognosy. It is the scientific study of the clinical use of herbal medicines and their effects. Phytotherapy is a field involving the study of alternative medical practices in which unrefined plant or animal extracts are used for treatment purposes in place of conventional medicine. Many of the modern drugs in the pharmacopoeia today are derived from plants. Quinine, aspirin, digitalis and opium are some herbal remedies that have a long history of use. Herbal remedies are quite prevalently used in patients with chronic illnesses, such as asthma, diabetes, cancer, etc. Herbal dietary supplements also fall under the field of phytotherapy. This book unfolds the innovative aspects of pharmacognosy and phytotherapy which will be crucial for the progress of these fields in the future. It presents researches and studies performed by experts across the globe. The readers would gain knowledge that would broaden their perspective about pharmacognosy and phytotherapy.

Various studies have approached the subject by analyzing it with a single perspective, but the present book provides diverse methodologies and techniques to address this field. This book contains theories and applications needed for understanding the subject from different perspectives. The aim is to keep the readers informed about the progresses in the field; therefore, the contributions were carefully examined to compile novel researches by specialists from across the globe.

Indeed, the job of the editor is the most crucial and challenging in compiling all chapters into a single book. In the end, I would extend my sincere thanks to the chapter authors for their profound work. I am also thankful for the support provided by my family and colleagues during the compilation of this book.

Editor

Antibacterial attributes of extracts of *Phyllantus amarus* and *Phyllantus niruri* on *Escherichia coli* the causal organism of urinary tract infection

Idayat Titilayo Gbadamosi

Department of Botany, University of Ibadan, Nigeria.

In view of the prevalence of urinary tract infection (UTI) worldwide, the increasing resistance of pathogenic bacteria to conventional antibiotics and their side effects, the aerial part and root of *Phyllanthus amarus* (Schum. and Thonn.) and *Phyllanthus niruri* (L.) were analysed for mineral and phytochemical constituents, and their ethanol extracts screened against five clinical isolates of *Escherichia coli* associated with UTI, to ascertain their effectiveness in UTI treatment, and provide basis for future clinical trials of the two plants. The isolates ($10^{-1} \times 10^{-6}$ cfu/ml) were tested against ethanol extracts (10 mg/ml) of plant parts using agar well diffusion method. Phytochemical and mineral analyses of the plant samples were done using standard protocols and all data were statistically analysed. The quantities of various phytochemical compounds and minerals were significantly ($P<0.05$) higher in *P. niruri* than *P. amarus*. At 10^{-6} cfu/ml inoculum concentration of all isolates, the inhibitory activities of extracts of *P. amarus* and *P. niruri* were the same, and significant ($P<0.05$) against isolates EC01, EC02, EC04 and EC05 compared to the control experiment. The inhibitory pattern varied against EC03, extract B (29.00 mm) was the most active, followed by extract C (24.00 mm), and extracts A and D gave the same diameter (19.00 mm) of inhibition. The two plants showed significant antibacterial activity against isolates and could be good alternatives to chemical antibiotics in the treatment of *E. coli* related UTI, however the mechanism of action of the plant extracts in treatment should be investigated.

Key words: Antibacterial activity, *E. coli*, *Phyllanthus amarus*, *Phyllanthus niruri*, urinary tract infection.

INTRODUCTION

A urinary tract infection (UTI) is a bacterial infection of the urinary tract consisting of the kidneys, ureters, bladder and the urethra. An infection of the lower urinary tract is a simple cystitis (bladder infection) of the upper tract pyelonephritis (a kidney infection). Common symptoms include burning with frequent urination (or an urge to urinate) in the absence of vaginal discharge and significant pain. These symptoms may vary from mild to severe and in healthy women lasting an average of six days (Nicolle, 2008; Lane and Takhar, 2011). People

*Corresponding author. E-mail: gita4me2004@yahoo.com.

having pyelonephritis, may experience flank pain, fever, or nausea, and vomiting in addition to the classic symptoms of a lower urinary tract infection (Colgan and William, 2011). Rarely the urine may appear bloody or contain visible pus (Lane and Takhar, 2011; Salvatore et al., 2011). Urinary tract infections occur more commonly in women than men, with half of women having at least one infection at some point in their lives. Recurrences of infection are common and risk factors include female anatomy, sexual intercourse and family history (Salvatore et al., 2011).

The main causal agent of cystitis and pyelonephritis is *Escherichia coli*, which causes of 80 to 90% of UTI (Nicolle, 2008; Salvatore et al., 2011). The increasing prevalence of antimicrobial resistance and side effects of antibiotics are major health problem worldwide. Results of multidrug resistance in *E.coli* isolates from many parts of the world have shown that the choice of drugs for the treatment of UTI is quite narrow today. Many drugs which are considered effective against uropathogens are now rarely prescribed as empirical therapy in areas where resistance rate to these antibiotics is high (Rawat and Umesh, 2010; Shalini et al., 2011). The side effects of antibiotics such as fever, nausea, diarrhoea and neurotoxicity have been reported in literature (www.bestnaturalremedies.net; Grill and Maganti 2011).

Phyllanthus amarus originates from tropical America, and has spread as a weed throughout the tropics and subtropics. In Africa, the plant is useful in the treatment of gonorrhoea, diarrhoea, dysentery, stomach-ache and haemorrhoids. A suppository of the leaf paste is applied to the vagina to treat amenorrhoea and polyps. Leaf sap, mixed with palm oil or not, is applied as ear drops to treat otitis and applied to abscesses, sores and wounds (Burkill, 1994). *Phyllanthus niruri* is a widespread tropical plant. It is an important plant of Indian Ayurvedic system of medicine used for problems of the stomach, genitourinary system, liver, kidney and spleen. The plant has also been used in Brazil and Peru as an herbal remedy for kidney stones (Patel et al., 2011).

In view of the prevalence of UTI in the world, the increasing resistance of pathogenic bacteria to antibiotics and side effects of antibiotics due to prolong use, this study screened *P. amarus* and *P. niruri* for phytochemical and mineral constituents. Also the ethanol extracts of aerial parts and roots of the two plants were tested against five clinical isolates of *E. coli* associated with UTI, to ascertain their efficacy in UTI treatment, and present them as alternatives to chemical antibiotics which could also be mammalian toxic and not easily biodegradable like the botanicals.

MATERIALS AND METHODS

Identification and preparation of plant materials

Whole plants of *P. amarus* and *P. niruri* were collected from the nursery of the Department of Botany, University of Ibadan, Nigeria.

The plant samples were identified and deposited in the University of Ibadan Herbarium (UIH). They were then thoroughly washed, separated into aerial parts and roots.

Phytochemical analysis of powdered plant samples

Powdered samples were screened for the presence of active compounds such as alkaloids, saponins, tannins, phenols and glycosides, using standard techniques (AOAC, 2005).

Mineral analysis of powdered plant samples

The method of Walsh (1971) was used for digestion of the two plant samples. After digestion calcium (Ca), magnesium (Mg), copper (Cu), zinc (Zn), iron (Fe), sodium (Na) and potassium (K) were analysed using Atomic Absorption Spectrophotometer (FC 210/211 VGP Bausch scientific AAS). Phosphorus was determined using Vanadomolybdate (Yellow method.). Percent transmittance was determined at 400 nm using Spectronic 20 (Bausch and Lomb) Colorimeter (AOAC, 2005).

Preparation of extracts

The fresh aerial parts (500 g each) and roots (500 g each) of *P. amarus* and *P. niruri* were macerated and extracted in 1000 ml of 80% ethanol for a week using cold extraction method. The extract was concentrated at 40°C, and stored in the refrigerator (4°C) prior to use. The extracts were coded as follows: A= *Phyllantus amarus* aerial parts; B= *P. amarus* roots; C= *P. niruri* aerial parts; D= *P. niruri* roots. 10 mg/ml of each extract was used for antibacterial screening against *E. coli* isolates.

Source of *E. coli* isolates

The test organisms were clinical urine isolates of *E. coli* associated with UTI in female patients, obtained through due process from University College Hospital (UCH), Ibadan, Nigeria.

Antibacterial assay

The isolates were maintained in cultures on nutrient agar (Difco Laboratories, USA). They were grown in nutrient broth (Difco Laboratories, USA) for 18 h at 35°C. Six concentrations of each isolate were prepared from the broth in sterile distilled water to give a range of concentrations at 10^{-1} to 10^{-6} cfu/ ml via serial dilution method prior to use. Exactly 1 ml of the inoculum was thoroughly mixed with 19 ml of sterile nutrient agar and poured into sterile Petri dish. The agar was left to solidify. Two wells of 6 mm in diameter were punctured in each agar plate and 60 µl of each extract was filled into the wells with the aid of a sterile micropipette. Sterile distilled water and ethanol were used instead of extract in the control experiment. Also, plates containing the test organisms in agar without extract were used as control. All experiments were done aseptically and each experiment was replicated three times. The plates were incubated at 37°C for 24 to 48 h. The zone of inhibition was measured and recorded in millimeters (mm).

Statistical analysis

Analysis of variance and comparison of means were carried out on all data using Statistical Analysis System (SAS). Differences between means were assessed for significance at P<0.05 by

Table 1. Phytochemical components of *P. amarus* and *P. niruri*.

Plant sample	Alkaloids (%)	Saponins (%)	Tannins (%)	Phenols (%)	Glycosides (%)
P. amarus	$0.096^b \pm 0.002$	$0.190^b \pm 0.002$	$0.022^b \pm 0.002$	$0.067^b \pm 0.002$	$0.077^b \pm 0.002$
P. niruri	$0.122^a \pm 0.002$	$0.214^a \pm 0.001$	$0.040^a \pm 0.001$	$0.079^a \pm 0.002$	$0.090^a \pm 0.002$

Values within a column followed by the same superscript are not significantly different at $P < 0.05$.

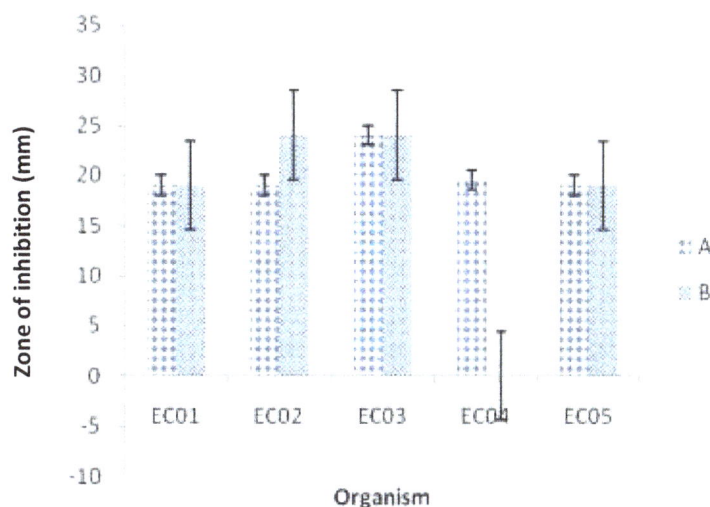

Figure 1. Comparative antibacterial activity of aerial part and root of *P. amarus* against *E. coli* (1×10^{-2} cfu/ml). A = aerial parts; B = roots.

Duncan's multiple range test (DMRT).

RESULTS

The two plants contained alkaloids, saponins, tannins, phenols and glycosides in varied quantity (Table 1). Saponin was the highest phytochemical in the two plants. The saponin content of *P. niruri* (0.214 %) was higher than *P. amarus* (0.190 %). Generally, the quantity of the various phytochemicals was significantly ($P<0.05$) higher in *P. niruri* than *P. amarus*. The mineral analysis revealed the presence of sodium (Na), potassium (K), calcium (Ca), phosphorus (P), magnesium (Mg), zinc (Zn), copper (Cu) and iron (Fe) in both plants (Table 2). *P. niruri* contained 46.35% of Zn whereas *P. amarus* had 28.20%. Copper was higher in *P. niruri* (5.60%) than *P. amarus* (2.20%). Overall, *P. niruri* was significantly richer in all minerals than *P. amarus*.

The extracts of the two plants showed antibacterial activity against the test organisms (Table 3). On isolate EC01, extract C was the most active (21.00 mm), followed by extract D (19.00 mm) and the least (11.00 mm) activity was observed in extract A at 10^{-1} cfu/ml. On isolate EC02, extract C gave the highest (19.00 mm)

inhibition, followed by extract D with 14.00 mm diameter of inhibition and the least (11.00 mm) activity was observed in extract B at 10^{-1} cfu/ml. The highest (24.00 mm) inhibitory activity against isolate EC03 at 10^{-1} cfu/ml was from extract B, followed by extracts A and C with 14.00 mm, extract D was inactive on isolate EC03 at 10^{-1} cfu/ml. At high concentration (10^{-1} cfu/ml) of inoculum of isolate EC04, extracts B and D were inactive, whereas extracts A and C gave the same diameter (19.00 mm) of inhibition. Although, extract B and D were inactive against isolate EC04 at high inoculum concentrations (10^{-1} and 10^{-3} cfu/ml), their activity increased along concentration gradient to 24.00 mm at 10^{-5} cfu/ml. All extracts (A, B, C and D) gave the same diameter (24.00 mm) of inhibition against EC04 at 10^{-5} cfu/ml. Isolate EC05 was susceptible to all extracts at 10^{-1} cfu/ml with the same diameter (24.00 mm) and extracts C and D were the most active (24.00 to 29.00 mm) against EC05 at all inoculum concentrations ($10^{-1} – 10^{-5}$ cfu/ml). Overall, the extracts (C and D) of *P. niruri* were more active than extracts (A and B) of *P. amarus* on isolates EC01, EC02, and EC05.

The comparative inhibitory effect of extracts of the aerial part and root of *P. amarus* showed that the root was inactive on isolate EC04 at 10^{-2} cfu/ml (Figure 1). The root extract of *P. niruri* was more active than the

Table 2. Mineral constituents of *P. amarus* and *P. niruri*.

Plant sample	%Na	%K	%Ca	%P	%Mg	%Zn	%Cu	%Fe
P. amarus	0.03±0.002	0.19[a]±.001	0.03[b]±0.001	0.19±0.001	0.26[b]±0.002	28.20±0.141	2.20[b]±0.141	12.65[b]±0.212
P. niruri	0.06±0.001	0.12[a]±0.001	0.07[a]±0.002	0.21±0.002	0.34±0.002	46.35±0.212	5.60[a]±0.141	37.40±0.282

Values within a column followed by the same superscript are not significantly different at $P < 0.05$.

aerial part extract on isolate EC04 at 10^{-4} cfu/ml (Figure 2). The collective antibacterial activity of all extracts of *P. amarus* and *P. niruri* against each isolate of *E. coli* at 10^{-6} cfu/ml is presented in Figure 3. The inhibitory activity of all extracts was the same against isolates EC01, EC02, EC04 and EC05. The inhibitory pattern of the extracts varied against EC03, extract B (29.00 mm) was the most active against it, followed by extract C (24. 00 mm) and extract A (19.00 mm) and D (19.00 mm) gave the same diameter of inhibition.

DISCUSSION

Although, *P. amarus* and *P. niruri* are often confused as the same plant species (Taylor, 2003), this study has shown clearly that the two plants are entirely different species. They differ in their phytochemical constituents. *P. niruri* contained significantly higher quantity of alkaloids, saponins, tannins, phenols and glycosides than *P. amarus*. Many valuable compounds isolated from the two plants have been reported to be responsible for their extensive pharmacological uses (Patel et al., 2011; Damle, 2008).

The mineral components of *P. niruri* were significantly higher than that of *P. amarus*. The occurrence of these minerals in both *Phyllanthus* species indicates that the plants have nutritional and therapeutic values. As an example Zn is an essential mineral required for normal growth and development, healthy skin, infection prevention

and wound healing. A zinc deficiency might cause delayed growth and development in children and adolescents, hair loss, diarrhoea, delayed wound healing, loss of appetite and weight loss. Children in developing countries who are zinc deficient might be at increased risk of infections such as pneumonia (Kirby, 2011). Zn has application in wound healing and ulcers (Patel et al., 2011). Zinc could also play a role in pneumonia prevention, and is recommended by the World Health Organization (WHO) and United Nations Children's Fund (UNICEF) as a treatment for acute diarrhoea (www.akilinitiative.org). Copper is an essential trace element that is vital to the health of all living things. In humans, copper is essential to the proper functioning of organs and metabolic processes (Johnson, 2008). Iron is an essential mineral needed for the formation of hemoglobin; an iron deficiency can lead to aneamia, a condition characterized by fatigue, shortness of breath, dizziness, weight loss and headaches (Kirby, 2011).

There is dearth of information in the literature on the use of *Phyllanthus* species in UTI treatment. As shown by the present study, the significant antibacterial activity of ethanol extracts of the two plants against *E. coli* is an indication of their therapeutic potential in management of UTI. Results obtained in this work agree with the findings of previous authors on antimicrobial status of *P. amarus* (Alli et al., 2011; Eldeen et al., 2011; Njoroge et al., 2012). Although, there is scarcity of information on the antimicrobial activity

of *P. niruri* in the literature, it has been reported to be effective against hepatitis B and other viral infections (Bhattacharjee and Sil, 2006; Bhattacharjee and Sil, 2007). The authors suggested that *P. niruri* species might inhibit proliferation of the virus by inhibiting replication of the genetic material of the virus (Thyagarajan et al., 1988). The lipid lowering activity of *P. niruri* has been reported (Chandra, 2000), as well as its antidiabetic, antimalarial, analgesic, and anti-spasmodic properties (Raphael and Sabu, 2000; Neraliya and Gaur, 2004; Santos, 1994). The therapeutic value of herbal remedies in UTI has been reported by previous authors. Ahmed et al. (2012) reported that the administration of aqueous extract of corn silk (*Zea mays*) significantly reduced the symptoms in patient with UTI in addition to reduction in the values of pus cells, red blood cells (RBCs), and crystals, without any reported side effect which indicated its efficacy and safety. Geetha et al. (2011) reported that *Vaccinium macrocarpon* (Cranberry), *Hydrastis canadensis* (Goldenseal), *Agathosma betulina* (Buchu), *Arctostaphylos uva-ursi* (Bearberry), *Echinaceae purpurea* (Cone flower) and *Equisetum arvense* (Horsetail) have been clinically proven for urinary tract infection cure as well as bladder infection treatment.

Mustard oils prepared with *Moringa oleifera* (horseradish) and nasturtium (Tropaelum), and grapeseed (*Vitis vinifera*) extract are effective in the treatment of UTI (www.naturalnews.com). Goldenrod (Asteraceae) is widely used in Europe

Table 3. *In-vitro* antibacterial activity of ethanol extracts of *P. amarus* and *P. niruri* against *E. coli* isolates implicated in UTI.

Plant extract	*E. coli* Isolate	Inoculum load (cfu/ml) / Zone of inhibition (mm)		
		1×10^{-1}	1×10^{-3}	1×10^{-5}
A		$11.00^e \pm 1.14$	$29.00^a \pm 1.14$	$29.00^a \pm 1.14$
B		$14.00^d \pm 1.14$	$29.00^a \pm 1.14$	$29.00^a \pm 1.14$
C	EC01	$21.00^b \pm 1.14$	$29.00^a \pm 1.14$	$29.00^a \pm 1.14$
D		$19.00^c \pm 1.14$	$29.00^a \pm 1.14$	$29.00^a \pm 1.14$
A		$14.00^d \pm 1.14$	$19.00^c \pm 1.14$	$19.00^c \pm 1.14$
B		$11.00^e \pm 1.41$	$24.00^b \pm 1.41$	$24.00^b \pm 1.41$
C	EC02	$19.00^c \pm 1.41$	$19.00^c \pm 1.41$	$24.00^b \pm 1.41$
D		$14.00^d \pm 1.41$	$19.00^c \pm 1.41$	$24.00^b \pm 1.41$
A		$14.00^d \pm 1.41$	$24.00^b \pm 1.41$	$19.00^c \pm 1.14$
B		$24.00^a \pm 1.41$	$24.00^b \pm 1.41$	$19.00^c \pm 1.14$
C	EC03	$14.00^d \pm 1.41$	$0.00^d \pm 0.00$	$29.00^a \pm 1.14$
D		$0.00^f \pm 0.00$	$24.00^b \pm 1.41$	$29.00^a \pm 1.14$
A		$19.00^c \pm 1.41$	$19.50^c \pm 0.70$	$24.00^b \pm 1.14$
B		$0.00^f \pm 0.00$	$0.00^d \pm 0.00$	$24.00^b \pm 1.14$
C	EC04	$19.00^c \pm 1.41$	$19.00^c \pm 1.41$	$24.00^b \pm 1.14$
D		$0.00^f \pm 0.00$	$19.00^c \pm 1.41$	$24.00^b \pm 1.14$
A		$24.00^a \pm 1.41$	$19.00^c \pm 1.41$	$29.00^a \pm 1.14$
B		$24.00^a \pm 1.41$	$19.00^c \pm 1.41$	$29.00^a \pm 1.14$
C	EC05	$24.00^a \pm 1.41$	$29.00^a \pm 1.41$	$29.00^a \pm 1.14$
D		$24.00^a \pm 1.41$	$29.00^a \pm 1.41$	$29.00^a \pm 1.14$

Values are mean ± SD of three replicates. Values within a column followed by the same superscript are not significantly different at $P < 0.05$. Daimeter of cork borer = 6 mm. A = *Phyllantus amarus* aerial parts; B = *Phyllantus amarus* roots; C= *Phyllantus niruri* aerial parts; D = *Phyllantus niruri* roots.

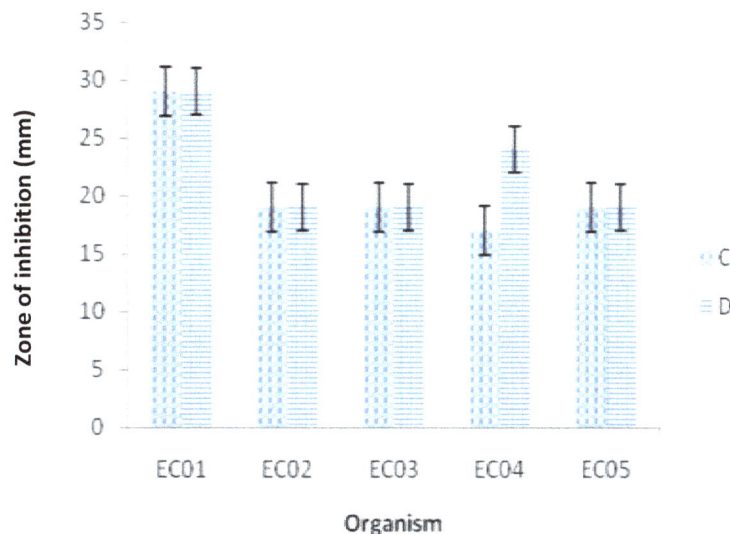

Figure 2. Comparative antibacterial activity of aerial part and root of *P. niruri* against *E. coli* (1×10^{-4} cfu/ml). C = aerial parts; D = roots.

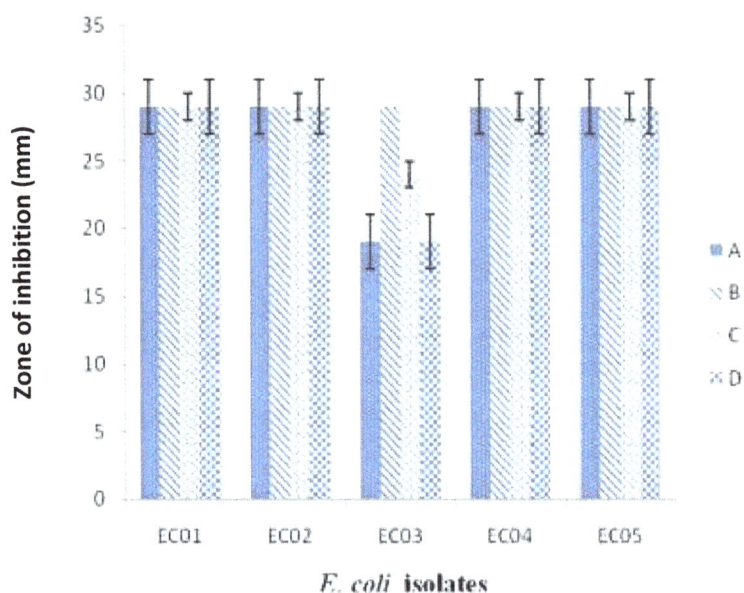

Figure 3. *In-vitro* antibacterial activity of ethanol extracts of *Phyllantus amarus* and *Phyllantus niruri* against *E. coli* (1×10^{-6} cfu/ml). A = *Phyllantus amarus* aerial parts; B = *Phyllantus amarus* roots; C = *Phyllantus niruri* aerial parts; D = *Phyllantus niruri* roots.

as an herb of choice for the treatment of urinary tract infections; it decreases inflammation and the painful spasms of bladder infections. Dandelion (*Taraxacum sp*) acts as a diuretic and flushes bacteria-causing microbes from the bladder. Dandelion also provides potassium, typically lost with diuretic use. Marshmallow (*Althaea officinalis*) root inhibits bacterial growth in urine by increasing its acidity (www.livestrong.com).

Conclusion

The ethanol extracts of aerial parts and roots of *P. amarus* and *P. niruri* showed significant antibacterial activity against isolates of *E. coli* (the main causative organism of UTI). Comparatively, there was no significant difference in the antibacterial activities of the extracts of the two plants; they differ significantly in their chemical and mineral constituents. The antibacterial activities of the extracts of the two plants could be attributed to their phytochemical and mineral components. The inhibitory activities of *P. amarus* and *P. niruri* extracts were the same against four of the five *E. coli* isolates, this shows that either plant species could be used in the treatment of UTI. It could be suggested that a decoction or an infusion of either of the two herbs could help in the treatment of UTI. However, an investigation of the mechanism of action of the two plants could enhance the understanding of their role in UTI treatment. Furthermore, this article provides basis for future clinical trials of compounds and extracts of the two plants in UTI patients.

REFERENCES

Ahmed SS, Mohammed IH, Hamdan SJ (2012). Use of aqueous extract of corn silk in the treatment of urinary tract infection. J. Intercult. Ethnopharmacol. 1(2):93-96.

Alli AI, Ehinmidu JO, Ibrahim YKE (2011). Preliminary phytochemical screening and antimicrobial activities of some medicinal plants used in Ebiraland. Bayero J. Pure Appl. Sci. 4:10-16.

AOAC (2005). Official Methods of Analysis, eighteenth ed. Association of Official Analytical Chemists, Washington, DC., USA.

Bhattacharjee R, Sil PC (2006). Hepatoprotective effect of aqueous extract of *Phyllanthus niruri* on nimesulide-induced oxidative stress *in vivo*. Indian J. Biochem. Biophys. 43(5):299-305.

Bhattacharjee R, Sil PC (2007). Protein isolate from the herb, *Phyllanthus niruri* L. (Euphorbiaceae), plays hepatoprotective role against carbon tetrachloride induced liver damage via its antioxidant properties. Food Chem. Toxicol. 45(5):817-826.

Burkill HM (1994). The useful plants of West Tropical Africa, second ed. Volume 2, Royal Botanic Gardens, Kew, Richmond, United Kingdom.

Chandra R (2000). Lipid lowering activity of *P. niruri*. J. Med. Arom. Plant Sci. 22(1):29-30.

Colgan R, Williams M (2011). Diagnosis and treatment of acute uncomplicated cystitis. Am. Fam. Physician 84(7):771-776.

Damle MC (2008). *Phyllanthus niruri*. Available at: http://www.pharmainfo.net/reviews/phyllanthus-niruri

Eldeen IMS, Seow EM, Abdullah R, Sulaiman SF (2011). *In vitro* antibacterial, antioxidant, total phenolic contents and anti-HIV-1 reverse activities of extracts of seven *Phyllanthus* sp. S. Afr. J. Bot. 77:75-79.

Geetha RV, Roy A, Lakshmi T (2011). Nature's weapon against urinary tract infections. Int. J. Drug Dev. Res. 3(3):85-100.

Grill MF, Maganti RK (2011). Neurotoxic effects associated with antibiotic use: management considerations. Br. J. Clin. Pharmacol. 72:381-393.

Johnson MD (2008). "Copper". Merck Manual Home Health Handbook. Merck Sharp & Dohme Corp., a subsidiary of Merck & Co., Inc. Available at: http://www.merck-manuals.com/404.html

Kirby S (2011). What are health benefits of micronutrients? Available at: www.livestrong.com/article/441906-what-are-health-benefits-of-micronutrients/

Lane DR, Takhar SS (2011). Diagnosis and management of urinary tract infection and pyelonephritis.Emerg. Med. Clin. North Am. 29(3):539-552.

Neraliya S, Gaur R (2004). Juvenoid activity in plant extracts against filarial mosquito Culex quinquefasciatus. J. Med. Arom. Plant Sci. 26(1):34-38.

Nicolle LE (2008). Uncomplicated urinary tract infection in adults including uncomplicated pyelonephritis. Urol. Clin. North Am. 35(1):1-12.

Njoroge AD, Anyango B, Dossaji SF (2012). Screening of Phyllanthus species for antimicrobial properties. Chem. Sci. J. 56:1-11.

Patel JR, Tripathi P, Sharma V, Chauhan NS, Dixit VK (2011). Phyllanthus amarus: Ethnomedicinal uses, phytochemistry and pharmacology: A review. J. Ethnopharmacol. 138(2):286-313.

Raphael KR, Sabu MC (2000). Antidiabetic activity of Phyllanthus niruri. Amala Res. Bull. 20:19-25.

Rawat V, Umesh PP (2010). Antibiotic resistance pattern of urinary tract isolates of Escherichia coli from Kumaun region. J. Comm. Dis. 42(1):63-66.

Salvatore S, Salvatore S, Cattoni E, Siesto G, Serati M, Sorice P, Torella M (2011). Urinary tract infections in women. Eur. J. Obstet. Gynecol. Reprod. Biol. 156(2):131-136.

Santos AR (1994). Analgesic effects of callus culture extracts from selected species of Phyllanthus in mice. J. Pharm. Pharmacol. 46(9):755-759.

Shalini JMC, Rashid MK, Joshi HS (2011). Study of antibiotic sensitivity pattern in urinary tract infection at a tertiary Hospital. Natl. J. Integr. Res. Med. (NJIRM) 2(3):43-46.

Taylor L (2003). Herbal secrets of the rainforest 2nd ed. Sage Press; Inc. USA.

Thyagarajan SP, Subramanian S, Thirunalasundar T (1988). Effect of Phyllanthus niruri on chronic carriers of hepatitis B virus. Lancet 2: 764-766.

Walsh LM (1971). Instrumental methods for the analysis of soils and plant tissue. Soil Science Society of America, Inc. Madison Wisconsin, USA.

www.bestnaturalremedies.net/antibiotics-associated-diarrhea. Antibiotics-Associated-Diarrhea-All you should know by Chris & Taylor. Accessed 1st March 2015.

www.livestrong.com. Herbs for urinary tract infection. Accessed 14th Dec. 2012.

www.naturanews.com. Use herbs to kill the bacteria that cause urinary tract infections. Accessed 14th Dec. 2012.

## 2

Phytochemical and zootechnical studies of *Physalis peruviana* L. leaves exposured to streptozotocin-induced diabetic rats

C. N. Fokunang[1]*, F. K. Mushagalusa[2], E. Tembe-Fokunang[1], J. Ngoupayo[3], B. Ngameni[3], L. N. Njinkio[4], J. N. Kadima[6], F. A. Kechia[4], B. Atogho-Tiedeu[5], W. F. Mbacham[6] and B. T. Ngadjui[3]

[1]Department of Pharmacotoxicology and Pharmacokinetics, Faculty of Medicine and Biomedical Sciences, University of Yaoundé I, P. O. Box 1634, Yaoundé Cameroon.
[2]Department of Pharmacy, Faculty of Medicine and Pharmacy, Official University of Bukavu, P. O. Box 570 Bukavu, Democratic Republic of Congo.
[3]Department of Pharmacognosy and Pharmaceutical chemistry, University of Bamenda, Cameroon.
[4]Department of Medical Laboratory Sciences, University of Bamenda, Cameroon.
[5]Department of Biochemistry, Faculty of Sciences; University of Yaounde I, P. O. Box 812 Yaounde, Cameroon.
[6]Department of Pharmacology, School of Medicine and Health Sciences, University of Rwanda, Rwanda.

This is a phytochemical and zootechnical study on *Physalis peruviana* leaves in streptozotocin induced diabetic rats. This was part of a scientific development program of plant resources used in Congolese traditional medicine for the treatment of diabetes mellitus in which individual and community consequences are well established. Different fractions with hexane, ethyl acetate and the residue were obtained from the hydroalcoholic extract of *P. peruviana* leaves. Phytochemical screening was focused on the usual reactions of characterization based on precipitation and coloration with general reagents. The diabetic conditions were induced in rats by a single administration of streptozotocin (50 mg/kg body weight) intravenously. The positive control group received glibenclamide (6.5 mg/kg body weight) and each test group received 100 mg/kg of body weight. Those groups were compared with a control group which received only a Tween 20 solution (1 ml per 100 g body weight). Zootechnical profiles were evaluated by weight monitoring as well as food and water consumption in rats. Phytochemical screening showed the presence of polyphenols, flavonoids, alkaloids, saponins, tannins, anthocyanins, mucilages, cardiac glycosides, coumarins and betalains in the hydroalcoholic extract and its fractions. A highly significant difference ($P < 0.001$) of water consumption in opposition to the food intake and weight changes was observed. This study suggested the isolation and characterization of compounds from hydroalcoholic extract from the leaves of *P. peruviana* L. and its fractions for an extensive antidiabetic investigation.

Key words: *Physalis peruviana*, phytochemical, antidiabetic activity, streptozotocin, zootechnical parameters.

INTRODUCTION

Several pathophysiological processes are involved in the development of diabetes mellitus. These range from autoimmune destruction of the β-cells of the pancreas with a consequent insulin deficiency to abnormalities that result in resistance to insulin action (Armelle et al., 2008; Arika et al., 2016).

Diabetes mellitus is the most prevalent disease in the world, affecting 25% of the population and afflicts 150 million people and is predicted to rise to 300 million by 2025 (WHO, 2002; Babu, 2016). Conventional management of diabetes is expensive and therefore not affordable by many patients, especially in developing nations. More so, conventional drugs are not readily available and have been found to have side effects with long term use (Arika et al., 2015; Deeni and Sadiq, 2002). The distinctive traditional medical opinions and natural medicines have shown a bright future in the therapy of diabetes mellitus and its complications (Ekramul et al., 2002; Arika et al., 2016).

The World Health Organization (WHO, 2002) recommended the use of medicinal plants for the management of DM and further encouraged the expansion of the frontiers of scientific evaluation of hypoglycemic properties of diverse plant species (WHO, 2002; Kwete et al., 2002; Chikezie et al., 2015).

Plants have potential sources of hidden phyto-constituents which can be responsible for solving various potential health problems (Noumi and Yomi, 2001; Kwete et al., 2007). Medicinal plants have curative properties due to the presence of various complex chemical substances of different composition, which are found as secondary plant metabolites in one or more parts of plants (Li et al., 2007; Patil, 2016). They are also associated with reduced risks of cancer, cardiovascular disease, diabetes and lower mortality rates of several human diseases (Momeni et al., 2005; Ozkan et al, 2016).

Physalis peruviana (Solanaceae) is a medicinal plant widely used in folk medicine for treating diseases such as malaria, asthma, hepatitis, dermatitis, cancer, diuretic, rheumatism, antispasmodic, diuretic, antiseptic, sedative, analgesic diseases, and has antioxidant, antifungal, antibacterial, anti-inflammatory, cataract-cleaning, antidiabetic and anti-parasitic properties (Mariotte et al., 2005; Kasali et al., 2013a; Çakir et al., 2014; Joshi and Joshi, 2015; Lashin et al., 2016; Higaki et al., 2016; Chang et al., 2016).

In a survey conducted in the Eastern part of the Democratic Republic of the Congo (DRC), a number of traditional healers pointed out the use of *P. peruviana* L. leaves for this purpose (Kasali et al., 2013b). The objectif of this study was to analyze the phytochemical composition and evaluate zootechnical parameters of a hydroalcoholic extract and its fractions in diabetic rats.

MATERIALS AND METHODS

Study sites

The present study was undertaken at the laboratory of Pharmacognosy, Faculty of Medicine and Pharmacy, Official University of Bukavu/Republic Democratic of Congo) and chemical study of medicinal plants, bacteria, fungi and endophytes was done at Faculty of Sciences, University of Yaounde 1/Cameroon; Phytochemical laboratory of Higher Teachers' Training College (Faculty of Sciences, University of Yaounde 1) and laboratory of Toxicological and Pharmacological Studies (Faculty of Medicine and Biomedical Sciences/ University of Yaounde 1). This study was conducted between September 2015 and April 2016.

Plant material

The leaves of *P. peruviana* L. (Solanaceae) were collected at Lwiro (Center for Research in Natural Sciences, Democratic Republic of Congo) situated at 50 km from Bukavu (South Kivu, Democratic Republic of Congo). They were identified a by Mr. Gentil IRAGI of Botany Department of this center and compared with voucher specimen No.2044. The leaves were air-dried and powdered for analysis.

Preparation of hydroalcoholic extract and its fractions

800 g of the powdered leaves of *P. peruviana* were macerated with 6 L of 70% EtOH (Jothi et al., 2015) for 48 h and the combined filtrate (using the Whatman filter paper No. 1) was evaporated under reduced pressure using a rotary evaporator. A dried extract with a yield of 28.95% was obtained. One part of the filtered hydroalcoholic extract was stored in a refrigerator at 4°C. Another part of this extract was soaked in hexane and decanted into a funnel. The hexane fraction was concentrated in a rotary evaporator (BÜCHI 461 water Bath). This operation was repeated several times until total exhaustion (the solution has become colorless). The same operations were carried out with ethyl acetate. The residue from this fraction was concentrated under reduced pressure using a rotary evaporator. The following yields were obtained: 3.19 and 25.06%, respectively, for hexane and ethyl acetate.

Animals

Healthy male albino Wistar rats (body weight 175 ± 10.6 g) aged 2-3 months, were used in the study. The rats were maintained under standard laboratory conditions at 27.75 ± 1°C, and normal photo period (12 h dark/12 h light) was used for the experiment. The rats were acclimatized to the laboratory conditions a week prior to the experiment.

The experimental protocol and the maintenance of the experimental animals was done in accordance with the regulations of the Organization for Economic Co-operation and Development (OECD) guide since in Cameroon, the ethics committee focuses only clinical studies. The animal experiment protocols were carried out in accordance with the guidelines of the ICH on preclinical pharmaceutical testing in mouse (OECD, 2001; Tsague et al., 2016).

Animal ethical regulatory consideration

Healthy male albino Wistar rats (body weight 150 to 250 g) were ethically required for use for the experiment according to

*Corresponding author. E-mail: charlesfokunang@yahoo.co.uk.

the ICH guidelines.

The experimental protocol and the maintenance of the experimental animals was done in accordance with the regulations of the OEDD guide, the EU parliament directives on the protection of animals used for scientific purposes, since in Cameroon, the ethics committee focuses only on clinical studies. The animal experiment protocols was carried out in accordance with the guidelines of the ICH on preclinical pharmaceutical testing in mouse (OECD, 2001; Akbarzadeh et al., 2007).

Phytochemical screening

Qualitative phytochemical tests of R. heudelotti methanolic extract were carried out according to Odebiyi and Sofowora (1978) methods to identify some components such as alkaloids, saponins, tannins, flavonoids, polyphenols and anthraquinones.

Test for alkaloids: 0.5 g of the sample was stirred with 5 ml of 1% aqueous HCl on a steam bath and then filtered. 1 ml of the filtrate was treated with a few drops of Mayer's reagent and a second 1 ml portion was treated similarly with Dragendroff reagent. Turbidity or precipitation with either of these reagents was taken as evidence for the presence of alkaloids in the extract.

Test for saponins: The ability of saponins to produce frothing in aqueous solution and to haemolyse red blood cells was used for the screening test. 0.5 g of plant extract was shaken with water in a test tube. Frothing which persisted on warming was taken as evidence for the presence of saponins.

Test for tannins: 0.5 g of dried extract was stirred with 5.0 ml of distilled water. This was filtered and ferric chloric reagent was added to the filtrate. A blue-black precipitate was taken as evidence for the presence of tannins.

Test for phenol and polyphenols: 0.5 g of plant extract was heated for 30 min in a water bath. 3 ml of 5% $FeCl_2$ was added to the mixture, then followed by the addition of 1 ml of 1.00% potassium ferrocyanide. The mixture was filtered and green (phenol) and blue (polyphenol) colours were observed.

Test for anthraquinones: 0.5 g of plant extract was shaken with 5 ml of benzene, filtered and 2 ml of 10% ammonia solution was added to the filtrate. The mixture was shaken and the presence of a pink or violet colour in the ammoniacal (lower) phase indicated the presence of free hydroxy anthraquinones.

Test for flavonoids: 0.5 g of plant extract was dissolved in 5 ml of NaOH at 1 N. The change of the yellow colour obtained after adding HCl 1 N indicated the presence of flavonoïds.

Zootechnical study in Streptozotocin-induced diabetic rats

Induction of diabetes

Diabetes was induced in fasted rats injecting 50 mg/kg streptozotocin (Sigma, France) in the tail vein. STZ was dissolved in 0.1 M citrate buffer (pH 4.5) (Tadjeddine et al., 2013). Streptozotocin induces diabetes within 3 days by destroying the beta cells (Ziane et al., 2015). After 48 h of STZ administration, blood glucose level of each rat was determined (Anthikat et al., 2016). Before induction, all rats were fasted 12 h (Ngueguim et al., 2016). Rats with serum glucose level above 300 mg/dl were considered as diabetic (Khathi et al., 2013).

Experimental protocol

The rats were divided into six groups of five rats in each group. Group 1: Untreated rats (control), received vehicle alone (1% tween 20, 1 ml per orally); Group 2: Rats treated with 6.5 mg/kg of glibenclamide, positive control; Group 3: Rats treated with 100 mg/kg of hydroalcoholic extract of P. peruviana; Group 4: Rats treated with 100 mg/kg of the hexane fraction of P. peruviana; Group 5: Rats treated with 100 mg/kg of the ethyl acetate fraction of P. peruviana; Group 6: Rats treated with 100 mg/kg of the residue fraction of P. peruviana.

All rats were administered single dose of drug (orally) daily for 28 days. Daily administration was through a gastric gavage by inducing a gastric tube (Gatierrez et al., 2014). The day of administration of first dose was considered the zero day of treatment.

At the end of the experimental period, all animals were deprived of food overnight and then sacrificed by cervical decapitation after anesthetizing by either inhalation (Saini and Sharma, 2013). One touch electronic Glucometer (One Touch Ultra®) was used for glucose measurement.

Water consumption and food intake

The body weight of each rat was measured once each week and the total amount of food consumed was recorded 3 times per week (Gutierrez et al., 2005).

Body weight monitoring

Body weights of all animals in each group were monitored using a top loader weighing balance throughout the experimental period (Ofusori et al., 2012).

Statistical analysis

All results were expressed as mean ± standard error (SE) for each sample. Statistical analysis was performed using GraphPad Prism 5.02 statistical package (GraphPad Software, USA). The data were analyzed by one way analysis of variance (ANOVA) followed by Turkey's multiple comparison post test. Differences between groups were considered to be significant at $P < 0.05$.

RESULTS

Phytochemical analysis

The results in the Table 1 represent the phytochemical analysis of some fractions from the hydroalcoholic extract of P. peruviana leaves. According to these results, the phytochemical analysis showed the presence of tannins and saponins in all fractions except in the hexane fraction. However, the method used did not show resins and oxalates. In addition, the highest percentage of positive tests were obtained from the hydroalcoholic extract (37.5%) respectively, followed by fractions with ethyl acetate residue (25%) and ethyl acetate (25 %), and finally the hexane fraction (12.5%).

Table 1. Phytochemical screening of *Physalis peruviana* leaves.

Metabolite	Reagent methods	HydAE	HexF	EthAF	ResEAF
Polyphenols	Ferric chloride	+	-	+	+
	Lead acetate				
Flavonoids	Iso amyl alcohol/Mg	+	-	+	+
	+ hydrochloric acid				
Alkaloids	Hodger	-	-	-	-
	Wagner	+	-	-	+
	Mayer	+	+	-	+
Cardiac glycosides	Glacial acetic acid/ $FeCl_3$	+	-	+	+
	+ Sulfuric acid				
Saponosides	Frothing test	+	-	+	+
Tannins	Ferric chloride	+	-	+	+
Anthocyanins	Sulfuric acid/Ammonia	+	+	+	-
Quinones	Sodium hydroxyde	-	-	-	-
Mucilages	Ethanol 95°	+	+	+	-
Resins	Glacial acetic acid/ H_2SO_4	-	-	-	-
Betalains	Sodium hydroxyde	+	+	-	-
Terpenoids and steroids	Liebermann-Burchard	+	-	-	-
Coumarins	Ferric chloride/NHO_3	+	-	+	+
Oxalates	Glacial acetic acid	-	-	-	-

+: Positive test, -: negative test, HydAE: hydroalcoholic extract, HexF: hexane fraction, EthAF: ethyl acetate fraction, ResEAF: residue ethyl acetate fraction.

Zootechnical evaluations

Water consumption and food intake

The water consumption showed a highly significant increase (*** = P > 0.001) in all animals treated against healthy animals (control), however intake food variation showed a highly significant decrease (P > 0.001) in all animals treated as compared to the healthy animals (Figure 1).

Body weight monitoring

There was a highly significant (p< 0.001) body weight changes in all treated rat groups as compared to the control the group (Figure 2). Between groups treated (with glibenclamide and plant extract/fractions), there was no significant difference (P<0.05). There was a significant difference (p< 0.05) between the control group and those treated with the aqueous alcoholic extract.

Assessment of weight variation of organs

From the study as shown in Table 2, there was no significant difference (p< 0.05) in the change of organ weight in all animals treated for heart, liver, brain, spleen and the two kidneys. However, a significant difference (p< 0.05) in weight variation of pancreas, liver, brain, lungs and testicles was noticed (Table 2).

DISCUSSION

There was an uneven distribution in this study of secondary metabolites in the hydroalcoholic extract and its fractions. Saponins and tannins tests were positive in the extract and in two of its fractions (ethyl acetate and its residue fractions), and having 25% of positive tests. Polyphenols compounds, flavonoids, anthocyanins, mucilage, cardiac glycosides and coumarin represented 9.4% in each category. This category is followed by grouping betalains (6.2%). Alkaloids represented 15.6% of positive tests for three different reagents used, which gave an average of 5.2% per reagent. Steroids and terpenes represented 3.1%. Quinones, resins and oxalates are not found (0%).

Many preceding studies reported the presence of some secondary metabolites in the fruit or the leaves of *P. peruviana*. Some studies indicated that cardiac glycoside, alkaloid, saponins, tannins, steroids and terpenoids and flavonoids were present while anthraquinones were absent

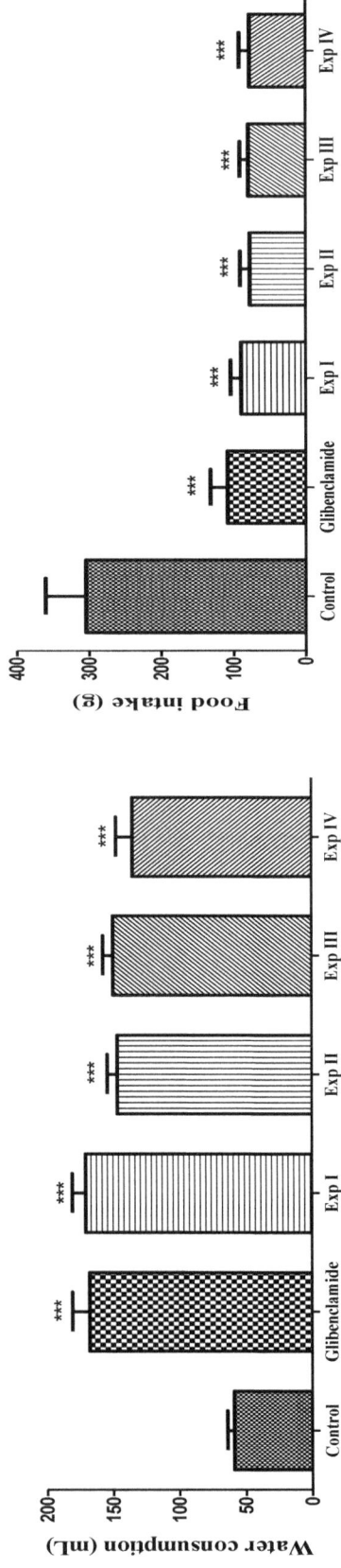

Figures 1. Water consumption and food Intake.

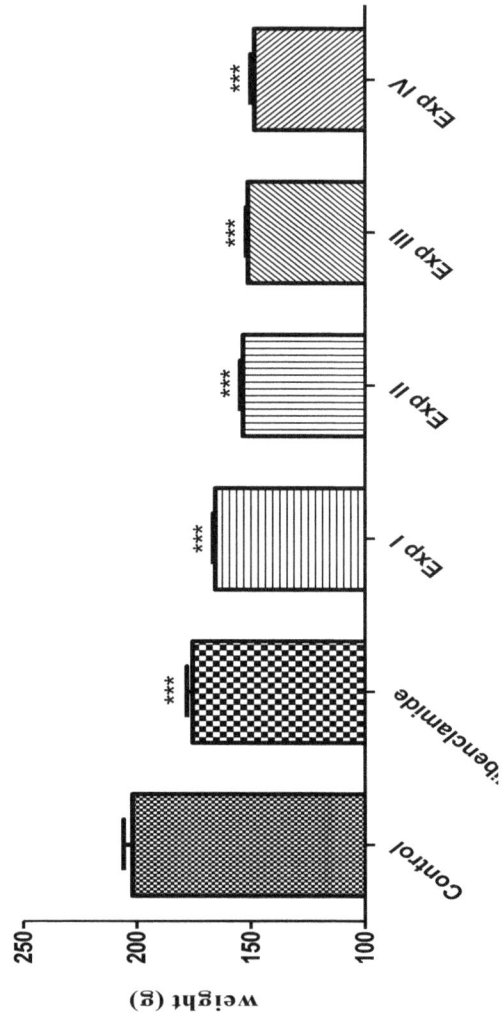

Figure 2. Body weight monitoring of test rats when compared with the control.

in the leaves (Moabe et al., 2013; Magambu et al., 2014). A phytochemical screening in regeneration plant, callus from seed, leaf and fruits from mother plants of *P. peruviana*, showed the present of alkaloids, glycosides, cardiac glycosides,

saponins, phenol, sterol, tannins, flavonoids and diterpene (Lashin and Elhaw, 2016). A phytochemical investigation of the crude ethanolic extract of *P. peruviana* L. revealed the presence of phenols, flavonoids, phytosterols, glycosides,

sterols, saponins, tannins and alkaloids (Ahmed, 2014). Previous phytochemical studies have isolated a number of compounds from *P. peruviana*, such as ticloidine, withanolides, phenolics and phytosterols (Gautam et al., 2015).

Table 2. Weight variation of organs.

Organs	Group 1	Reference	Exp. I	Exp. II	Exp. III	Exp. IV
Heart	0.66±0.09	0.73±0.04	0.57±0.10	0.59±0.06	0.48±0.06	0.55±0.14
Lung	2.20±0.27	2.57±0.08	1.06±0.19**	1.78±0.58	1.05±0.1**	1.90±0.14
Liver	5.33±0.5	7.40±0.56**	5.72±0.58	5.68±0.62	5.58±0.39	5.69±0.64
Brain	1.62±0.05	1.52±0.07	1.52±0.12	1.4±0,13*	1.55±0.08	1.55±0.08
Pancreas	0.77±0.09	0.48±0.04**	0.57±0.05*	0.45±0.1**	0.55±0.01**	0.52±0.1*
Spleen	0.76±0.14	0.71±0.15	0.69±0.15	0.65±0.09	0.50±0.10	0.96±0.07
Right kidney	0.67±0.06	0.85±0.01	0.79±0.11	0.67±0.11	0.62±0.06	0.63±0.02
Left kidney	0.73±0.05	0.84±0.03	0.77±0.11	0.69±0.14	0.62±0.09	0.63±0.05
Right testicle	1.52±0.41	1.39±0.03	1.03±0.46	0.72±0.2**	0.62±0.03**	0.62±0.01*
Left testicle	1.54±0.33	1.42±0.01	1.08±0.41*	0.71±0.1**	0.56±0.01**	0.61±0.02*

The values are expressed as mean ± SEM of the respective groups (n=5). The weight values of groups are compared with normal control animals, value *p< 0.05 and **p< 0.01. Exp. I: Group treated with 100 mg/kg of hydroalcoholic extract of the plant; Exp. II: Group treated with 100 mg/kg of the hexane fraction of plant; Exp. III: Group treated with 100 mg/kg of the ethyl acetate fraction of plant, Exp. IV: Group treated with 100 mg/kg of the residue fraction of the plant.

P. peruviana contain the pseudo-steroids (physalines) and glycosides which show the anticancer activity. From the aerial parts of *P. peruviana*, various withanolide glycosides have been isolated. From the whole plant material, there is isolation of two withanolides (Sharma et al., 2015). Three new physalin steroids, physalinIII, physalin IV, 3-O-methylphysalin X, together with five known physalins were isolated from the 80% EtOH extract of calyces of *P. alkekengi* var. franchetii (Yu et al., 2013).

Withanolides are natural steroidal lactones produced mainly by plants in the Solanaceae that often have many health benefits such as anti-inflammatory activity (Ahmed, 2014). *Physalis* (L.) species contains various carbohydrates, lipids, minerals, vitamins and phytosteroles (Sharma et al., 2015). This genus contains calystegins, alkaloids from nortropane, and steroidal glycoalcalkaloids from spirosolane (Jouzier et al., 2005; Xu et al., 2013).

A number of phytochemical are known, some of which include: alkaloids, saponins, flavonoids, tannins, glycosides, anthraquinones, steroids and terpenoids. They do not only protect the plants but have enormous physiological activities in humans and animals. These include cancer prevention, antibacterial, antifungal, antioxidative, hormonal action, enzyme stimulation and many more. Phytochemicals are responsible for the medicinal activity of plants and they have protected human from various diseases (Savithramma et al., 2011). Many classes of plants secondary metabolites, such as alkaloids, terpenoids, polyphenols, flavonoids and many others show promising antidiabetic potentials. These natural constituents may act as a promising source of delivering oral hypoglycemic effect with minimal side effects (Singab et al., 2014).

According to the results, the administration of a single dose of Streptozotocin (50 mg/kg weight body) increased water consumption. Other studies have shown that diabetes mellitus is characterized by classical symptoms such as polyphagia, and

polydipsia which are exhibited in HFD-STZ diabetic rats and this may be attributed to the impaired glucose homeostasis as a result of insulin inefficiency (Akbarzadeh et al., 2007). Water consumption was inversely related to food intake, this was an indication that the decrease in food intake in diabetic animals was linked to the significant amount of sugars in the blood that had an impact on the index of satiety. High levels of sugars were associated with decreased appetite and short-term food intake as has been reported also (Anderson and Woodend, 2003). Oral treatment with the fruit extract of *P. peruviana* to diabetic group of rats decreased food and fluid consumptions which could be due to improved glycemic status (Sathyadevi et al., 2014).

This study showed a significant decrease in final weight, weight gain at p< 0.001 and also food intake at p< 0.05 as compared to control group. Both *Physalis* powder and juice treated groups showed a significant decrease in final weight (p< 0.01 and 0.05, respectively), weight gain and FER at p< 0.05 as compared to the control group. Aqua *Physalis* extract and methanol *Physalis* extract treated groups showed non-significant difference in these parameters as compared to the control group. *Physalis* powder, juice, aqua *Physalis* and methanol extract treated groups showed a significant increase in final weight, weight gain, food intake as compared to reference group (Hafez et al., 2011). This study also showed differences in some changes in organ weight and body weight Diabetic condition has been known to be associated with weight loss as reported by Anderson and Woodend (2003). The weight loss recorded in untreated diabetic animals could be a symptom of ill health, which may have been caused by the release of free radicals (Abdelmoaty et al., 2010).

The streptozotocin-induced diabetes rats showed significant loss of body weight with respect to the extract treated and controlled groups. Kumar et al. (2011) reported that antidiabetic and antihyperlipidemic effects is best induced in rat models using streptozotocin-induced rat models for better comparison with test plants, and give a better result profile of the test battery. With respect to the reference group, the inability of the plant to improve the animals' weight, at the end of treatment was observed, although a stabilization of weight was recorded at the end of treatment.

Conclusion

The result of this present study showed that the hydroalcoholic extract of *P. peruviana* and its fractions contains many secondary metabolites which will be used against diabetes. It is interesting to isolate and characterize some compounds of this plant and to extend their antidiabetic potential investigations.

ACKNOWLEDGEMENTS

The authors thank Intra-ACP program through AFIMEGQ Project. Also, they are grateful to all personal of Chemical Study of Medicinal Plants, Bacteria, Fungi and Endophytes Laboratory (Faculty of Sciences of University of Yaounde 1/Cameroon), Phytochemical Laboratory of Higher Teachers' Training College (Faculty of Sciences, University of Yaounde 1), Laboratory of Toxicological and Pharmacological Studies (Faculty of Medicine and Biomedical Sciences/ University of Yaounde 1) and Mr. Gentil Iragi of Department of Biology (Center for Research in Natural Sciences, NSRF/Lwiro) in Democratic Republic of Congo, for authentication of the plant.

REFERENCES

Abdelmoaty MA, Ibrahim MA, Ahmed NS, Abdelaziz MA (2010). Confirmatory studies on the antioxidant and antidiabetic effect of quercetin in rats. Indian J. Clin. Biochem. 25(2):188-192.

Ahmed LA (2014). Renoprotective Effect of Egyptian Cape Gooseberry Fruit (*Physalis peruviana* L.) against Acute Renal Injury in Rats. Sci. World J. Article ID 273870, 7 http://dx.doi.org/10.1155/2014/273870.

Akbarzadeh A, Norouzian D, Mehrabi MR, Jamshidi SH, Farhangi A, Verdi AA, Mofidian SMA, Rad BL (2007). Induction of diabetes by streptozotocin in rats. Indian J. Clin. Biochem. 22(2):60-64.

Anderson G, Woodend D (2003). Effect of glycemic carbohydrate on short term satiety and food intake. Nutr. Rev. 61(Supl 5):S17-S26.

Anthikat RNR, Michael A, Vageesh S, Balamurugan R, Ignacimuthu S (2014). The effect of *Areca catechu* L., extract on streptozotocin Induced hyperglycaemia in wistar rats. Int. J. Pharm. Bio. Sci. 5(4):316-321.

Arika WM, Abdirahman YA, Mawia MM, Wambua KF, Nyamai DM (2015). Hypoglycemic Effect of Lippia javanica in Alloxan Induced Diabetic Mice. J. Diabetes Metab. 6:624.

Arika WM, Ogola PE, Nyamai DW, Mawia AM, Wambua FK, Kiboi NG, Wambani JR, Njagi SM, Rachuonyo HO, Emmah KO, Lagat RC, Muruthi CW, Abdirahman YA, Agyirifo DS, Ouko RO, Ngugi MP, Njagi, ENM (2016). Mineral Elements Content of Selected Kenyan Antidiabetic Medicinal Plants. Adv. Tech. Biol. Med. 4(1):160.

Armelle MT, Ngameni B, Kuete V, Ingrid SK, Ambassa P, Roy R, Bezabih M, Xavier EF, Bonaventure NT, Berhanu AM, Marion MJJ, Namrita L, Veronique PB (2008). Antimicrobial activity of the crude extracts and five flavonoids from the twigs of *Dorstenia barteri* (Moraceae). J. Ethnopharmacol. 116:483-489.

Babu NR (2016). Studies on the evaluation of antidiabetic and antioxidant activities using some selected medicinal plants. Int. J. Herbal Med. 4(2):21-24.

Çakir Ö, Pekmez M, Çepni E, Candar B, Fidan K (2014). Evaluation of biological activities of *Physalis peruviana* ethanol extracts and expression of Bcl-2 genes in HeLa cells. Food Sci. Technol. Campinas 34(2):422-430.

Chang LC, Sang-ngern M, Pezzuto JM (2016). Poha Berry (*Physalis peruviana*) with Potential Anti-inflammatory and Cancer Prevention Activities. Haw J. Med. Publ. Health 75 (11):353-359.

Chikezie PC, Ojiako OA, Nwufo KC (2015). Overview of Anti-Diabetic Medicinal Plants: The Nigerian Research Experience. J. Diabetes Metab. 6:546.

Deeni Y, Sadiq N (2002). Antibacterial properties and phytochemical constituents of the leaves of African mistletoe (*Tapinanthus dodeneifolius* (DC) Danser) (Loranthaceae): and ethno medicinal plants of Hausaland, Northern Nigeria. J. Ethnopharmacol. 83:463-480.

Ekramul IM, Naznin KA, Ekramul HM (2002). In *vitro* antibacterial activity of the extracts and glycoside from *Sida rhombilfolia* Linn. J. Med. Sci. 2(3):134-136.

Gautam SK, Dwivedi DH, Kumar P (2015). Preliminary studies on the bioactive phytochemicals in extract of Cape gooseberry (*Physalis Peruviana* L.) fruits and their Products. JPP 3(5):93-95.

Gutierrez RMP, Ahuatzi DM, Horcacitas MDC, Baez EG, Victoria TC, Mota-Flores JM (2014). Ameliorative Effect of Hexane Extract of *Phalaris canariensis* on High Fat Diet-Induced Obese and Streptozotocin-Induced Diabetic Mice. eCAM. doi.org/10.1155/2014/145901.

Hafez DA, El-safty SMS, Al-shammari AM (2011). Therapeutic effect of Physalis consumption on liver necrosis in experimental rats. Res. J. Spec. Educ. 2(23):1368-1383.

Higaki R, Chang LC, Inouye DK, Sang-ngern M (2016). Antibacterial Activity of Extracts from *Physalis peruviana* (Poha Berry). J. Health Disp. Res. Pract. 9(1):57-58.

Joshi K, Joshi I (2015). Nutritional composition and biological activities of rasbhari: An overview. Int. J. Recent Sci. Res. 6(11):7508-7512.

Jothi MA, Kumar BSV, Parameswari CS, Vincent S, Sivasubramanian S (2015). Antidiabetic activity of Cinnamomum macrocarpum Hook.f. leaves on alloxan-induced diabetic swiss albino mice. Int. J. Plant. Anim. Env. Sci. 5(3):16-19.

Jouzier E (2005). Solanacées médicinales et philatélie. Bull. Soc.

Pharm. Bordeaux. 144:311-332.

Kasali FM, Kadima NJ, Mpiana PT, Ngbolua JPK, Tshibangu DS (2013a). Assessment of antidiabetic activity and acute toxicity of leaf extracts from Physalis peruviana (L.) in guinea-pig. Asian Pac J. Trop. Biomed. 3(11):885-890.

Kasali FM, Mahano AO, Bwironde FM, Amani AC, Mangambu JD, Nyakabwa DS, Wimba LK, Tshibangu DST, Ngbolua KN, Kambale JK, Mpiana PT (2013b). Ethnopharmacological survey of plants used against diabetes in Bukavu city (D.R. Congo). J. Ethno. Trad. Med. 119:538-546.

Khathi A, Serumula MR, Myburg RB, Heerden FRV, Musabayane TC (2013). Effects of Syzygium aromaticum-Derived Triterpenes on Postprandial Blood Glucose in Streptozotocin-Induced Diabetic Rats Following Carbohydrate Challenge. Plos One. 8(11).

Kumar S, Kumar V, Prakash O (2011). Antidiabetic and antihyperlipidemic effects of Dillenia indica (L.) leaves extract. Br. J. Pharm. Sci. 47(2):374-378.

Lashin II, Elhaw MH (2016). Evaluation of Secondary Metabolites in Callus and Tissues of Physalis peruvianna. Int. J. Mod. Bot. 6(1):10-17.

Li HB, Cheng KW, Wong CC, Fan KW, Chen F, Tian Y (2007). Evaluation of antioxidant capacity and total phenolic content of different fraction of selected microalgae. Food Chem. 102:771-776.

Momeni J, Djoulde RD, Akam MT, Kimbu SF (2005). Chemical constituents and antibacterial activities of the stem bark extracts of Ricinodendron heudelotii (Euphorbiaceae). Indian J. Pharm. Sci. 67:386-399.

Ngueguim FT, Esse EC, Dzeufiet PDD, Gounoue RK, Bilanda DC, Kamtchouing P, Dimo T (2016). Oxidised palm oil and sucrose induced hyperglycemia in normal rats: effects of Sclerocarya birrea stem barks aqueous extract. BMC Complement Altern. Med. 16:47.

Noumi E, Yomi A (2001). Medicinal plants used for intestinal diseases in Mbalmayo Region, Central Province, Cameroon. Fitoterapia 72:246-254.

Ofusori DA, Komolafe OA, Adewole OS, Obuotor EM, Fakunle JB, Ayoka AO (2012). Effect of ethanolic leaf extract of Croton zambesicus (Müll. Arg.) on lipid profile in streptozotocin-induced diabetic rats. Diabetol. Croatica 41(2):69-76.

Organisation of Economic Co-operation and Development (OECD) (2001). The OECD guideline for testing of chemical: 420 Acute Oral Toxicity. OECD, Paris. pp. 1-14.

Ozkan G, Kamiloglu S, Ozdal T, Boyacioglu D, Capanoglu E (2016). Potential Use of Turkish Medicinal Plants in the Treatment of Various Diseases. Molecules 21:257.

Patil MB (2016). Anti-Diabetic Activity of Some Medicinal Plants. Ind. J. Appl. Res. 6(1):641-642.

Saini S, Sharma S (2013). Antidiabetic effect of Helianthus annuus L., seeds ethanolic extract in streptozotocin- nicotinamide induced type 2 diabetes mellitus. Int. J. Pharm. Pharm. Sci. 5(1):382-387.

Sathyadevi M, Suchithra ER, Subramanian S (2014). Physalis peruviana Linn. fruit extract improves insulin sensitivity and ameliorates hyperglycemia in high-fat diet low dose STZ-induced type 2 diabetic rats. J. Pharm. Res. 8(4):625-632.

Savithramma N, Rao ML, Suhrulatha D (2011). Screening of medicinal plants for secondary metabolites. MEJSR. 8:579-584.

Sharma N, Bano A, Dhaliwal HS, Sharma V (2015). Perspectives and possibilities of indian species of genus (Physalis peruviana L) - a comprehensive review. Eur. J. Pharm. Med. Res. 2(2):326-353.

Singab AN, Youssef FS, Ashour ML (2014). Medicinal Plants with Potential Antidiabetic Activity and their Assessment. Med. Aromat Plants 3:151.

Tadjeddine AL, Kambouche N, Medjdoub H, Meddah B, Dicko A, Saidi S, Derdour A (2013). Antidiabetic effect of Anacyclus valentinus L. aqueous extract in normoglycemic and streptozotocin induced-diabetic rats. Am. J. Phytomed. Clin. Ther. 1(5):424-431.

Tsague MV, Fokunang NC, Tembe AE, Mvondo AM, Afane EA, Oben EJ, Ngadjui TB, Ntchapda F, Sokeng DS, Nyangono BCF, Dimo T, Minkande JZ ((2016). Hydroethanolic Extract of Eribroma oblongum (Malvaceae) Stem Bark Prevents Hypertension, Oxidative Stress and Dyslipidemia in L-NAME Induced Hypertension in Wistar Rats. J. Dis. Med. Plants 2(4):43-50.

World Health Organization (WHO) (2002). Stratégie de l'OMS pour la médecine traditionnelle pour 2002-2005. WHO/EDM/TRM/2002. Genève: OMS: P 65.

Xu WX, Chen JC, Liu JQ, Zhou L, Wang YF, Qiu MH (2013). Three new physalins from Physalis alkekengi var. franchetii. Nat. Prod. Bioprospect. 3:103-106.

Ziane N, Dahamna S, Aouachria S, Khanouf S, Harzallah D (2015). Pistacia atlantica, nouvelle substance utilisée contre le diabète associé au stress oxydant. Diabet. Metab. 41(1):46-47.

## 3

Comparative study between effects of ethanol extract of Zingiber officinale and Atorvastatine on lipid profile in rats

Abdelkrim Berroukche*, Abdelkrim Attaoui and Mustafa Loth

Laboratory of BioToxicology, Pharmacognosy and Biological Recycling of Plants Biology Department, Faculty of Sciences, Moulay Tahar University, Saida 20000, Algeria.

Zingiber officinale is known for its cholesterol-lowering and antioxidant properties. The use of traditional medicine reduces the use of drugs with a risk of toxicity. This study aims to assess the effects of ethanol extract of *Z. officinale* and atorvastatin on lipid parameters in rats fed with high-fat diet. The experiment was carried out on 40 rats during 9 weeks. The animals were divided into 4 groups; group 1 (normal healthy controls), group 2 (hypercholesterolemic diet controls), group 3 (treated with ethanol extract of *Z. officinal* at 500 mg / kg / day) and group 4 (treated with Atorvastatin at 20 mg/kg/day). It has been shown, respectively in groups 3 and 4, a stable body weight (289 vs 282 g) and a highly significant reduction of cholesterol (295.9 vs 275.1 mg/dl), total triglycerides (46.8 vs 41.9 mg/dl) and LDL (278.2 vs 259.1 mg/dl), but not a significant increase in HDL (8.6 vs 7.8 mg/dl). Results showed that *Z. officinale* is similar to Atorvastatin as a cholesterol-lowering agent in the treatment of patients exposed to risk of obesity and cardiovascular disease. Therefore, combination regimens containing ginger and low dose of statins could be advantageous in treating hypercholesterolemic patients.

Key words: *Zingiber officinale*, cholesterol, antioxidant, Atorvastatine, cardiovascular disease.

INTRODUCTION

Metabolic syndrome, including obesity and dyslipidaemia that predisposes type 2 diabetes, is becoming more prevalent in many countries (Ascaso and Carmena, 2015). In developed countries metabolic syndrome appears to affect around 25 % of the population (Salas et al., 2014). The modern lifestyle of increased intake of high-calorie food contributes to the rising prevalence of obesity and type 2 diabetes (Isordia-Salas et al., 2012; Salas et al., 2014). Epidemiological studies also revealed that 90% of all patients with type 2 diabetes have been overweight, and indicated that obesity is a strong risk factor, and cause of type 2 diabetes and associated with metabolic disturbances (Salas et al., 2014). The therapeutic options such as dietary modification or a

*Corresponding author. E-mail: kerroum1967@yahoo.fr.

combination of synthetic antidiabetic, hypolipidaemic drugs have their own limitations and undesirable side-effects (Heeba and Abd-Elghany, 2010). There is an increased demand to search and evaluate traditional approaches for the treatment of metabolic disorders, particularly the use of herbal medicines. *Zingiber officinale* is widely used around the world in foods as a spice (Das et al., 2012). For centuries, it has been an important ingredient in herbal medicines for the treatment of rheumatism, nervous diseases, asthma, stroke, and diabetes (Kim et al., 2012). The major chemical constituents of essential oil *Z. officinale* rhizome include various terpenoids such as shogaols, paradols and zingerone (Jelled et al., 2015).

In laboratory experiments, ethanolic extract of *Z. officinale* has been shown to reduce plasma lipids in cholesterol-fed hyperlipidaemic rabbits (Zhang et al., 2011). It has been shown previously that long term dietary feeding of ginger has hypoglycemic and hypolipidemic effects in rats (Zhang et al., 2011). Besides, *Z officinale* has also been shown to reduce lipid parameters in streptozotocin induced diabetic rats (Ibrahim and Shathly, 2015).

Statins are group of drugs that have been recognized as the most efficient drugs for the treatment of hyperlipidemia. Atorvastatin differs from other statins in that it has a longer action and presents active metabolites which are biotransformed mainly by cytochrome P3A4 in the liver. Previous studies have reported severe AT-induced hepatotoxicity (Heeba and Abd-Elghany, 2010). Natural products and their active principles, as sources for new drug discovery and treatment of diseases, have attracted attention in recent years. Herbs and spices are generally considered safe and proved to be effective against various human ailments (Heeba and Abd-Elghany, 2010). *Zingiber officinale* is one of the commonly used medicinal plants around the world (Heeba and Abd-Elghany, 2010). In this study, we aim to compare the effects of *Zingiber officinale* and Atorvastaine on lipid profile in rats fed with high fat diet.

MATERIAL AND METHOD

Plant material and extraction

Zingiber officinale rhizomes were purchased from a local market in Saida, Algeria, during February 2013, and authenticated by Prof. M. Terras of the Biology Department, Moulay Tahar University, Saida, Algeria. The plant was dried in the shade. The dried rhizomes were powdered mechanically. Pulverised *Z. officinale* rhizomes (3 kg) were added to 5 L of 95% ethanol at room temperature for 7 days. The ethanol extract of *Zingiber officinale* rhizomes (EEZO) was evaporated to dryness under reduced pressure, for the total elimination of alcohol, followed by lyophilisation, yielding 500 g of dry residue. The EEZO was kept at - 20 °C until use and suspended in distilled water.

Preparation of animals

Male Wistar rats, 2 months of age and with mean weight of 180 g, were obtained from the Laboratory Animal of Biology Department (University of Oran, Algeria). They were maintained in a temperature-controlled room (25 ± 1°C) on a 12:12 h light–dark cycle in the Biology Department, University of Saida, Algeria. The rats were divided into four groups (10 rats / group); group 1 as a normal healthy control (NHC), group 2 as pathogenic hypercholesterolemic diet control (HDC), group 3 as HDC and treated with EEZO, and group 4 as HDC treated with Atorvastatine (ATV). Food and water were available ad libitum. Regular rat diet with 19% protein, 58% carbohydrate, and 7% fat was used as the maintenance and control diet. Hypercholesterolemia was induced by force feeding orally of 0.5 g cholesterol in 5 ml hydrogenated vegetable oil (Hemn et al., 2015) for 9 weeks along with normal rats feed in groups 2, 3 and 4. All animal procedures were performed according to the Guide for the Care and Use of Laboratory Animals as well as the guidelines of the Animal Welfare Act. The EEZO (500 mg / kg b.w. in 2 % water) and ATV (20 mg / kg b.w.) were administrated daily orally from the 7th week to groups 3 and 4, respectively. Group 2 served as pathogenic hypercholesterolemic diet control (HCD) and group 1 was kept as a normal healthy control (NHC).

Body weight data and biochemical parameter analysis

The daily body weights were recorded in all groups of rats during 9 weeks. After having heated the tail of the animal to cause vasodilation of the veins, an incision was practiced at the extremity of the tail (Sanchez et al., 2010). The blood samples were collected after every week during all the period of experimentation. Diagnostic kits (VIDAS) for the measurement of total cholesterol (TC) and total triglycerides (TG) were purchased from Bio Merieux Company (Lyon, France). Lipid parameters as TC, TG and high density lipoprotein-cholesterol (HDL-C) were measured using the semi-automatic analyzer mini-VIDAS, while low density lipoprotein-cholesterol (LDL-C) and very low density lipoprotein-cholesterol (VLDL-C) were measured using the Friedewald equations:

$$LDL = TC - HDL - \left(TG/5\right)$$
$$VLDL = TG/5$$

Statistical analysis

Data are expressed as the difference between the initial and final values (± SD) with a value of *p < 0.05* considered statistically significant. Statistical evaluation was performed by one way analysis of variance (ANOVA). The Tukey-test was used for all pairwise multiple comparisons of the mean ranks of the treatment groups. All analysis was carried out with the statistical software SigmaPlot *version 11.0.*

RESULTS

The changes in the mean body weight of the experimental groups of rats during 9 weeks treatment period are shown in Table 1. During the period of experimentation, there was no significant difference in the body weight in

Table 1. Weight and biochemical parameters of pathogenic hypercholesterolemic diet control (HDC) and normal healthy control (NHC) rats.

Parameters (Mean ± SD)	Group 1 (NHC)	Group 2 (HDC)	Group 3 (HCD+EEZO)	Group 4 (HDC+ATV)
Body weight (g)	226.33±22.68	282.22±69.6	289.44±57.75	280.55±54.34
Serum TC (mg/dL)	186.1±8.01	*327.84±105.83	295.9±84.71	275.16±85.57
Serum HDL-C (mg/dL)	***14.75±0.84	8.01±1.93	8.26±2.5	7.86±2.33
Serum LDL-C (mg/dL)	*166±6.74	307.7±101.1	287.26±83.82	259.08±86.38
Serum VLDL-C (mg/dL)	5.32±0.83	*10.42±4.63	9.36±3.37	8.38±3.11
Serum TG (mg/dL)	26.63±4.18	*52.14±23.67	46.84±16.87	41.93±15.55

SD: standard deviation; NHC: normal healthy control; HDC: hypercholesterolemic diet control; EEZO: ethanol extract *Zingiber officinale*; ATV: atorvastatine, TC: total-cholesterol; HDL-C: high density lipoprotein-cholesterol; LDL-C: low density lipoprotein-cholesterol, VLDL-C: very low density lipoprotein-cholesterol; TG: total-triglyceride.***: $p = 0,0009$ (highly significant different). *: $p = 0.02$ (statistically different).

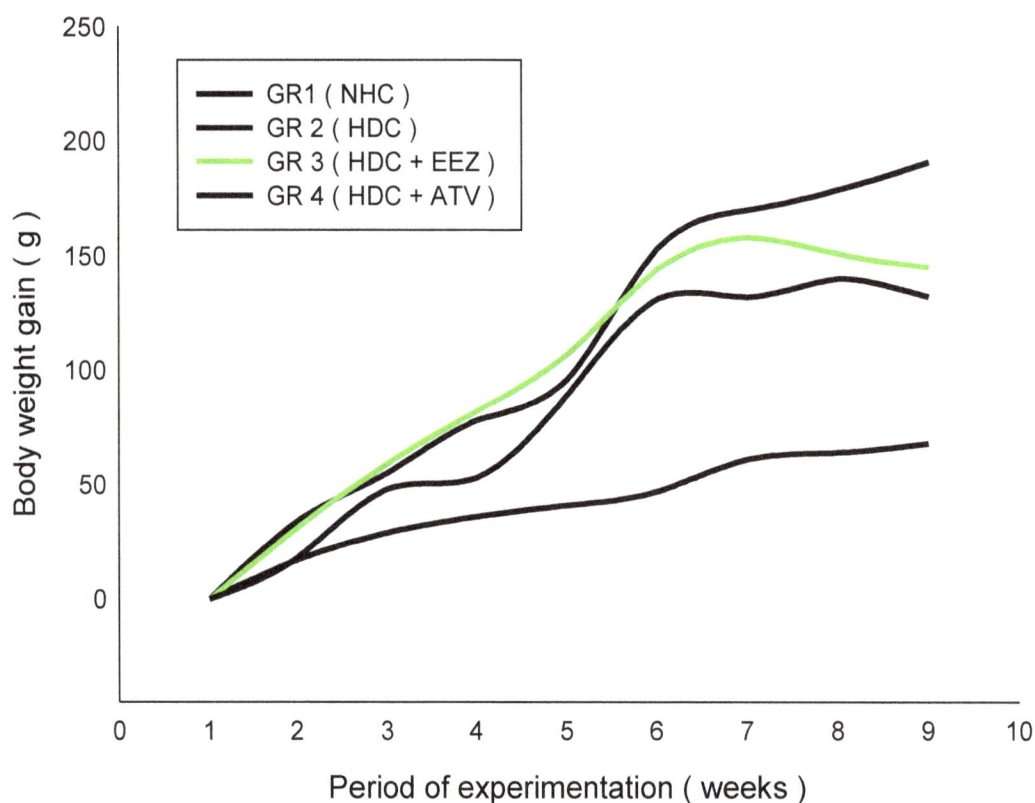

Figure 1. Variation of body weight gain in rats feed high fat diet and treated with ethanol extract of *Zingiber officinale* rhizomes (EEZO) and Atorvastatine (ATV).

different groups ($p = 0.08$) (Figure 1). Table 1 shows that serum T-cholesterol concentration was higher in three groups of rats (HDC, HDC+EEZO and HDC+ATV) than NHC rats, whereas these concentrations were not significantly different among the 3 groups of rats mentioned previously. The solution of the EEZO (500 mg / kg b.w. / day), administrated to rats from the 7th week, had induced a significantly decrease of serum T-C in comparison with hypocholesterolemic diet control rats untreated with OOZE ($p = 0.008$) (Figure 2).

Atorvastatine drug (20 mg / kg b.w./ day), administrated to animals from the 7th week, caused a high significantly reduction of serum TC level in comparison with the HDC rats, but the decrease of this parameter was not higher than that of HDC rats treated with OOZE. The mean values of serum HDL-C concentrations observed in

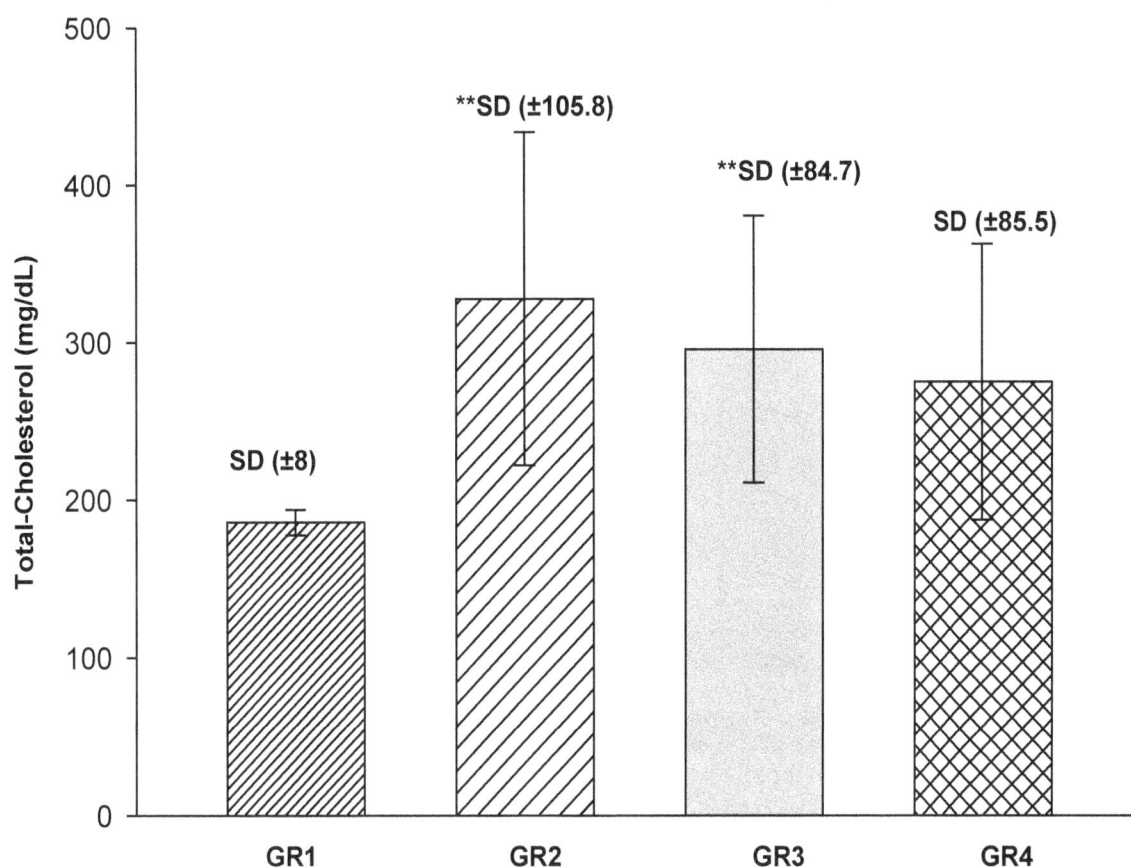

Figure 2. Variation of serum Total-Cholesterol concentration in rats feed high fat diet and treated with ethanol extract of *Zingiber officinale* rhizomes (EEZO) and Atorvastatine (ATV). GR1: NHC, GR2: HDC, GR3: HDC+EEZO and GR4: HDC+ATV.

different groups of rats are shown in Table 1. The serum HDL concentrations before the treatments were not significantly different among the HDC, (HDC+EEZO) and (HDC+ATV) groups of rats (Figure 3). Serum HDL-C levels, among 3 groups of animals cited previously, were significantly lower than that of NHC rats. The treatment of hypercholesterolemic diet animals of groups 3 and 4, respectively with EEZO (500 mg / kg b.w./day) and ATV (20 mg / kg / day) from the 7th week, had significantly caused an increased serum HDL-C level in comparison with the group 2 (HDC untreated) ($p = 0.0009$). Whereas NHC rats, fed with low-fat diet, showed significantly increased serum HDL-C levels (Figure 3). The levels of LDL-C as calculated by Friedewald's equation in various groups of experimental rats are shown in Table 1. The serum LDL-C concentrations, before the treatments, were not statistically different among the groups 2, 3 and 4 (Figure 4). Rats fed high-fat diet (HDC) showed significant elevation of serum LDL-C compared with the serum LDL of normal control rats ($p = 0.002$) at the end

of 6 weeks treatment. But the pathogenic hyper-cholesterolemic diet rats, treated separately with EEZO and ATV from the 7th week of experimental period, showed high significant reduction in LDL-C compared with the high-fat diet-fed control (HDC). Furthermore, the serum LDL-C concentrations, in EEZO treated group, were not significantly different from the normal control group at the end of the treatment. The EEZO and ATV produced significant anti-hyperlipidaemic action. The test drug and standard drug significantly reduced the levels of serum VLDL-C ($p = 0.025$) (Figure 5) and total-triglycerides (TG) ($p = 0.026$) (Figure 6) when compared with group 2, that is, pathogenic hypercholesterolemic diet control (HDC).

DISCUSSION

In this study, we investigated the protective effects of ethanolic extract of *Z. officinale* in high-fat diet-fed rats, a

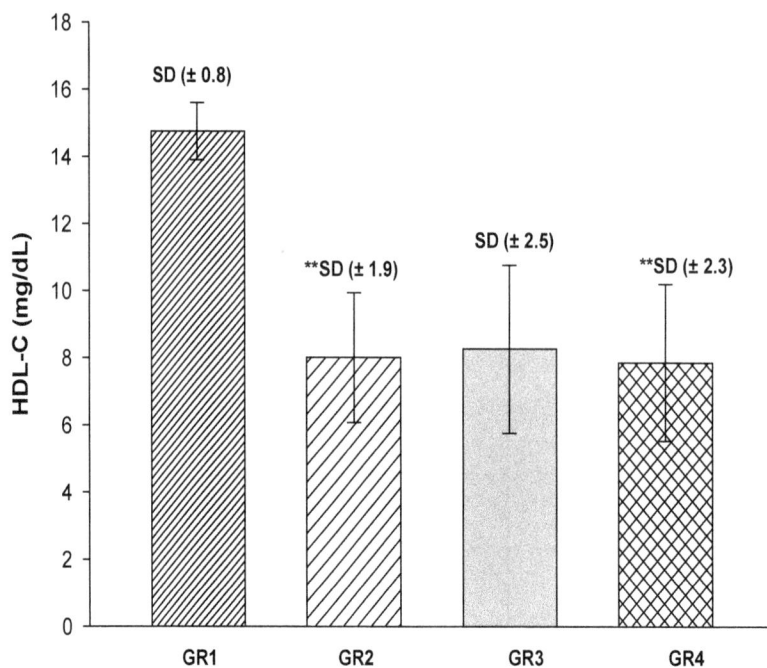

Figure 3. Variation of serum HDL-Cholesterol concentration in rats feed high fat diet and treated with ethanol extract of *Zingiber officinale* rhizomes (EEZO) and Atorvastatine (ATV).

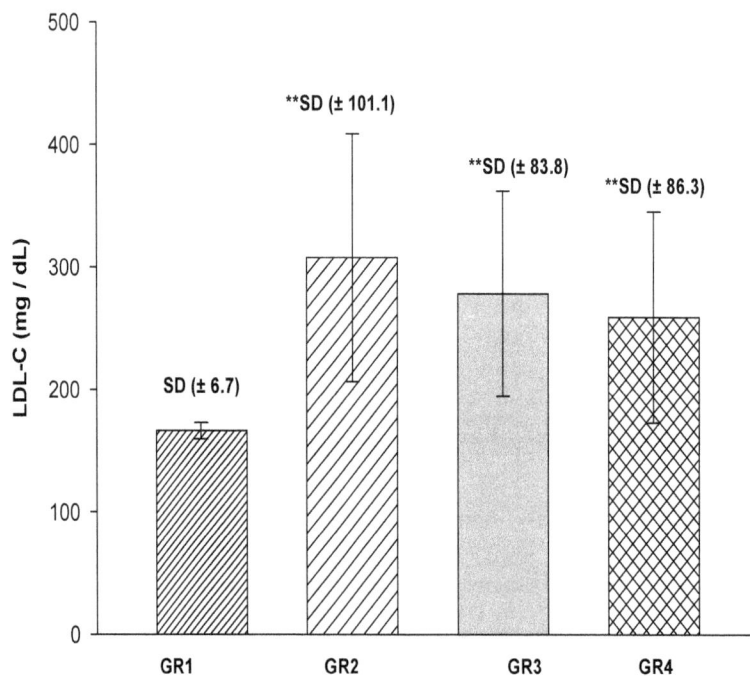

Figure 4. Variation of serum LDL-Cholesterol concentration in rats feed high fat diet and treated with ethanol extract of *Zingiber officinale* rhizomes (EEZO) and Atorvastatine (ATV).

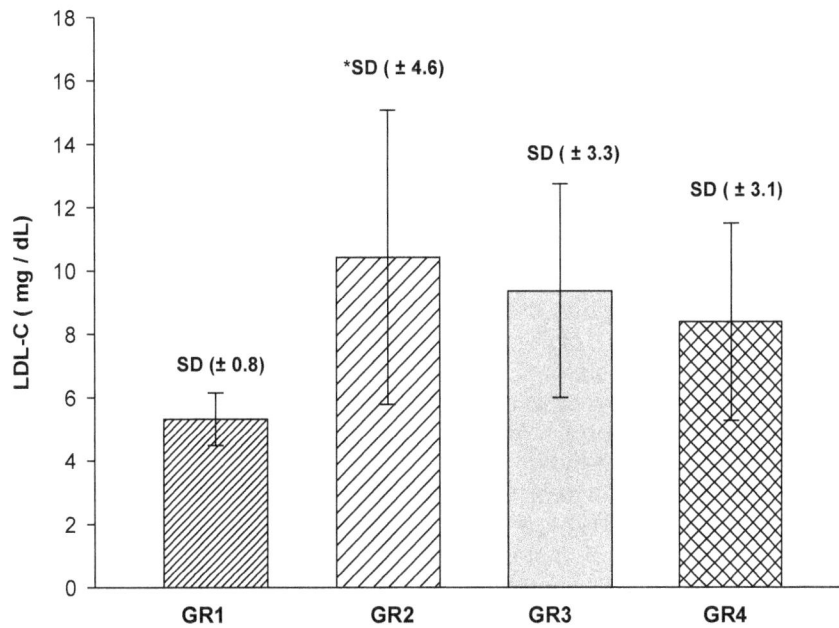

Figure 5. Variation of serum VLDL-Cholesterol concentration in rats feed high fat diet and treated with ethanol extract of *Zingiber officinale* rhizomes (EEZO) and Atorvastatine (ATV).

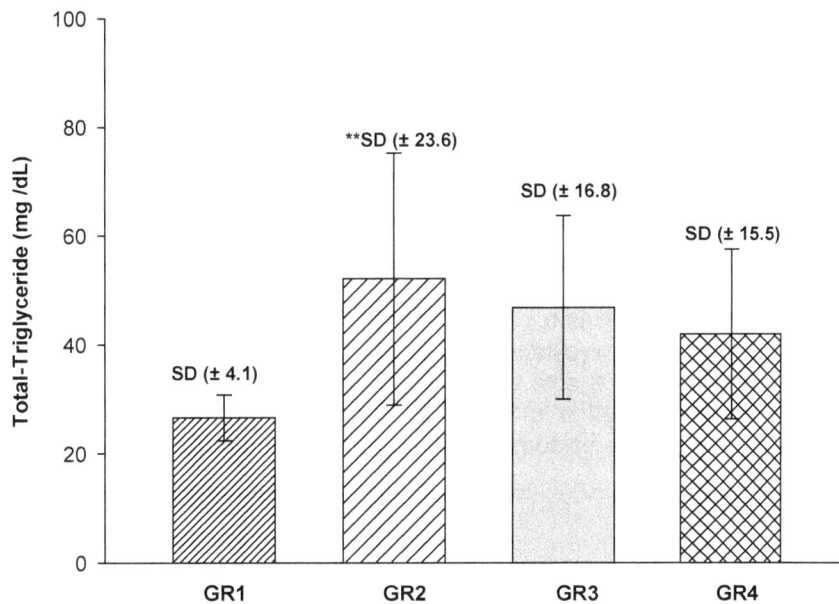

Figure 6. Variation of serum Total-Triglyceride concentration in rats feed high fat diet and treated with ethanol extract of *Zingiber officinale* rhizomes (EEZO) and Atorvastatine (ATV).

metabolic model of hyperlipidaemia, which according to Heeba and Abd-Elghany (2010), is similar to human metabolic syndrome. Dyslipidaemia is the most important risk factor contributing to the development of atherosclerosis in type 2 diabetes (Meaney et al., 2013). The development of metabolic syndrome is influenced by a combination of genetic and environmental factors. Among the environmental factors, long-term high-fat intake is most intensively studied because of its contribution to the development of metabolic syndrome in human beings and rodents (Salas et al., 2014).

Results of this study are consistent with results of previous research works that have shown the anti-hypercholesterolemic effects of Z. officinale (Prasad et al., 2012). The ethanolic extract of Zingiber officinale rhizome, administered to animals with the high-fat diet effectively reduced the serum total cholesterol, LDL-C, total triglycerides and raised HDL-C. Earlier studies (Al-Noory et al., 2013) have demonstrated that Z. officinale through its activity on hepatic cholesterol-7α-hydroxylase, stimulates the conversion of hepatic cholesterol to bile acids. More recently, Poorrostami et al. (2014) found that Z. officinale increased the faecal excretion of cholesterol, suggesting that this species may block the absorption of cholesterol in the gut. The increase in LDL-C may be due to the reduced expression or activity of the LDL-receptor sites in response to high-fat diet treatment as advocated by Brown and Goldstein (2012). Essential oil of Z. officinale is rich in antioxidants and anti-inflammatory components as α-zingiberene, β-sesquiphellandrene, curcumene, β-phellandrene, β-bisabolene and camphene (Yanagisawa et al., 2012). The powdered Z. officinale rhizomes contains aromatic components mainly gingerol and shogaols (Li et al, 2012; Asami et al., 2010). Pharmacological activities, mainly hypolipidimic effects, have been attributed to molecules of gingerol (Yanagisawa et al., 2012). Statins, overhung by Atorvastatin, slow the progression of hyperlipidemia. It has been suggested as an association of low HDL-C with a greater cardiovascular risk. This drug, as inhibitor of transfer of cholesteryl ester protein, increases from 40 to 60% of serum HDL-C and moderately reduces the serum LDL-C (Larach et al., 2013) . Although atorvastatin drug is rich in synthetic bioactive molecules and acts quickly and precisely at specific molecules, Zingiber officinale showed comparable effects on hyperlipidemia or hypercholesterolemia.

Conclusion

The ethanolic extract of Zingiber officinale protects from the high-fat diet induced metabolic disorders by strongly decreasing the body weight gain, protection from hyperlipidaemic conditions. The results confirm that Z. officinale is an antihyperlipidaemic agent, and possesses a potential medicinal value. Its traditional consumption in foods as a spice is beneficial in the prevention of metabolic disorders caused by high-fat diet. However,

further detailed clinical studies are required to establish its application.

ACKNOWLEDGEMENT

We thank the medical team of Biology Analysis Laboratory, which under the leadership of Dr. Z. HADDI had enabled us to establish all the serum assay tests for biochemical parameters. Our thanks also go to members of the administration of our Biology Department (Faculty of Sciences, University of Saida, Algeria) for their help, which materialized by putting at our disposal animals and their breeding.

REFERENCES

Al-Noory AS, Amreen AN,Shatha Hymoor S (2013). Antihyperlipidemic effects of ginger extracts in alloxan-induced diabetes and propylthiouracil-induced hypothyroidism in (rats). Pharmacogn. Res. 5(3):157-161.

Asami A, Shimada T, Mizuhara Y, Asano T, Takeda S, Aburada T, Miyamoto K, Aburada M (2010). "Pharmacokinetics of [6]-shogaol, a pungent ingredient of Zingiber officinale Roscoe (Part I)," Jr. Nat. Med. 64(3):281-287.

Ascaso JF, Carmena R (2015). Importance of dyslipidaemia in cardiovascular disease: A point of view. Clin. Investig. Arterioscler. 15:111-114

Brown MS, Goldstein JL (2012). Scientific Side Trips: Six Excursions from the Beaten Path. J. Biol. Chem. 287(27):22418-22435.

Das L, Bhaumik E, Raychaudhuri U, Chakraborty R (2012). Role of nutraceuticalsin human health. J. Food Sci. Technol. 49:173-183.

Heeba GH, Abd-Elghany MI (2010). Effect of combined administration of ginger (Zingiber officinale Roscoe) and atorvastatin on the liver of rats. Phytomedicine 17:1076-1081

Hemn HO, Noordin MM, Rahman HS, Hazilawati H, Zuki A, Chartrand MS (2015). Antihypercholesterolemic and antioxidant efficacies of zerumbone on the formation, development, and establishment of atherosclerosis in cholesterol-fed rabbits. Drug Des. Dev. Ther. 9:4173-4208.

Ibrahim AAE, Al-Shathly MR (2015). Herbal Blend of Cinnamon, Ginger, and Clove Modulates Testicular Histopathology, Testosterone Levels and Sperm Quality of Diabetic Rats. Int. J. Pharm. Sci. Rev. Res. 30(2):95-103.

Isordia-Salas I, Santiago-German D, Rodrıguez-Navarro H, Almaraz-Delgado M, Leanos-Miranda A (2012). Prevalence of metabolic syndrome components in an urban Mexican sample: comparison between two classifications. Exp. Diabetes Res. 2025-2040.

Jelled A, Fernandesb A, Barrosb L, Chahdourab H, Achourc L Ferreira I, Ben Cheikh H (2015). Chemical and antioxidant parameters of dried forms of gingerrhizomes. Ind. Crops Prod. 77:30-35.

Kim IL, Yang M, Goo TH, Jo C, Ahn DU, Park JH, Lee OH, Kang SN (2012). Radical scavenging-linked antioxidant activities of commonly used herbs and spices in Korea. Int. J. Food Sci. Nutr. 63:603-609.

Larach DB, Cuchel M, Rader DJ (2013). Monogenic causes of elevated HDL cholesterol and implications for development of new therapeutics. Clin. Lipidol. 8(6):635-648.

Li Y, Tran VH, Duke CC, Roufogalis BD (2012). Preventive and Protective Properties of Zingiber officinale (Ginger) in Diabetes Mellitus, Diabetic Complications, and Associated Lipid and Other Metabolic Disorders: A Brief Review. Evid Based Complement. Altern. Med. 516870.

Meaney A, Ceballos-Reyes G, Gutierrez-Salmean G, Samaniego-Mendez V, Vela-Huerta A, Alcocer L, Zarate-Chavarria E, Mendoza-Castelan E, Olivares-Corichi I, Garcia-Sanchez R, Martinez-Marroquin Y, Ramirez-Sanchez I, Meaney E (2013) Cardiovascular risk factors in a Mexican middleclass urban population. The Lindavista Study. Baseline data. Arch. Cardiol. Mex. 83(4):249-256.

Poorrostami A, Farokhi F, Heidari R (2014). Effect of hydroalcoholic extract of *ginger* on the liver of epileptic female rats treated with lamotrigine. Avicenna J. Phytomed. 4(4):276-286.

Prasad SS, Kumar S, Vajpeyee SK, Bhavsar VH (2012). To establish the effect of ginger-juice *Zingiber officinale* (Zingiberaceae) on important parameters of lipid profile. Int. J. Pharm. Sci. Res. 3(4):352-356.

Salas R, Bibiloni Mdel M, Ramos E, Villarreal JZ, Pons A, Tur JA, Sureda A (2014). Metabolic syndrome prevalence among Northern Mexican adult population. PLoS One 9:e105581.

Sanchez VC, Pietruska JR, Miselis NR, Hurt RH, Kane AB (2010). Biopersistence and potential adverse health impacts of fibrous nanomaterials: what have we learned from asbestos? Wiley Interdiscip Rev. Nanomed. Nanobiotechnol. 1(5):511-529.

Yanagisawa M, Sugiya M, Iijima H, Nakagome I, Hirono S, Tsuda T (2012). Genistein and daidzein, typical soy isoflavones, inhibit TNF-α-mediated downregulation of adiponectin expression via different mechanisms in 3T3-L1 adipocytes. Mol. Nutr. Food Res. 56(12):1783-1793.

Zhang Z, Wang X, Zhang J, Zhao M (2011). Potential antioxidant activities in vitro of polysaccharides extracted from ginger (*Zingiber officinale*). Carbohydr. Polym. 86:448-452.

## 4

Biochemical and antioxidants activity of crude, methanol and n-hexane fractions of *Vernonia calvoana* on streptozotocin induced diabetic rats

Iwara Arikpo Iwara*, Godwin Oju Igile, Friday Effiong Uboh, Kelvin Ngwu Elot and Mbeh Ubana Eteng

Department of Biochemistry, Faculty of Basic Medical Sciences, University of Calabar, P. M. B. 1115, Calabar, Nigeria.

This study is aimed at evaluating the biochemical effects and antioxidants activity of extracts of *Vernoia calvoana* Hook. f (V.C) on STZ induced diabetic rats. Thirty-six rats weighing (100 to 150 g), were divided into 6 groups of 6 animals each. Groups 1 and 2 representing normal and diabetic controls (NC and DC), respectively, receiving placebo, while groups 3 to 6 represented diabetic treated, receiving 500 mg/kg body weight (b.w.) metformin, 400 mg/kg b.w. crude, n-hexane and methanol fractions of V.C, respectively. Treament with drug and extracts of V.C showed a decrease in fasting blood glucose (FBG) in all experimental groups and was significant ($p<0.05$) on the 7th day of the experimental period, compared to diabetic control. Progressive increase in body weight was observed in all experimental groups compared to DC group. A significant ($p<0.05$) increase in glutathione peroxidase (GPX) and catalase (CAT) activities were recorded in all experimental treated animal compared to DC and NC. Malondialdehyde (MDA) concentration was observed to decrease significant ($p<0.05$) in all experimental groups compared to DC. Histopathologically, the changes in pancreatic integrity were consistent with that of biochemical findings. It may be concluded that, extracts of V.C possess potent ameliorative activity against STZ-induced diabetes, via a potential free radical mopping activity.

Key words: *Vernonia calvoana*, extracts, diabetes mellitus, antioxidants.

INTRODUCTION

Deep rooted in the cultures of rural dwellers is the use of plants and plant-parts as first point of call for both their daily primary health care and nutritional needs. According to World Health Organization (WHO), about 65 to 80% of the world's population in developing countries depends essentially on plants and plant derived compounds for their primary healthcare and as source of nutrition (WHO, 2014).

Report by WHO globally, estimated that approximately 5 to 8% of the global population is affected by diabetes mellitus (Chakraborty and Rajagopalan, 2002). Diabetes now is becoming the third "killer" of mankind along with cancer, cardiovascular and cerebrovascular disease (Donga et al., 2011). It has also been predicted that by

*Corresponding author E-mail: iwaraarik@yahoo.com or iwaraiwara83@gmail.com.

the year 2025, more than 75% of people with diabetes will reside in developing countries (King, 2012). Significant amount of synthetic antidiabetic drugs like glybenclamide, metformin, and thiazolindiones are well known today not only to be expensive but also produces serious side effects (Venkatesh et al., 2003). Therefore, there has been a growing interest in the ethnobotanical approach to screen the anti-diabetic properties of plants traditionally used in our locality and other parts of the world.

Vernonia (Asteraceae) plant species is the largest genus in the tribe Vernoniae, with close to 1000 species (Keeley and Jones, 1979). The genus *Vernonia* has several species, some which are useful as food, medicinal agents and industrial raw materials. *Vernonia calvoana* and *Vernonia colorata* species are both eaten as leafy vegetables (Burkill, 1985; Iwu, 1993).

V. calvoana (Hook f) belongs to the family of Asteraceae. It is found locally in mountainous and high plateau regions of West, Central, East and Southern Africa. The plant is also known as *Vernonia hymenolepis* A. Rich, *Vernonia leucocalyx* or *Baccharoides calvoana*. In English, it is called sweet bitter leaf or bitter leaf. In France, it is called *Vernonie douce* or *Vernonie*. The Cameroonians call it Bayangi or Ndole. It is also known as "Ekeke leaf" among the indigenous people of the central senatorial district of Cross River State of Nigeria (Igile et al., 2013). It serves as a green-leafy vegetable and is also used for ethno-medical purposes in Nigeria and Cameroun (Focho et al., 2009). It is popularly eaten raw and fresh as a local delicacy with or without palm oil in pepper sauce because the vegetable imparts a sweet taste like sugar in the tongue after its consumption. It serves as a component of traditional salad among the indigenous consumers. It may also be cooked in native soups. Its consumption is based on the belief that the plant is use in the management and cure of heart diseases, blindness, diabetes, malaria, stomach ache, as an anti-helminthic agent, and to prevent constipation. The vegetable is less bitter than the sister plant (*Vernonia amygdalina*), and yet both plants are used for the same ethno-medicinal purposes both as food and for traditional treatment of diseases in some part of south-south of Nigeria (Igile et al., 2013). Preliminary pharmacological studies carried out in experimental models have validated the plant to have hypoglycemic and hypolipidemic activity (Iwara et al., 2015). Chemical evaluations of these plants by Igile et al. (2013) have revealed high levels of antioxidant vitamins (A, C, E and B-complex), mineral elements (Fe, Se, Zn, Cu, Cr and Mn) and phytochemical compounds (polyphenols, flavonoids and tannins) in the leaves of *V. calvoana*. These antioxidant and phytochemicals compounds have been reported widely to ameliorate free radical mediated disease like cancer, mutagenesis, cardiovascular disease, and diabetes by neutralizing the ROS generated (Atangwho et al., 2013). The observed pharmacological activities of this plant

extract may be due to the presences of bioactive phytochemicals. Therefore, this study was designed to investigate the biochemical effect and anti-oxidant activity of crude extract and fractions of *V. calvoana* in streptozotocin (STZ) induced diabetic rats.

MATERIALS AND METHODS

Sample collection and preparation

Fresh leaves of *V. calvoana* were harvested from a farm in Ugep, in Yakurr L.G.A of Cross River State, Nigeria. The leaves were collected in the early hours of the day, cleaned and air dried for 7 days after which they were ground into powder form. A measured quantity of 5 kg of powder leaves were extracted via cool maceration in 8 L of 80% ethanol for 48 h. The extract was further double filtered with chess cloth, then with filtered paper (Whatman 4 filtered paper) and the residue obtained was further extracted with 4 L of 80% ethanol. The filtrate was then concentrated at 45°C in rotary evaporator to 10% volume and then to complete dryness using water bath yielding 310.3 g (6.2%) of crude extract. The crude extract obtained was subjected to fractionation.

Fractionations of plant extract using column chromatography

The crude extract (251.8 g) was chromatographically eluted with two different solvents: n-hexane and methanol in a column packed with silica gel of mesh 60 to 120. The fractions were collected and evaporated in rotary evaporator at 50°C to 10% of its original volume and further evaporated to paste form in a water bath at 50°C. The percentage yield for the fractions were 12 g (4.8%) methanol fraction and 20 g (8.10%) n-hexane fraction. The fractions and the remaining crude extract were stored in a freezer at -4°C for further experiments.

Acute toxicity testing

Acute toxicity level of the fractionated extracts was carried out in mice (Mus Musculus) to determine the dose levels to be administered to the experimental animal using Lorke's method (Lorke, 1983).

Animal handling/design

Thirty-six Wistar rats of both sexes weighing 100 to 150 g were obtained from the animal house of the Department of Zoology and Environmental Biology, University of Calabar, Calabar. The animals were allowed to acclimatize for three weeks in the animal house of the Department of Biochemistry and were housed in well ventilated cages (wooden bottom and wire mesh top), and kept under normal environmental conditions of room temperature and relative humidity. Administration of extract was twice daily in 6 h cycle. The animals were divided into six groups of six animals each (Table 1). The protocol was in accordance with the guidelines of the National Institute of Health (NIH) publication (1985) for laboratory Animal Care and Use and approved by the College of Medical Sciences Animal Ethics Committee, University of Calabar, Nigeria (Atangwho et al., 2013).

Induction of diabetes

Diabetes was induced with 45 mg/kg body weight of STZ in 0.1 M

Table 1. Experimental design.

Group	Number of animal	Treatment	Dose
Normal control	6	Placebo	0.2 ml 10% DMSO
Diabetic control	6	Placebo	0.2 ml 10% DMSO
Diabetic treated	6	Metformin	500 mg/kg
Diabetic treated	6	Methanol fraction	400 mg/kg
Diabetic treated	6	n-Hexane fraction	400 mg/kg
Diabetic treated	6	Crude fraction	400 mg/kg

sodium citrate buffer (pH 4.4). Animals with fasting blood glucose >7.8 mmol/l or > 180 mg/dl were enrolled for the study (Ebong et al., 2008).

Experimental protocol

Animals were grouped as shown in the aforementioned scheme and also accordingly treated with extracts of V.C and metformin. The dosages of the plant extracts were as determined from preliminary work in our laboratory (Iwara et al., 2015). Metformin (Glucophage) (500 mg/kg b.w. S.C.) was as previously used by Atangwho et al. (2013). The plant extracts and glucophage was administered via oral gastric intubation, twice per day (10.00 am: 4.00 pm). Treatment lasted for 21 days and throughout this period animals were maintained on pallets prepared with Growers feed from Vital Feeds, Jos, Plateau state, Nigeria, and tap water. Both feed and water were provided *ad libitum.*

Measurement of fasting blood glucose and body weight

Fasting blood glucose was determined at interval of 7 days during the 3 week experimental period using glucometer (one touch). Body weight of animals was determined also at interval of 7 days using weighing balance.

Collection of samples for analysis

After 21 days experimental period, food was withdrawn from the rats and fasted overnight with access to water. The rats were then anaesthetized over chloroform vapor and sacrificed. Whole blood was collected via cardiac puncture using sterile syringes and needles, and emptied into EDTA bottle, allowed for 2 h stored in a refrigerator at 4°C. The refrigerated blood sample was then centrifuged at 3000 rpm for 10 min to recover the plasma from cells. Plasma was separated with sterile syringes and needle and stored frozen until used for biochemical analysis.

Pancreas was removed and blotted with Whatman No. 1 filter paper to clean the excess blood on the organs, and then weighed using weighing balance. Thereafter, a portion of the tissue was sliced and suspended in 10% fixative (formal saline) for histological analysis.

Biochemical analyses

Analytical kits for glucose analysis were purchased from Agappe diagnostics. GPX, MDA and CAT kit where purchase from Biovision incorporated.

Histopathology

The histological examination of the pancreas of the induced models and the control was carried out using differential staining procedure described by Drury and Wallinggton (1967).

Statistical analysis

The results were analyzed for statistical significance by one way analysis of variance (ANOVA) with a post hoc Dunnet at ($p < 0.05$ t) using SPSS software and Microsoft Excel. All data were expressed as mean ± standard error of mean (SEM; n = 6 replications).

RESULTS

Effect of crude extract, methanol and n-hexane fractions of V.C on blood glucose

Hourly changes in fasting blood glucose for 4 h, changes in plasma blood glucose (PBG) and weekly fasting blood glucose (FBG) were determined in this study during the 21 days experimental period. The results obtained are presented in Figures 2 and 3 and Tables 2 and 3. From the result, the PBG (Figure 1) of diabetic coontrol (DC) groups was observed to be significantly ($p<0.05$) increased, compared to the normal control (NC) group. Upon treatement with test drug/sample (Metformin, crude extract, methanol and n-hexane fractions of V.C), significant ($p<0.05$) decrease in PBG was observed in all treated groups, compared to both DC and NC groups; with crude extract, methanol and n-hexane fractions treated groups showing close activity to that of metformin treated groups. Also from Table 2, the weekly FBG levels of diabetic control groups were observed to be significantly ($p<0.05$) increased, compared to NC groups at the beginning of the experiment with constant level till the end of the experimental period. However, on treament with test drug and the fractions, decrease in FBG was observed in all experimental groups. The decrease was more significant on the 7th day of the experimental period, compared to the diabetic control, and thereafter increased on day 14, and then reduced on day 21. Moreso, the hourly changes in FBG (Table 3) within 4 h of the first day of experiment showed increase in the glucose levels within 1 h in the DC and methanol

Table 2. Effect of crude extract, methanol, n-hexane fractions of V.C leaves and metformin on weekly Fasting blood glucose of STZ-induced Diabetic rats.

Treatment group	Basal (mg/dl)	Day 7 (mg/dl)	Day 14 (mg/dl)	Day 21 (mg/dl)	% Change
NC	81±7.31	112±5.2	100±4.4	72±2.7	-12.5
DC	284±2.1*	393±8.5	395±10.7*	387±7.4*	26.6
Met	278±4.6*	226±8.2*	195±4.4[a]	106±3.1[a]	-162
V.C Crude	254±4.4*	192±9.6*	259±8.8*	267±1.3*	4.7
V.C Met	252±5.6*	67±10.8*,[a]	190±6.4[a]	155±1.8[a]	-62.6
V.C-Hex	285±9.1*	183±7.3[a]	352±1.2*	230±1.2*	-23.9

Values are expressed as Mean ±SEM (n= 6). *Significantly different from NC at p<0.05. a=p<0.05 vs. DC.

Table 3. Effect of crude extract, methanol, n-hexane fractions of V.C leaves and metformin on hourly Fasting blood glucose of STZ-induced Diabetic rats.

Treatment group	Basal (mg/dl)	1 h (mg/dl)	2 h (mg/dl)	4 h (mg/dl)	% Change in FBG (mg/dl)
NC	81±7.31	102±1.7	95±2.3	72±2.7	-12.5
DC	284±2.1*	550±2.6*	450±4.3*	430±3.2*	33.9
Met	278±4.6*	184±4.0*,[a]	160±1.7*,[a]	159±2.1*,[a]	74.8
V.C Crude	254±4.4*	284±3.8*	250±3.2*,[a]	253±1.8*,[a]	3.9
V.C Met	252±5.6*	483±4.6*	485±2.1*	281±2.4*,[a]	10.3
V.C-Hex	285±9.1*	258±7.2*,[a]	258±2.5*,[a]	272±3.1*,[a]	-4.7

NC: Normal control, DC: diabetic control, MET: metformin, V.C _CRUDE: *Vernonia calvoana* crude, V.C MET: *Vernonia calvoana* metformin, V.C_nHEX: *Vernonia calvoana* hexane. Values are expressed as Mean ± SEM (n= 6). *Significantly different from NC at p<0.05. [a]p<0.05 vs. DC.

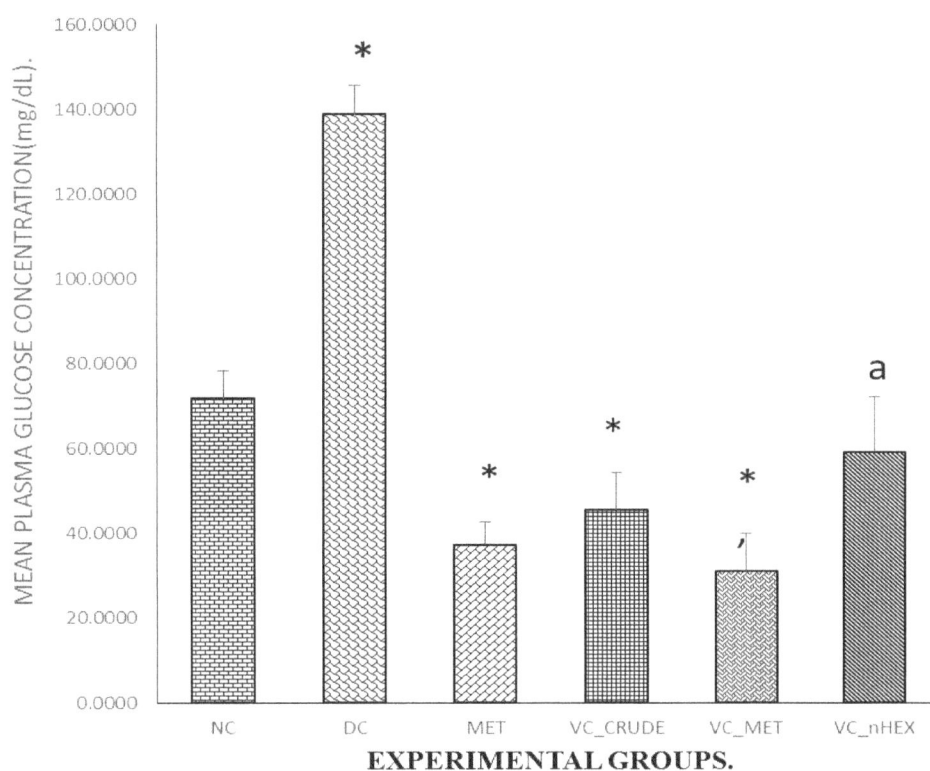

Figure 1. Plasma glucose concentrations of the different experimental groups. Values are expressed as Mean±SEM (n= 6). *Significantly different from NC at p<0.05. [a]p<0.05 vs. DC, [b]p<0.05 vs. VC_MET.

Table 4. Effect of crude extract, methanol, n-hexane fractions of V.C leaves and metformin on body weight changes of STZ-induced diabetic rats.

Treatment group	Basal (g)	Day 7 (g)	Day 14 (g)	Day 21 (g)	% Change in BW (g)
NC	88±1.7	112±8.5	131±10.2	119±6.6	26
DC	145±7.4	138±6.9	124±3.7	138±2.8	-5.1
Met	101±3.8	106±3.8	124±4.6	148±9.7	31.8
V.C Crude	108±5.2	108±9.0	123±8.4	128±11.7	15.6
V.C Met	109±2.8	107±0.8	117±0.9	125±2.7	12.8
V.C-Hex	122±5.5	112±3.8	131±6.7	128±2.6	4.7

NC: Normal control, DC: diabetic control, MET: metformin, V.C _CRUDE: *Vernonia calvoana* crude, V.C MET: *Vernonia calvoana* metformin, V.C_nHEX: *Vernonia calvoana* hexane. Values are expressed as Mean ± SEM (n= 6). *Significantly different from NC at $p < 0.05$. [a]$p < 0.05$ vs. DC.

fraction treated experimental groups. The NC, metformin and n-hexane fractions of V.C showed marked reduction in FBG 1 h after first administration.

Effect of crude extract, methanol and n-hexane fractions of V.C leaves on body weight changes

The results of changes in the body weight of experimental animal after 21 days period are presented in Table 4. Observed from these result was a significant ($p < 0.05$) reduction in body weight of DC, compared to NC groups. On treament with test drugs/fractions after 7th day period, progreassive increase in body weight was observed in all experimental groups compared to the DC group, and the steady body weight increase was maintained till the 21st day. However, at 14th day period, the DC groups showed an increased body weight that was also sustain till the last day.

Effect of crude extract, methanol, n-hexane fractions of V.C leaves and metformin on oxidative oxidative stress marker and antioxidant enzyme

The levels of antioxidant enzymes and oxidative stress maker are shown in Figures 2, 3 and 4. Results obtained showed a significant ($p < 0.05$) decrease in the activities of glutathione peroxidase (GPX) and catalase (CAT) (Figures 2 and 3) in DC, compared to NC. A significant ($p < 0.05$) increase in GPX and CAT activities were recorded on administration of the diabetic rats with n-hexane and methanol fractions of V.C, compared to DC and NC. Also, an insignificant ($p > 0.05$) increase in the concentration of MDA was observed in DC, compared to the NC (Figure 4). On administration of V.C crude extract, methanol, n-hexane fractions and metformin, the MDA concentrations was observed to reduce with the n-hexane fraction showing the most significant ($p < 0.05$) reduction.

Effect of treatment on the histology of pancreatic tissues

Presented in Figures 3a, b, c, d, e and f are the cellular architecture of pancreas. Photomicrograph of a section of the pancreas of NC group (Figure 3a) showed compact islets consist of round to oval, well circumscribed collections of endocrine cells. The cells have uniform round nuclei with coarsely clumped chromatin and inconspicuous nucleoli. The cytoplasm is pale. The cells are separate by small capillaries into lobules. The insulin producing cells are located centrally and the glucagon cells peripherally located. The surrounding pancreatic acinar have abundant cytoplasm and basally located nuclei. Induction for diabetes (DC group, Figure 3b), showed a compact islet surrounded by pancreatic acinar cells. The islet cells are oval to round separated by blood capillaries. The cells are sparsely populated with scanty cytoplasm and clumped chromatin pattern. The acinar are unremarkable. On treatment with metformin (Figure 3c) showed a hyperplasia of islet of Langerhans surrounded by pancreatic acinar cells. The islets are compact consisting of uniform round to oval cells with regular outline, scanty cytoplasm and clumped chromatin pattern. In the methanol treated group (Figure 3d), the islets consisted of a densely packed round to oval, collections of deeply stained endocrine cells; having a round nuclei with coarsely clumped chromatin and inconspicuous nucleoli. The cells are separate by small capillaries. The surrounding pancreatic acinar are lined by tall cuboidal cells with basally located. Also, the n-hexane treated group (Figure 3e) showed islets consisting of round to oval, collections of sparsely populated endocrine cells. These cells are loosely packed with round nuclei having coarsely clumped chromatin and inconspicuous nucleoli. The cells are separate by small capillaries into lobules. There cytoplasm are pale while that of the crude extract (Figure 3f) was observed to consist of an islet having a sparsely populated endocrine cells. The cells have oval to round nuclei with coarse chromatin patterns and are separated by thin walled capillaries. These cells are more at the

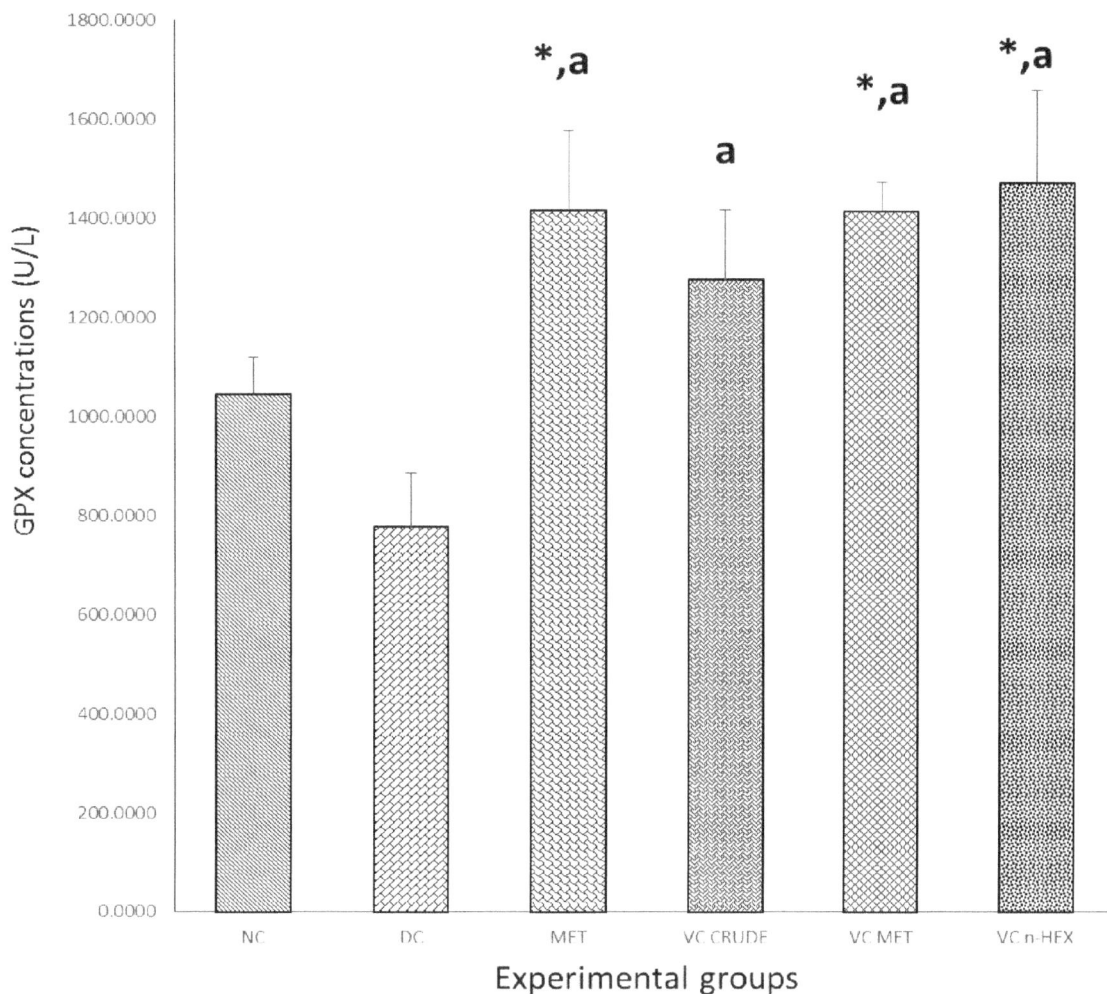

Figure 2a. GPX concentration in the different experimental groups. Values are expressed as mean ± SEM (n=5). *Significantly different from NC at $p < 0.05$. [a]$p < 0.05$ vs. DC, [b]$p < 0.05$ vs. MET, [d]$p < 0.05$ vs. crude VC. NC: Normal control, DC: diabetic control, MET: metformin, V.C _CRUDE: *Vernonia calvoana* crude, V.C MET: *Vernonia calvoana* metformin, V.C_nHEX: *Vernonia calvoana* hexane.

DISCUSSION

From time immemorial, nature has been a source of medicinal agents. Significant number of modern drugs have been isolated and characterized from natural sources. Medicinal plants have been used for centuries as remedies for human and animal diseases as they contain phyto-chemicals of therapeutic value. Green plants are known to represent a reservoir of effective chemotherapeutic agents with more systemic and easily biodegradable potentials (Atangwho et al., 2013).

The administration of streptozotocin at recommended therapeutic dose to animals induces a response in the concentration of glucose in the blood with an accompanying change in the insulin concentration as well as sequential change in the architecture of the beta cells (Mythili et al., 2004). Streptozotocin, being a diabetogenic agent, inhibits insulin secretion and causes a state of insulin-dependent diabetes mellitus by selectively causing necrosis of the pancreatic beta cell, and this can be related to alkylating potential of STZ. Consequently, in the present study, it was observed that injection of 45 mg/kg b.w of STZ caused an increase in fasting and plasma blood glucose of diabetic control (DC) compared to that of normal; with result of the test extracts comparing favorable with metformin (a known standard diabetic drug). These results were in agreement with the earlier report by Iwara et al. (2015) on the hypoglycemic and hypolipidemic potentials of *V. calvoana* in alloxan-induced diabetic rats. However, from the observed results, it may be assumed that the n-hexane extract of *V. calvoana* is less likely to have hypoglycemic activity;

central portion and the surrounding acinar are closely packed and lined cuboidal epithelium.

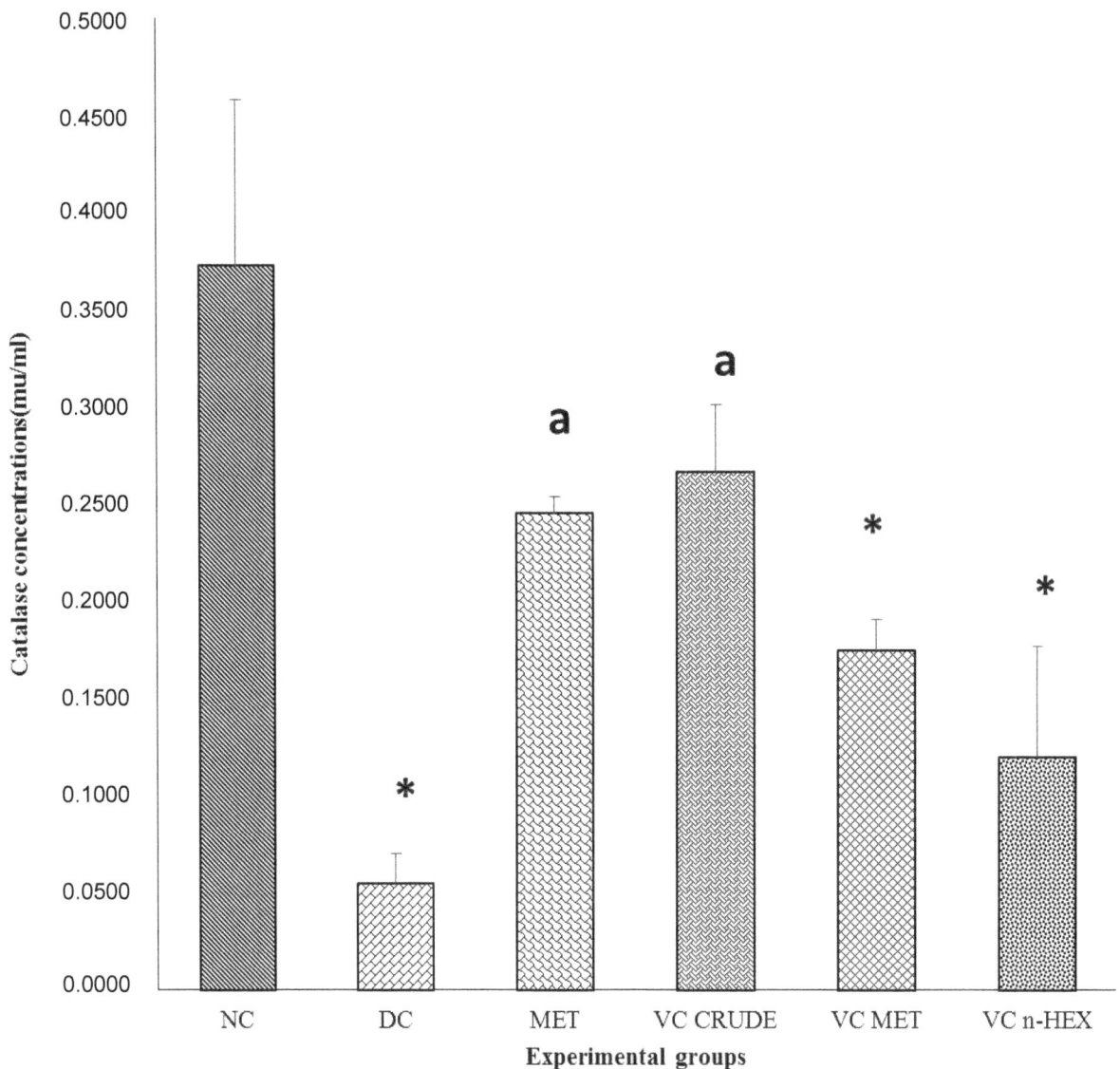

Figure 2b. Catalase concentrations of the different experimental groups. Values are expressed as mean ± SEM (n=5). *Significantly different from NC at $p<0.05$. [a]$p<0.05$ vs. DC, [b]$p<0.05$ vs. MET, [d]$p<0.05$ vs. crude VC. NC: Normal control, DC: diabetic control, MET: metformin, V.C _CRUDE: *Vernonia calvoana* crude, V.C MET: *Vernonia calvoana* metformin, V.C_nHEX: *Vernonia calvoana* hexane.

thus giving it more desirable antidiabetic features of medicinal plants. It can also be further deduced from the present study that both the methanol and n-hexane fractions of *V. calvoana* contain long-term glycemic constituents which will be of great use for future studies.

Tissue wasting is one of the observable features of untreated diabetic condition in experimental rat models (Ahmed, 2005). This occurs as a result of lack of uptake of glucose by the tissues which serve as the primary source of energy for the body due to insufficient insulin that signals glucose uptake in the body. As a result, the body starts burning fat and muscles for energy production thus leading to lost in weight. In the present study, a significant decrease in body weight of diabetic control animals, compared to normal control, was observed; showing a clear indication of the deterioration of the glucose control mechanism, which progresses in stages and would probably climax in the death of the animal if left untreated (Atangwho et al., 2012). Upon treatment of the diabetic rats with extracts of *V. calvoana* and metformin, a significant increase in body weight was observed. This implies that treatment with experimental drugs helps to enhance availability of glucose to the tissues, both for supply energy and to build tissue materials needed for growth.

Increased oxidative stress has been postulated to play a key role in the pathogenesis of diabetes mellitus associated complications like neuropathy, nephropathy,

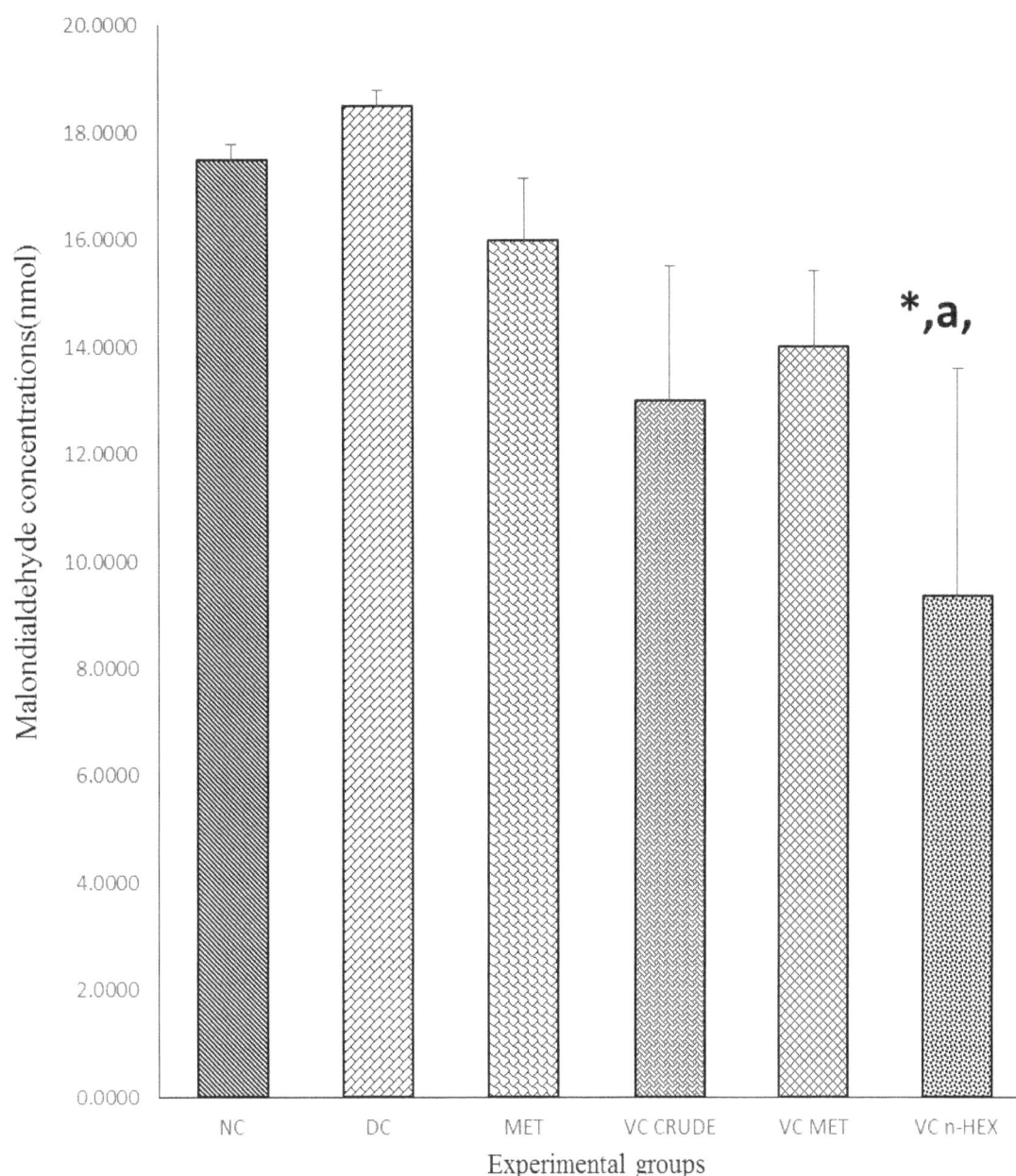

Figure 2c. Malondialdehyde concentrations of the different experimental groups. Values are expressed as mean ± SEM (n=5). *Significantly different from NC at p<0.05. [a]p<0.05 vs. DC, [b]p<0.05 vs. MET, [d]p<0.05 vs. crude VC. NC: Normal control, DC: diabetic control, MET: metformin, V.C _CRUDE: *Vernonia calvoana* crude, V.C MET: *Vernonia calvoana* metformin, V.C_nHEX: *Vernonia calvoana* hexane.

cardiomyopathy, and retinopathy (Williams et al., 2013). Basically, hyperglycemic conditions are associated with elevated reactive oxygen species (ROS) production, predominantly through mitochondrial electron transport chain and nicotinamide adenine dinucleotide phosphate oxidase (Ray and Shah, 2005). The possible sources of ROS include autoxidation of glucose, shifts in redox balance, decreased tissue concentration of glutathione and vitamin E, as well as impaired activity of superoxide dismutase (SOD) and catalase (CAT). Oxidative stress has been widely established as a major contributory factor in the development and progression of diabetes and its complications. It has been suggested that insulin resistance may be accompanied by intracellular production of free radicals. Thus, a vicious cycle between hyperinsulinemia and free radicals could be operating in the early stages of diabetes pathogenesis. Insulin resistance induced elevated plasma free radicals, in turn,

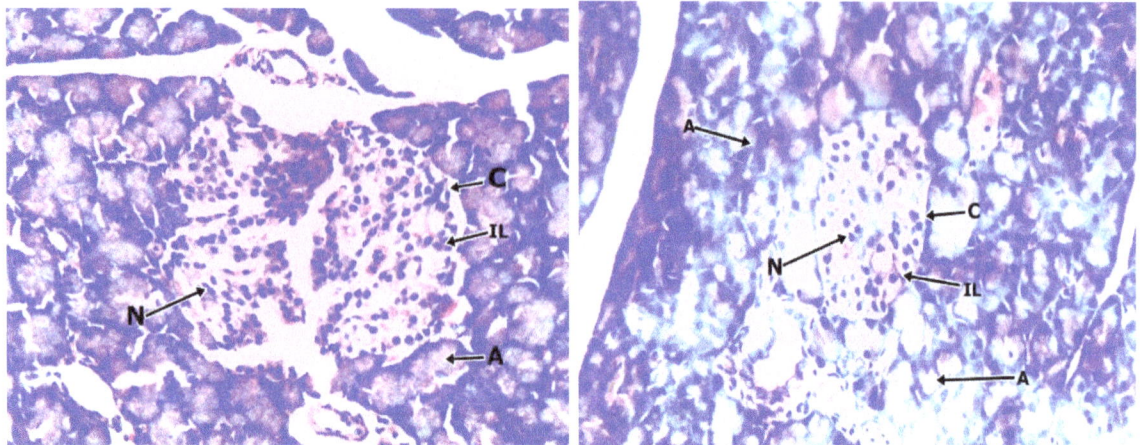

a: Normal control

b: diabetic control

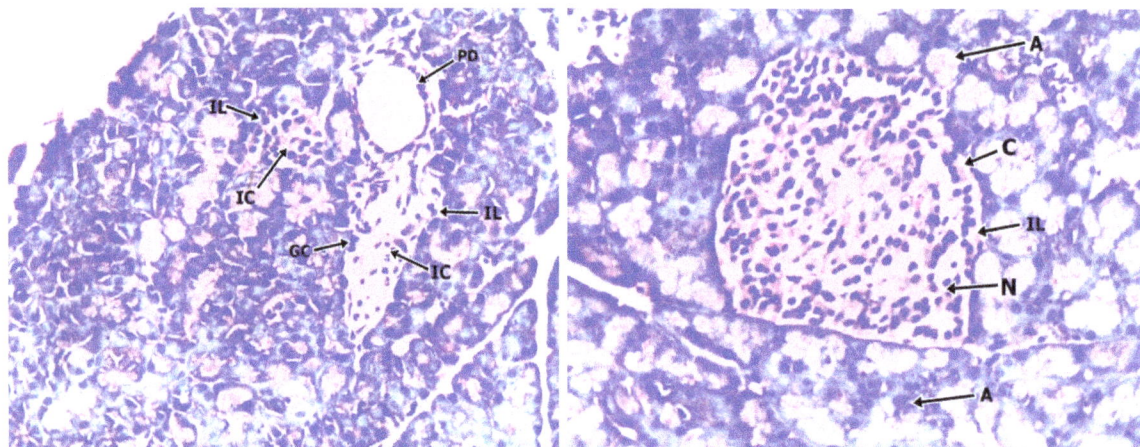

c: metformin

d: methanol

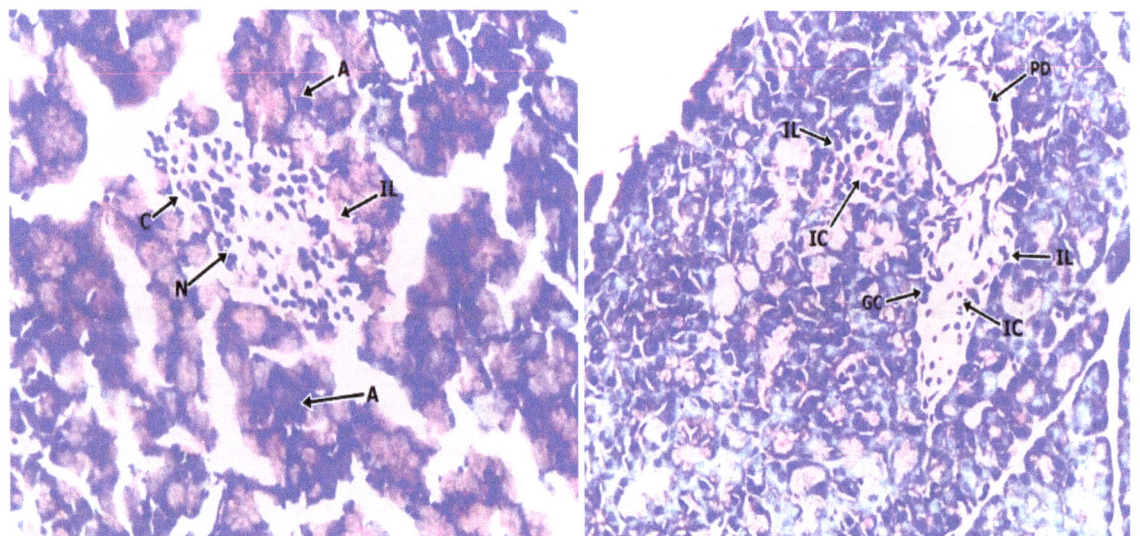

e: n-hexane group

f: crude extract group

Figure 3. (a, b, c, d, e, f) Photomicrographs of pancreas (normal and diabetic control) and (metformin and methanol group) (X 400). H&E = Haematoxilin and Eosin. IL=islet of Langerhans, IC=islet cell, PC=pancreatic cell, A=acinar, N=nucleus. Photomicrographs of pancreas (normal and diabetic control) and (n-hexane and crude extract group) (X 400). H&E = Haematoxilin and Eosin, G=Gomeri stains. IL=islet of Langerhans, IC=islet cell, PC=pancreatic cell, A=acinar, N=nucleus.

may cause a deterioration of insulin action, with hyperglycemia being a contributory factor (Ceriello, 2000). Other mechanisms by which increased oxidative stress is involved in the diabetic complications include activation of several transcription factors, protein kinase C, and advanced glycated end products (AGEs). In the present study, decrease in antioxidant enzymes, including glutathione peroxidase (GPx) and CAT) activities, and increase in MDA concentration recorded for DC were reversed upon treatment with the leaves' extracts and standard drug. This effect may be attributed to the presence of bioactive components reported in this study for this plant such as 2-furanmethanol, 2-tridece-1-ol, phytol, n-hexadecanoic acid, 9, 12, 15-octadecatrien-1-ol for the n-hexane extract and 2-butanone, 1-hydroxy-3-methyl-2-butanone, hexadecanoic acid, oleic acid, e-11-teradecenoic acid and cyclohexane propanol for the methanol fraction. Probably, these compounds may by reacting with a free radical, donates hydrogen atoms with an unpaired electron (H·), converting free radicals into less reactive species (Iwara et al., 2016). This may also contributed to the observed antioxidant activities reported in this study for VC leaves' extracts. The observation agrees with the earlier reports by Igile et al. (2013) and Iwara et al. (2015).

Streptozotocin is known to induce chemical diabetes (type 1) by selective destruction of pancreatic beta cells through three processes, including deoxyribonucleic acid alkylation, nitric oxide production and free radical generation (Szkudelski, 2001). The selective pancreatic beta cell toxicity of s STZ and the resulting diabetic metabolic state are clearly related to the glucose moiety in its chemical structure, which enables streptozotocin to enter the beta cell via the low affinity Glut 2 glucose transporter in the plasma membrane (Elsner et al., 2000). This condition was observed in this study, as diabetic control rat pancreas showed a compact islet surrounded by pancreatic acinar cells. The observation is consistent with the literature reports on STZ-induced pancreas damage (Noor et al., 2010). However, these lesions were slightly reversed or ameliorated after treatment with met and extracts of V. calvoana indicating a recovery effect. The recovery may be attributed to the phytochemicals that has been reported by Igile et al. (2013) and in this research. Moreover, it was observed in this study that components in the extract of methanol fractions appears to mimic the standard drugs in the following parameters plasma blood glucose, fasting blood glucose, body weight changes, GPX and MDA and may follow the same mechanism of action.

Conclusion

Conclusively, findings in this study suggests for the first time that extracts V. calvoana possess potent ameliorative activity against STZ-induced diabetes, potentially due to free radical mopping activity of the extract and thus ameliorate metabolic complications of diabetic state.

ACKNOWLEDGEMENTS

The authors are grateful to Professor Patrick Ekong Ebong of the Department of Biochemistry, University of Calabar, Nigeria, for making available the facilities in his Endocrine and Phytomedicine Laboratory for successful completion of this research work.

REFERENCES

Ahmed N (2005). Advanced glycation endproducts-role in pathology of diabetic complications. Diabetes Res. Clin. Pract. 67(1):3-21

Atangwho IJ, Ebong PE, Eyong EU, Asmawi MZ, Ahmad M (2012). Synergistic antidiabetic activity of Vernonia amygdalina and Azadirachta indica: Biochemical effects and possible mechanism. J. Ethnopharmacol. 141(3):878-887.

Atangwho IJ, Egbung GE, Ahmad M, Yam MF, Asmawi MZ (2013). Antioxidant versus anti-diabetic properties of leaves from Vernonia amygdalina Del. growing in Malaysia. Food Chem. 141(4):3428-3434.

Burkill HM (1985). The Useful Plants of West Tropical Africa, (2nd Ed). London: Royal Botanic Gardens Kew, pp. 510.

Ceriello A (2000). Oxidative stress and glycemic regulation. Metabolism 49(2):27-29.

Chakraborty R, Rajagopala R (2002). Diabetes and insulin resistance associated disorders-disease and the terapy. Curr. Sci. 83:1533-1538.

Donga JJ, Surani VS, Sailor GU, Chauhan SP, Seth AK (2011). A systematic review on natural medicine used for therapy of diabetes mellitus of some Indian medicinal plants. Pharma Science Monitor-An Int. J. Pharm. Sci. 1(2):36-72.

Drury RAB, Wallington EA (1967). Carleton's histological technique, (4th Ed). London: Oxford University Press.

Ebong PE, Atangwho IJ, Eyong EU, Egbung GE (2008). The antidiabetic efficacy of combined extracts from two continental plants: Azadirachta indica (A. Juss) (Neem) and Vernonia amygdalina (Del.) (African Bitter Leaf). Am. J. Biochem. Biotechnol. 4(3):239-244.

Elsner M, Guldbakke B, Tiedge M, Munday R, Lenzen S (2000). Relative importance of transport and alkylation for pancreatic beta-cell toxicity of streptozotocin. Diabetologia 43(12):1528-1533.

Focho DA, Nkeng EAP, Lucha CF, Ndam WT, Afegenui A (2009). Ethnobotanical survey of plants used to treat diseases of the reproductive system and preliminary phytochemical screening of some species of Malvaceae in Ndop Central Sub-Division, Cameroon. J. Med. Plants Res. 3:301-314.

Igile GO, Iwara IA, Mgbeje BIA, Uboh FE, Ebong PE (2013). Phytochemical, Proximate and Nutrient Composition of Vernonia calvaona Hook (Asterecea): A Green-Leafy Vegetable in Nigeria. J. Food Res. 2(6).

Iwara IA, Igile GO, Uboh FE, Eyong EU, Ebong PE (2015). Hypoglycemic and hypolipidemic potentials of extract of Vernonia Calvoana on Alloxan –Induce Diabetics Albino Wistar rats. Eur. J. Med. Plant 8(2):78-86.

Iwara IA, Uboh FE, Igile GO, Edward JM, Eteng MU (2016). Bioactive components and in vitro antioxidants activity of extracts of Vernonia calvoana leaves. J. Trop. Med. (In press).

Iwu MM (1993). Handbook of African medicinal plants. London: CRC Press, P 415.

Keeley SC, Jones SB (1979). Distribution of pollen types in Vernonia (Vernonieae: Compositae). Syst. Bot. 4:195-202.

King AJ (2012). The use of animal models in diabetes research. Brit. J. Pharmacol. 166(3):877-894.

Lorke DA (1983). New Approach to Practical Acute Toxicity Testing. Arch Toxicol 53:275-287.

Mythili M, Vyas R, Akila G, Gunasekaran S (2004). Effect of streptozotocin on the ultrastructure of rat pancreatic islets. Microsc. Res. Tech. 63(5):274-281.

Noor AS, Jilani PS, Sharique A, Ahamad I, Durga KR (2010). Increased frequency of micronuclei in diabetes mellitus patients using pioglitazone and glimepiride in combination. Food Chem. Toxicol. 48:3432-3435.

Ray R, Shah AX (2005). NADPH oxidase and endothelial cell function. Clin. Sci. 109:217-226.

Szkudelski T (2001). The mechanism of alloxan and streptozotocin action in B cells of the rat pancreas. Physiol. Res. 50:536-546.

Venkatesh S, Reddy GD, Reddy BM, Ramesh M, Rao AA (2003). Antihyperglycemic activity of *Caralluma attenuata*. Fitoterapia 74(3):274-279.

Williams M, Hogg RE, Chakravarthy U (2013). Antioxidants and diabetic retinopathy, Curr. Diabetes Rep. 13(4):481-487.

World Health Organization (WHO) (2014). Global health estimates: Deaths by cause, age, sex and country, 2000-2012. Geneva, WHO.

## 5

Phytochemical and biological investigation of *Eugenia uniflora* L. cultivated

Riham O. Bakr[1], Shaza A. Mohamed[2] and Nermien E. Waly[3]*

[1]Department of Pharmacognosy, Faculty of Pharmacy, MSA University, Giza 11787, Egypt.
[2]Department of Pharmacognosy, Faculty of Pharmacy, Al-Azhar University (Girls), Cairo, Egypt.
[3]Department of Physiology, Faculty of Medicine, Helwan University, Helwan 11795, Egypt.

Eugenia uniflora L. (Myrtaceae) is a plant species used in folk medicine for treatment of various disorders. This study aims to quantify the phenolic and flavonoid contents of *E. uniflora* aqueous methanolic extract (AME), identification of its major constituents, as well as the evaluation of its biological activity. Quantification was performed using colorimetric assays. Column chromatographic separation was used for isolation of the major phenolic constituents while their structures were elucidated by 1D- and 2D Nuclear magnetic resonance spectroscopy (NMR) spectra. Alkaloids were identified using gas chromatography-mass spectrometry (GC-MS) analysis. The antidepressant activity of *E. uniflora* AME in mice was evaluated using the tail suspension test (TST). The weight control effect was evaluated by serial weighing. The results showed high phenolic and flavonoid contents of *E. uniflora* AME. The chromatographic investigation identified a new flavonoid, myricetin 3-*O*-(4'', 6''-digalloyl) glucopyranoside, for first time in this genus, along with four flavonoids and phenolic acids. Integerrimine alkaloid was identified through GC/MS analysis. Administration of *E. uniflora* AME significantly reduced the immobility time in mice (P value of < 0.0001) in a dose- dependent manner for doses of 1, 10, 50 and 100 mg/kg. Also, a non-significant weight reduction in mice chronically treated with the *E. uniflora* AME was observed. Our study reports the isolation of myricetin 3-*O*- (4'', 6''-digalloyl) glucopyranoside from *E. uniflora*. It confirms that *E. uniflora* leaf extract has an antidepressant and anti-obesity effect.

Key words: *Eugenia uniflora*, flavonoid, alkaloid, depression, obesity.

INTRODUCTION

Obesity and depression are escalating global and societal problems (McArdle et al., 2013; WHO, 2006). Associated environmental factors such as poor dietary habits, and sedentary lifestyle, that impair hormone secretion and metabolism result in obesity (McArdle et al., 2013). There is an increasing interest by researchers to identify food items or dietary components that may control weight. On the other hand, conventional therapy

*Corresponding author. E-mail: nwaly@icloud.com.

of depression has been reported to be effective only in 50% of cases due to this, thus the necessity for a new treatment has risen (Kessler et al., 2003). The use of herbal therapy may be preferred in depression as it could provide a safer and potentially a more effective therapeutic option (Elhwuegi, 2004; Halliwell, 2006).

The genus *Eugenia* is considered one of the largest genera belonging to family Myrtaceae with about 500 species of trees and shrubs in tropical and subtropical America (Faqueti et al., 2013). *Eugenia uniflora* L. (Pitanga cherry or Brazilian cherry) is a putative candidate for management of both diseases. *E. uniflora* L. is a semi-deciduous shrubby tree with edible, cherry-like fruits, native to Brazil. The leaves and fruits of *E. uniflora* have been used in folk medicine for treatment of diarrhea, inflammation, rheumatic pains, fever, stomach problems and hypertension (Almeida et al., 1995; Consolini et al., 1999). In addition, it was reported to possess a wide range of medicinal properties including alleviation of mood disorders, antibacterial, antifungal, cytotoxic as well as radical scavenging activities (Alves, 2008; Auricchio et al., 2007; Auricchio and Bacchi, 2003; Franco and Fontana, 2004; Rattmann et al., 2012; Samy et al., 2014a; Saravanamuttu, 2012; Schapoval et al., 1994).

Among its wide range of biological activities, *E. uniflora* showed hypoglycemic as well as hypolipidemic effects (Saravanamuttu, 2012). Also, oral administration of essential oils (EO) from other *Eugenia* species (*E. brasiliensis*, *E. catharinae* and *E. umbelliflora*) produced antidepressant-like effects in mice (Colla et al., 2012; Victoria et al., 2013).

The leaves of *E. uniflora* were the subject of many phytochemical reports and the plant itself is deemed of interest as it is rich in tannins, flavonoids, triterpenpoids and alkaloids. The identified alkaloids have been correlated with its anti-diabetic activity (Auricchio and Bacchi, 2003; Consolini et al., 1999; Fortes et al., 2015; Lee et al., 1997; Samy et al., 2014a; Saravanamuttu, 2012).

Our objectives were to identify the major constituents of *E. uniflora* aqueous methanolic extract (AME) using different chromatographic techniques, quantifying its phenolic and flavonoid contents, as well as investigating its antidepressant and weight control activity in mice.

MATERIALS AND METHODS

General experimental procedure

The NMR spectra were recorded at 400 (^{1}H) and 100 (^{13}C) MHz, on Varian Mercury 300, Bruker APX-400 and JEOL GX-500 NMR spectrometers and δ-values are reported as parts per million. (ppm) relative to TMS in the convenient solvent. For column chromatography, Sephadex LH-20 (Pharmacia, Uppsala, Sweden), microcrystalline cellulose (E. Merck, Darmstadt, Germany) was used. For paper chromatography, Whatman No. 1 sheets

(Whatman Ltd., Maidstone, Kent, England) were used. The solvent systems were: S1: n-BuOH-HOAc-H$_2$O (4:1:5, upper layer) and S2: 15 % aqueous HOAc. All solvents used for separation processes were of analytical grade.

Plant material

Fresh leaves of *E. uniflora* L. were harvested in April 2014 from El Zohria garden, Cairo, Egypt and were identified according to *Prof.* Abdel-Haleem Abdel-Mogaly, Department of Plant Taxonomy, Herbarium of Horticultural Research Institute, Agricultural Research Centre, Dokki, Cairo, Egypt. A voucher specimen (RS 0018) was deposited in the herbarium of the Faculty of Pharmacy, MSA University.

Extraction and isolation

Fresh leaves of *E. uniflora* (1 kg) were dried, ground and defatted in petroleum ether under reflux. The extracts were combined and dried under vacuum, while the leaves were refluxed with 70% methanol till exhaustion. The extracts were filtered off, combined, and dried under reduced pressure, giving rise to a crude aqueous methanolic extract (AME) (110 g). Seventy grams of the AME were applied on a cellulose column (1.5 m × 10 cm, 1000 g), elution being carried out with water-methanol mixtures of decreasing polarity and monitored by paper chromatography and detection by UV light. Fractions of 100 mL each were collected. The similar fractions were gathered yielding four main fractions according to their chromatographic properties (fluorescence-UV light, and responses towards different spray reagents on PC). Fraction I (0-20% MeOH, 15 g) was phenolic free. Fraction II (30-40% MeOH, 4 g) was subjected to Sephadex LH-20 column using 50% MeOH to yield compound 1 (20 mg). Fraction III (40-60% MeOH, 2 g) was purified on a Sephadex column using saturated butanol for elution, to yield compound 2 (15 mg). Fraction IV (80-100% MeOH, 2.5 g) was chromatographed on a Sephadex column with 50% MeOH to yield compounds 3, 4 and 5 (7 mg, each). For alkaloid estimation, ten grams of the AME extract was mixed with 200 mL distilled water, acidified with 5% sulfuric acid solution, and then fractionated with dichloromethane. The aqueous extract was further alkalinized with ammonia, then extracted with dichloromethane. The process was repeated until the dichloromethane extract was negative to Dragendorff's reagent (Yubin et al., 2014). The combined dichloromethane extract was concentrated under vacuum and kept for GC/MS analysis. 0.25 g of total alkaloid extract was obtained with a percentage yield 2.5%.

GC/MS analysis

The analysis was carried out using a GC (Agilent Technologies 7890A) interfaced with a mass-selective detector (MSD, Agilent 7000) equipped with a nonpolar Agilent HP-5ms (5%-phenyl methyl poly siloxane) capillary column (30 m × 0.25 mm i.d. and 0.25 μm film thickness). The carrier gas was helium with the linear velocity of 1 mL/min. The identification of components was based on the comparison of their mass spectra and retention time with those of the authentic compounds and by computer matching with NIST and WILEY libraries as well as by comparison of the fragmentation pattern of the mass spectral data with those reported in the literature (Santana et al., 2013).

Quantitative colorimetric estimation of phenolic and flavonoid contents

The total phenolic content of *E. uniflora* AME was quantified using

Folin-Ciocalteau Reagent (FCR) and gallic acid as standard (Sellappan et al., 2002) measured at λ_{max} of 765 nm. Calculations were based on gallic acid calibration curve where the total phenolics were expressed as milligram of gallic acid equivalents (GAE) per gram dry extract. The total flavonoid content was determined using aluminum chloride colorimetric assay (Kosalec et al., 2004) where the measurement was performed at λ_{max} of 415 nm. Calculations were based on quercetin calibration curve and the total content was expressed as milligram of quercetin equivalent (QE) per gram dry extract. All measurements were carried out in triplicate.

HPLC analysis

Identification of flavonoids in *E. uniflora* AME was performed using HPLC (Mattila et al., 2000). Dry plant extract (0.1 g) was mixed with 5 mL methanol and centrifuged at 10,000 rpm for 10 min and the supernatant was filtered through a 0.2 μm Millipore membrane filter, after which then 1 to 3 mL was collected in a vial for injection into HPLC Hewlett-Packard (series 1050) equipped with auto-sampling injector; solvent degasser, ultraviolet (UV) detector set at λ_{max} of 330 nm and quarter horsepower pump (series 1050). The column temperature was maintained at 35°C. Gradient separation was carried out with methanol and acetonitrile as a mobile phase at flow rate of 1 mL/min. Phenolic compounds were determined according to Goupy et al.,(1999) with the same sample preparation with the exception that the UV detector was set at λ_{max} of 80 nm and quarter HP pump (series 1100). Flavonoids and phenolic acid standards from Sigma Co. were dissolved in a mobile phase and injected into HPLC. Retention time and peak area were used for calculation of flavonoids and phenolic acid concentrations by the data analysis of Hewlett-Packard software.

Antidepressant activity

Animals

Forty male albino mice (4 to 5 weeks) were used for this study. Animals were housed randomly in-groups of 4 rats per cage, kept at room temperature and provided with rodent chow and water ad libitum. Mice were kept under a 12:12 h light: dark cycle (lights on at 07:00 h). Mice were allowed to acclimatize to the holding room for at least 24 h before the behavioral procedure. All manipulations were conducted in the light phase, with each animal used only once (n = 7 animals per group). Animal care and handling was performed in conformance with approved protocols of the MSA research ethics committee.

Treatment

The *E. Uniflora* AME was dissolved in distilled water and administered orally acutely (just once at the beginning of the experiment) or chronically (for 10 days) at doses 1, 10, 50 and 100 mg/kg by oral route (p.o.) 60 min before the tail suspension test. A control group received distilled water only.

Tail suspension test (TST)

The total duration of immobility induced by tail suspension was measured according to the method described previously (Steru et al., 1985). Mice were suspended about 50 cm above the floor by adhesive tape placed around 1 cm from the tip of the tail. Immobility time was recorded during a 6 min period. Mice were considered immobile only when they hung passively or stay completely

motionless. Conventional antidepressants decrease the immobility time in this test (Cunha et al., 2008; Steru et al., 1985).

Statistical analysis

All experimental results are given as the mean ± S.E.M. Comparisons between experimental and control groups were performed using one-way ANOVA. A value of P of 0.05 was considered to be significant.

RESULTS

Phytochemical investigation

Column chromatographic investigation of *E. uniflora* AME results in the isolation of five compounds identified as: Myricetin 3-O-(4", 6"-digalloyl glucopyranoside (1), myricetin 3-O-glucopyranoside (2) (Figure 1), quercetin (3), gallic acid (4) and ellagic acid (5). Compounds (1) and (2) were identified by comparing their spectroscopic data with that reported (Samy et al., 2014b) while compounds 3 to 5 were identified using Co-chromatography, by comparing with standards.

Myricetin 3- O-(4", 6"-digalloyl glucopyranoside (1)

Yellow amorphous powder, purple fluorescent turned into yellow by long UV light. ^{1}H NMR (400 MHz, CD$_3$OD): ppm 3.2-4.3 (sugar protons), 5.3 (1H, br s, H-1"), 6.12 (1H, d, J=2Hz, H-6), 6.31 (1 H, d, J=2Hz, H-8), 7.14 (2H, d, J=2Hz, H-2'-6'), 7.22 (2 H, s, H-2"/6"'), 7.29 (2H, s, H-2"'/6"'),. ^{13}C-NMR (100 MHz, CD$_3$OD): 63 (C-6"), 71.5 (C-4"), 72.1 (C-2"), 74 (C-5"), 75 (C-3"), 94.6 (C-8), 99.8(C-6), 101 (C-1"), 107.06 (C-10), 109.6 (C-2'-6'), 109.6 (C-2"'-6"'), 121 (C-1"'), (122 (C-1'), 136 (C-3), 137 (C-4'), 141.1 (C-4"'), 143.4 (C-3'-5'), 143.4 (C-3"'-5"'), 156.92 (C-9), 159 (C-2), 163 (C-5), 165 (C-7), 168 (C-7"'), 168.2 (C-7"'), 179 (C-4).

Myricetin 3-O-glucopyranoside (2)

Yellow amorphous powder, purple fluorescent turned into yellow by long UV light. ^{1}H NMR (400 MHz, CD$_3$OD):3.2-4.3 (sugar protons), 5.05 (1H, d, J=7.6 Hz, H-1"), 6.1 (1H, d, J=2Hz, H-6), 6.31 (1 H, d, J=2Hz, H-8), 7.23 (2H, d, J=2Hz, H-2'-6'), ^{13}C-NMR (100 MHz, CD$_3$OD):61 (C-6"), 70 (C-4"), 72 (C-2"), 73 (C-5"), 76 (C3"), 94 (C-8), 99 (C-6), 104 (C-1"), 105 (C-10), 109 (C2',6'), 109 (C-2"'-6"'), 122 (C-1'), 136 (C-3), 138 (C-4'), 146 (C-3'-5'), 158 (C2, C-9), 162 (C-5), 166 (C-7), 179 (C-4).

Compound 3, 4 and 5

These were identified as quercetin, gallic acid and ellagic acid by Co-PC.

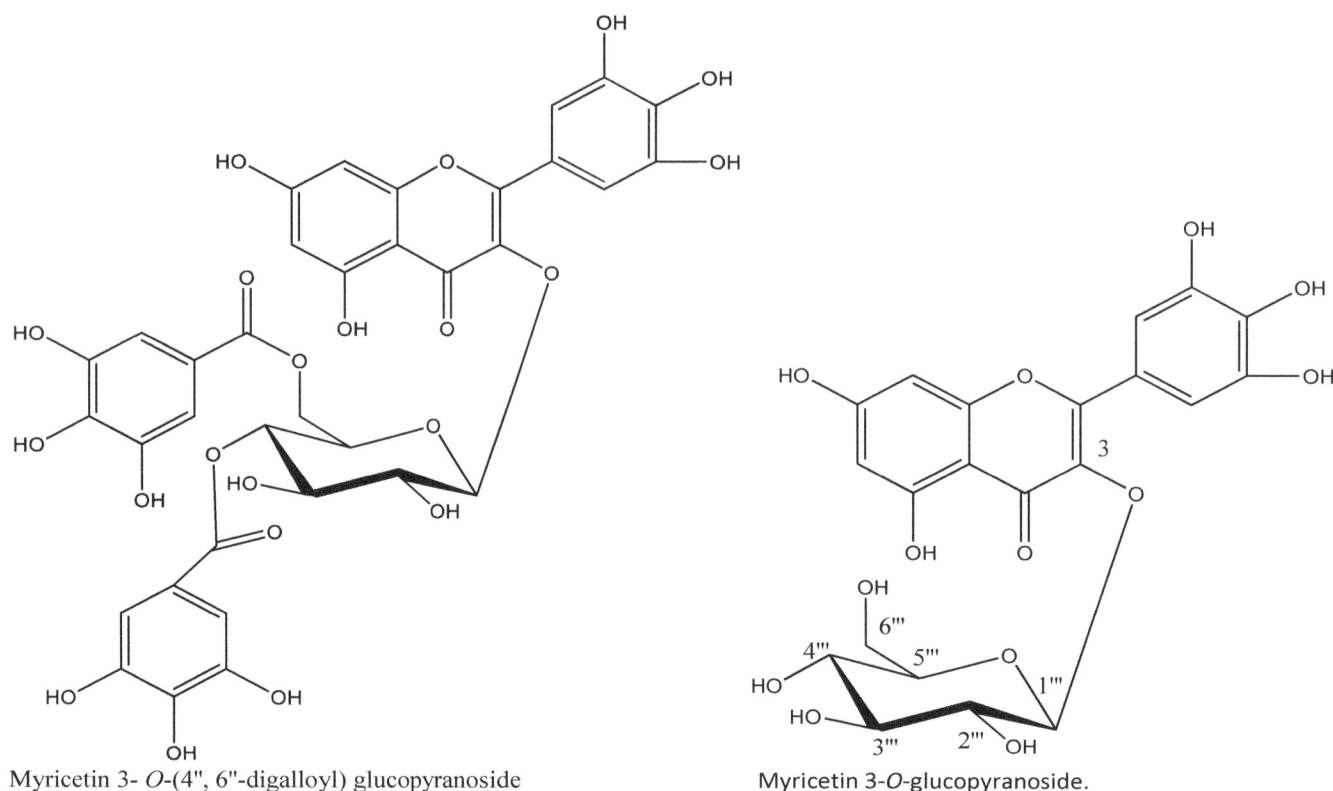

Myricetin 3- *O*-(4", 6"-digalloyl) glucopyranoside

Myricetin 3-*O*-glucopyranoside.

Figure 1. Chemical structures of *E. uniflora* main constituents.

GC/MS analysis

Investigation of the dichloromethane fraction resulted in the identification of ten compounds (Figure 2 and Table 1) including one main alkaloid, nitrogenated derivatives and some fatty acids. The identification was based on comparison of the MS characteristics and molecular weight (MW) with the mass spectra of the available databases and previous reports. Dodecanoic, oleic acid, in addition to hexadecanoic, heptadecanoic and octadecanoic acid derivatives have been identified. Compound 10 was identified as Integerrimine according to its fragmentation pattern (Figure 3).

Quantitative colorimetric estimation of phenolic and flavonoid contents

E. uniflora appeared rich in phenolic content expressed as 98.17±0.35 mg/g GAE (standard curve equation: y = 0.0011x + 0.0009, r^2 = 0.9867). In addition, flavonoid content represented 8.1±0.27 mg/g QE (standard curve equation: y = 0.005x - 0.0198, r^2 = 0.9774).

HPLC analysis

HPLC analysis was employed to identify the main phenolic and flavonoid contents based on comparison of spectra with those of available standards. Results were presented in Tables 2 and 3. The results showed that gallic acid (10.85 mg/g) was the most abundant phenolic acid followed by benzoic acid (5.23 mg/g) then isoferulic acid (2.96 mg/g), while flavonoid analysis revealed quercetrin (2.17 mg/g) as the main identified flavonoid followed by naringin (1.92 mg/g).

Antidepressant activity

Administration of *E. uniflora* AME reduced the immobility time in the TST in a dose-dependent manner for doses 1 and 10 mg/kg. The average immobility time for control mice was 3.7 ± 0.4 seconds, while it was 2.3 ± 0.8 and 0.9 ± 0.3 s for doses 1 and 10 mg/kg consequently. This reduction was statistically significant with the P value of < 0.0001. At doses of 50 and 100 mg/kg the extract still significantly reduced (P value of < 0.0001) the immobility time to 1.6 ± 0.4, and 2.4 ± 0.3 seconds respectively (Figure 4).

On the other hand, administering *E. uniflora* AME chronically for 10 days significantly (P <0.0001) reduced the immobility time in TST at all doses tested. The immobility times for doses 1, 10, 50 and 100 mg/kg were 1.4 ± 0.2, 2.3±0.3, 2.9 ± 0.5 and 2.1 ± 0.4 s, respectively.

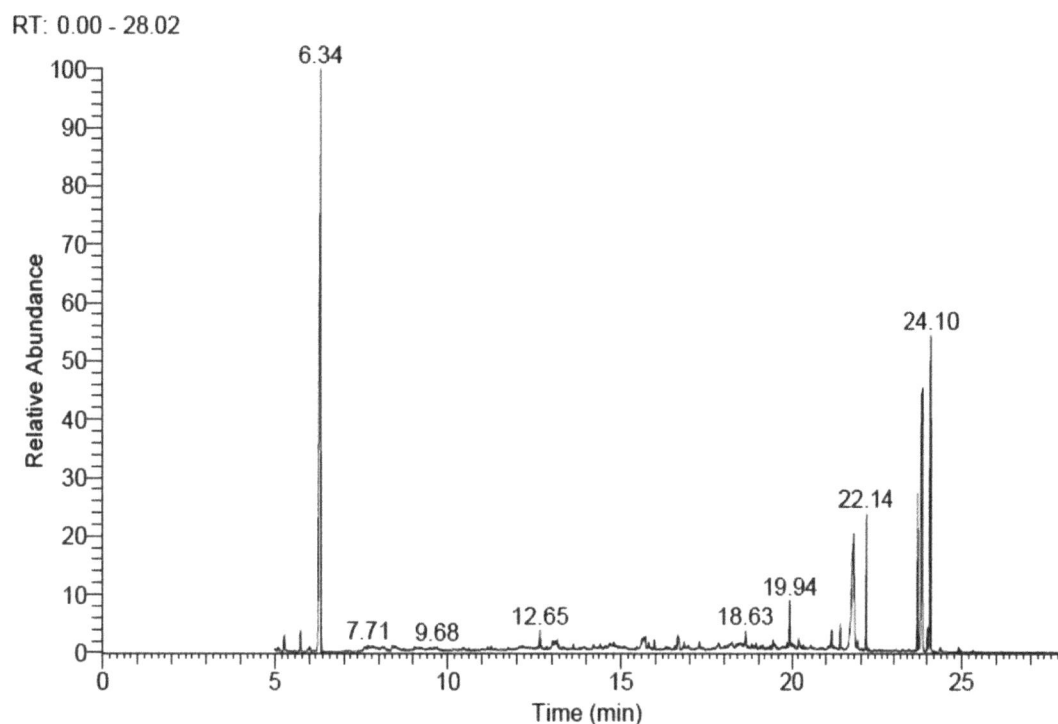

Figure 2. Fragmentation pattern of integerrimine identified in *E. uniflora* dichloromethane fraction.

Table 1. Identification of the main constituents in the dichloromethane fraction (GC/MS analysis).

S/N	Rt[1]	Constituent	M+	Mass spectral data (m/z[2], intensity %)
1	5.28	Pyridine	79	79 (100%) 52 (80%) 51 (60%) 50 (48%)
2	5.75	3 methyl Pyrrol	81	81 (75%) 80.1 (100%) 53 (30%)
3	6.33	2 butoxy ethanol	118	57.1 (100%) 45 (46%) 87.1 (30%) 75 (15%) 100 (10%)
4	15.70	Dodecanoic acid	200	55.1 (100%) 43 (92%) 73 (90%) 60 (85%) 129 (30%) 85 (30%)
5	16.66	Dihydromethyl jasmonate	226	83 (100%) 55 (30%) 67 (20%) 105 (20%) 155 (15%)
6	21.38	Heptadecanoic acid methyl ester	298	74 (100%) 87.1 (80%) 43 (60%) 55 (50%) 298.3 (30%) 143.1 (10%) 109 (10%)
7	21.76	Oleic acid	282	55.1 (100%) 69 (70%) 83 (69%) 97.1 (50%) 111.1 (30%) 129 (15%) 264.2 (15%) 226.1 (10%)
8	22.14	Octadecyl acetate	312	43 (100%) 83.1 (90%) 97.1 (80%) 111.1 (50%) 125.1 (20%) 252.2 (10%) 139.1 (10%) 165.1 (10%)
9	23.73	Hexadecanoic acid bis (2ethylhexyl)ester	370	129 (100%) 57 (50%) 112 (50%) 70.1 (30%) 83 (27%) 147 (27%) 241 (8%) 259.1 (8%)
10	23.86	Integerrimine	335	120.1 (100%) 136 (98%) 94.1 (80%) 80.1 (50%) 43 (22%) 67 (20%) 220.1 (20%) 335.1 (20%) 246 (18%)

Rt = Retention time; m/z = Mass to charge ratio; M+ = Molecular ion.

The immobility time for the control was 2.1±0.8 s (Figure 5).

In addition, a non-significant weight reduction in mice chronically treated with the *E. uniflora* AME was observed. The average weight for the control mice was 17.75 ± 0.7 while for the treated groups it was 16.8 ± 0.9, 18.3 ± 0.6, 17.1 ± 0.8 and 16.4 ± 0.8 g for doses of 1, 10, 50 and 100 mg/kg respectively (Figure 6). For all

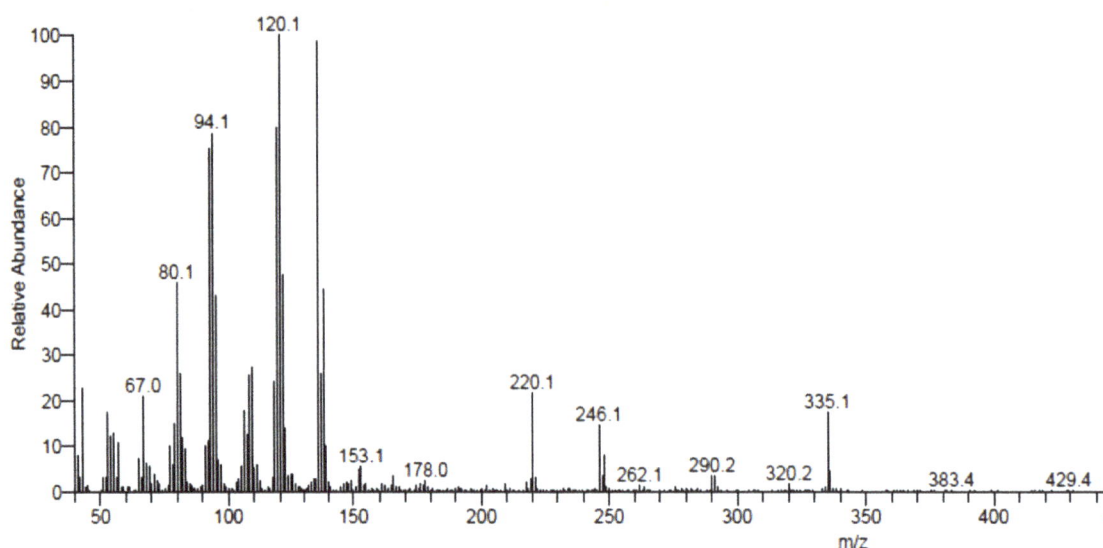

Figure 3. Fragmentation pattern of integerrimine identified in *E. uniflora* dichloromethane fraction using HPLC.

Table 2. Phenolic acid identified in *E. uniflora* AME using HPLC analysis.

Phenolic compound	Concentration (mg/g)
Gallic acid	10.85
Protocatechuic acid	0.238
Chlorogenic acid	1.364
Catechol	0.474
Catechin	0.289
P- hydroxy-benzoic acid	0.26
Caffeic acid	0.019
Vanillic acid	0.969
Ferulic acid	0.433
Isoferulic acid	2.96
Ellagic acid	1.383
Alpha coumaric acid	0.169
Benzoic acid	5.23
Salicylic acid	0.441
3, 4, 5 methoxy-cinnamic acid	0.066
P-Coumaric acid	0.162
Cinnamic acid	0.037

Table 3. Flavonoid content in *E. uniflora* AME using HPLC analysis.

Flavonoid	Concentration (mg/g)
Naringin	1.92
Rutin	0.38
Hesperidin	0.196
Quercetrin	2.17
Quercetin	0.024
Naringenin	0.069
Hesperetin	0.38
Apigenin	0.023
7-OH- flavone	0.007

experiments N=7 for each experimental group.

DISCUSSION

This study confirmed high phenolic and flavonoid contents evaluated through HPLC and colorimetric assays, in agreement with reported literature (Suhendi et al., 2011). Beside the previously tentatively identified constituents, five compounds were isolated and identified.

Compound 1, Myricetin 3- O-(4", 6"-digalloyl) glucopyranoside was identified for first time in this species, compared with myricetin 3-O-(4"-O-galloyl) α-L-rhamnopyranoside, previously identified (Samy et al. 2014a). ^{1}H-NMR and ^{13}C-NMR showed closely related data to myricetin 3 O-glucopyranoside (compound 2) except for the presence of additional signals at δ 7.22 and 7.29 ppm referring to the galloyl moieties. The location was determined to be at C-6" and C-4" on the basis of the downfield shift of C-6" and C-4" glucose compared with the resonance of the corresponding carbon in the spectrum of the free glucopyranose present in compound 2. The two equivalent Galloyl protons H-2 and H-6 appeared as sharp singlet integrated for two protons at δ 7.22 and 7.29 ppm. Our data are similar to previous literature (Suhendi et al., 2011).

Integerrimine, the main alkaloid identified through its fragmentation pattern (Figure 3), was compared with the

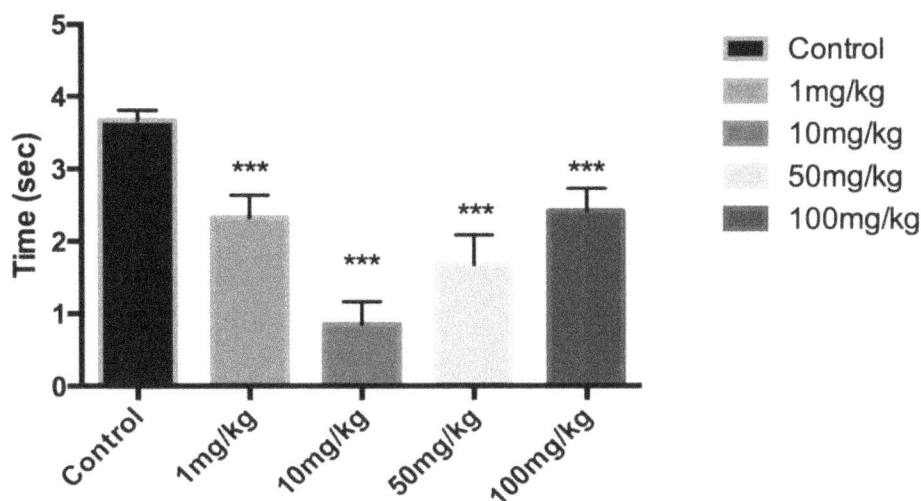

Figure 4. The effect of acute treatment with *E. uniflora* AME on the tail suspension test (TST) in mice. Administration of *E. uniflora* AME significantly reduced the immobility time in TST in mice treated for 60 min before the test at doses of 1, 10, 50 and 100 mg/kg. Results expressed as mean ± SEM and analyzed using one-way ANOVA; (*** = P value was < 0.0001).

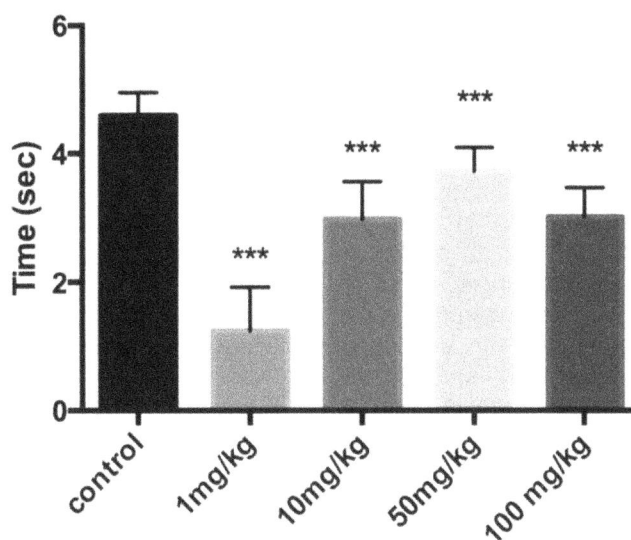

Figure 5. The effect of chronic treatment with *E. uniflora AME* on tail suspension test (TST) in mice. Administration of *E. uniflora* AME significantly reduced the immobility time in TST in mice treated for 10 days before the test at doses of 1, 10, 50 and 100 mg/kg. Results expressed as mean ± SEM and analyzed using one-way ANOVA; (*** =P value was < 0.0001).

reported literature (El-Shazly et al., 1996; Zhu et al., 2015). The series of ions at *m/z* 136, 120, 119, 93, 94 and 80, are characteristic of 1, 2- unsaturated pyrrolizidine diesters. While the presence of a base peak at *m/z* 120 and 138 is denoting a retronecine-type of pyrrolizidine alkaloid, where the ion fragment at *m/z* 220 is due to the cleavage of the weak allylic ester bond.

Gallic acid was identified with HPLC analysis in high concentration in agreement with Schumacher et al. (2015), while benzoic acid derivatives have been

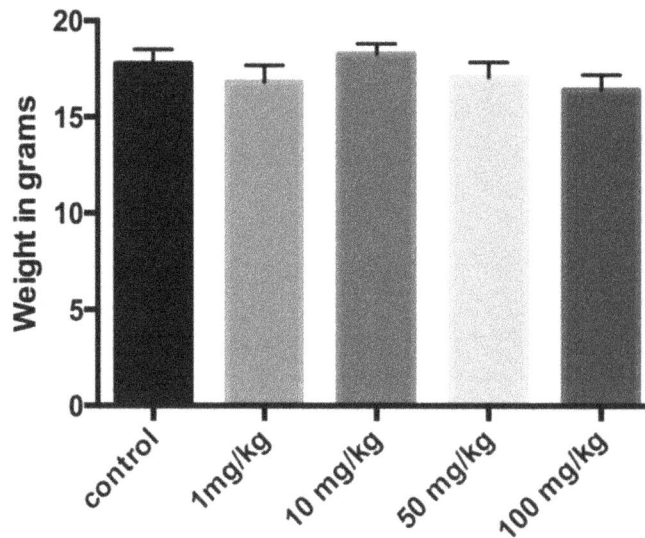

Figure 6. The effect of chronic treatment with *E. uniflora* AME on weight in mice. Administration of *E. uniflora* AME reduced the weight in TST in mice treated for 10 days at doses of 1, 10, 50 and 100 mg/kg. Results expressed as mean ± SEM and analyzed using one-way ANOVA.

identified in *E. polyantha* (Lelono et al., 2013). Quercetrin which was the highest identified flavonoid was previously identified by Rattmann *et al.* (2012).

With respect to the antidepressant activity of *E. uniflora* AME extract the result of this study show that the extract significantly reduced the immobility time in a dose-dependent manner at the doses of 1 and 10 mg/kg. At higher doses the effect was less pronounced although the reduction was still significant when compared with the control. Our results come in agreement with Victoria et al., (Victoria et al., 2013) where they studied the antidepressant-like effect of *E. uniflora* essential oil in the TST at doses of 10 and 50 mg/kg. Furthermore, the administration of *E. uniflora* extract for one month still had antidepressant like activity (Figure 4) with the dose 1 mg/kg being highly significant compared to the other doses. These results could explain the traditional use of *E. uniflora* in folk medicine for the treatment of symptoms related to depression, as well as its use by Guarani Indians as a tonic stimulant (Alonso, 1998; Greinger, 1996). The stepwise fashion of the decrease in the reduction of immobility time at higher doses than 10 mg/kg could in fact support a receptor mediated mechanism for the antidepressant effect of *E. uniflora* AME (Colla et al., 2012).

The antidepressant activity demonstrated by *E. uniflora* AME can be attributed to its myricetin content. Previous report suggested the ability of myricetin to attenuate the depressant-like behaviors in mice exposed to repeated restraint stress by restoring the brain derived neurotropic

factor (BDNF) levels and attributed to the myricetin-mediated anti-oxidative stress in the hippocampus (Ma et al., 2015). Further studies however are needed to confirm this suggestion.

On the other hand, the different results obtained by Colla et al. (2012) who studied the hydro-alcoholic extract of different *Eugenia* species could be attributed to the difference in the plant constitution. Also, we used different species of mice and only male mice, which can account for different responses to the extract. Further studies are required to confirm the effective dose required for the antidepressant activity of the *E. uniflora* in different animal species as well as in human to detect the difference in response between males and females.

Although statistically non-significant, the *E. uniflora* AME produced a degree of weight loss in animals that received the extract for one month. This result could suggest a potential role for this extract in treatment of obesity especially that it has been reported that it has anti-hyperlipidemic and hypoglycemic effect (Ramalingum and Mahomoodally, 2014).

Conclusion

This study reports for the first time the identification of myricetin 3- O-(4'', 6''-digalloyl) glucopyranoside and confirmed the high phenolic and flavonoid contents of Egyptian grown *E. uniflora* AME, beside the presence of alkaloid and fatty acids. In addition, this work supports the role for *E. uniflora* AME in the management of depression and obesity. Further studies are required to correlate myricetin derivatives with the biological activities of *E. uniflora,* determine the effective dose, and the exact mechanism through which these effects are achieved.

FUNDING

This research is not supported by any funding agency.

ACKNOWLEDGEMENT

The authors would like to acknowledge Prof. Richard Hallworth, PhD, Biomedical Sciences Department at Creighton University, Omaha, NE, USA, for his invaluable editorial assistance.

REFERENCES

Almeida CE, Karnikowski M, Foleto R, Baldisserotto B (1995). Analysis of antidiarrhoeic effect of plants used in popular medicine. Rev. Saúde Públ. 29:428-433.

Alonso JR (1998).PhytomedicineTreaty-Clinical and Pharmacological Basis, ISIS Ediciones S. R. L., Buenos Aires, Argentina.

Alves EO, Mota JH, Soares TS, Vieira MC, Silva CB (2008). Etnobotanical survey and medicinal plants characterization in forest fragments in Dourados-MS.Ciência e Agrotecnologia, Lavras 32:651-658.

Auricchio MT, Bugno A, Barros SBM, Bacchi EM (2007). Antimicrobial and antioxidant activities and toxicity of *Eusenia uniflora*. Latin Am. J.Pharm. 26:78-81.

Auricchio MT, Bacchi EM (2003). Eugenia uniflora L. "Brazilian cherry" leaves: pharmacobotanical, chemical and pharmacological properties. Rev. Inst. Adolfo Lutz 62:55-62.

Colla AR, Machado DG, Bettio LE, Colla G, Magina MD, Brighente IM, Rodrigues AL (2012). Involvement of monoaminergic systems in the antidepressant-like effect of *Eugenia brasiliensis* Lam. (Myrtaceae) in the tail suspension test in mice. J. Ethnopharmacol. 143:720-731.

Consolini AE, Baldini OA, Amat AG (1999). Pharmacological basis for the empirical use of *Eugenia uniflora* L. (Myrtaceae) as antihypertensive. J. Ethnopharmacol. 66:33-39.

Cunha MP, Machado DG, Bettio LE, Capra JC, Rodrigues AL (2008). Interaction of zinc with antidepressants in the tail suspension test. Prog Neuropsychopharmacol. Biol. Psychiatr. 32:1913-1920.

El-Shazly A, Sarg T, Ateya A, Abdel Aziz A, El-Dahmy S (1996). Pyrrolizidine Alkaloids from *Echium setosum* and *Echium vulgare*. J . Nat. Prod. 59(3):310-313.

Elhwuegi AS (2004).Central monoamines and their role in major depression. Prog Neuropsychopharmacol. Biol. Psychiatr. 28:435-451.

Faqueti LG, Petry CM, Meyre-Silva C, Machado KE, Cruz AB, Garcia PA, Cechinel-Filho V, San Feliciano A, Monache FD (2013). Euglobal-like compounds from the genus Eugenia. Nat. Prod. Res. 27:28-31.

Fortes GAC, Carvalho AG, Ramalho RRF, da Silva AJR, Ferri1 PH, Santos SC (2015). Antioxidant Activities of Hydrolysable Tannins and Flavonoid Glycosides Isolated from Eugenia uniflora. L. Rec. Nat. Prod. 9:251-256.

Franco IJ, Fontana VL, (2004). Herbs and Plants-Medicine of the Simple, eleventh ed. Editora Livraria Vida LTDA, Brazil.

Goupy P, Hugues M, Biovin P, Amiot M (1999). Amiot J. Antioxidant composition and activity of barley (Hordeum vulgare) and malt extracts and of isolated phenolic compounds. J. Sci. Food Argic. 79:1625-1634.

Greinger CR (1996). Medicinal plants of Seychelles. J. Royal Soc. Health 116(2):107-109.

Halliwell B (2006).Oxidative stress and neurodegeneration: where are we now? J. Neurochem. 97(6):1634-1658.

Kessler RC, Berglund P, Demler O, Jin R, Koretz D, Merikangas KR, Rush J, Walters EE, Wan PS (2003). The epidemiology of major depressive disorder: results from the National Comorbidity Survey Replication (NCS-R). JAMA 289(23): 3095-3105.

Kosalec H, Bakmaz M, Pepeljnjak S, Vladimir-kne S (2004). Quantitative analysis of the flavonoids in raw propolis from Northern Croatia. Acta Pharm. 54:65-72.

Lee MH, Nishimoto S, Yang LL, Yen KY, Hatano T, Yoshida T, Okuda T (1997). Two macrocyclic hydrolysable tannin dimers from Eugenia uniflora. Phytochemistry 44:1343-1349.

Lelono R, Arthur A, Sanro T (2013). Preliminary studies of Indonesian *Eugenia polyantha* leaf extracts as inhibitors of key enzymes for type 2 diabetes . J. Med. Sci. 13(2):103.

Ma Z, Wang G, Cui L, Wang Q (2015). Myricetin attenuates depressant-like behavior in mice subjected to repeated restraint stress. Int. J. Mol. Sci. 16:28377-28385.

Mattila P, Astola J, Kumpulainen J (2000). Determination of flavonoids in plant material by HPLC with diode-array and electro-array detections. J. Agric. Food Chem. 48:5834-5841.

McArdle MA, Finucane OM, Connaughton, RM, McMorrow AM, Roche HM, (2013). Mechanisms of obesity-induced inflammation and insulin resistance: insights into the emerging role of nutritional strategies. Front Endocrinol (Lausanne) 4: Article 52, 1-23.

Ramalingum N, Mahomoodally MF (2014). The therapeutic potential of medicinal foods. Adv. Pharmacol. Sci. 2014:1-18 Article ID.,354264.

Rattmann YD, De Souza, LM, Malquevicz-Paiva SM, Dartora N, Sassaki GL, Gorin PA, Iacomini M (2012). Analysis of flavonoids from Eugenia uniflora leaves and Its protective effect against Murine Sepsis. Evid. Based Complement. Alternat. Med. 2012:1-9, Article ID 623940,

Samy MN, Sugimoto S, Matsunami K, Otsuka H, Kamel MS (2014a). Bioactive compounds from the leaves of *Eugenia uniflora*. J. Nat. Prod. 7:37-47.

Samy MN, Sugimoto S, Matsunami, K Otsuka H, Kamel, MS (2014b). Taxiphyllin 6'-O-gallate, actinidioionoside 6'-O-gallate and myricetrin 2"-O-sulfate from the leaves of Syzygium samarangense and their biological activities. Chem. Pharm. Bull. 62(10):1013-1018.

Santana PM, Miranda M, Payrol JA, Silva M, Hernández V, Peralta E (2013b). Gas chromatography-mass spectrometry study from the leaves fractions obtained of *Vernonanthura patens* (Kunth) H. Rob. Int. J. Org. Chem. 3:105-109.

Saravanamuttu S, Sudarsanam D (2012). Antidiabetic plants and their active ingredients. IJPSR 3(10): 3639-3650.

Schapoval EE, Silveira SM, Miranda ML, Alice CB, Henriques AT (1994). Evaluation of some pharmacological activities of Eugenia uniflora L. J. Ethnopharmacol. 44:137-142.

Schumacher NS, Colomeu TC, De Figueiredo D, Carvalho Vde C, Cazarin CB, Prado, MA, Meletti LM, Zollner Rde L, (2015). Identification and antioxidant activity of the extracts of Eugenia uniflora Leaves. characterization of the anti-Inflammatory properties of aqueous extract on diabetes expression in an experimental Model of spontaneous type 1 diabetes (NOD Mice). Antioxidants (Basel) 4(4): 662-680.

Sellappan S, Akoh CC, Krewer G (2002). Phenolic compounds and antioxidant capacity of Georgia-grown blueberries and blackberries. J. Agric. Food Chem. 50:2432-2438.

Steru L, Chermat R, Thierry B, Simon P (1985). The tail suspension test: a new method for screening antidepressants in mice.Psychopharmacol. (Berl) 85:367-370.

Suhendi A, Ibtisam, Hanwar I, (2011). Determination of flavonoid and phenolics compounds in Dewandaru (*Eugenia uniflora* L.) by colorimetric method . Proceedings of the 2nd International Seminar on Chemistry, pp. 231-233.

Victoria FN, De Siqueira Brahm A, Savegnago L, Lenardao EJ (2013). Involvement of serotoninergic and adrenergic systems on the antidepressant-like effect of *E. uniflora* L. leaves essential oil and further analysis of its antioxidant activity. Neurosci. Lett. 544:105-109.

## 6

Study of chemical composition of *Foeniculum vulgare* using Fourier transform infrared spectrophotometer and gas chromatography - mass spectrometry

Hussein J. Hussein[1], Mohammed Yahya Hadi[2] and Imad Hadi Hameed[1]*

[1]Department of Biology, Babylon University, Iraq.
[2]College of Biotechnology, Al-Qasim Green University, Iraq.

Medicinal plants are potential sources of natural compounds with biological activities and therefore attract the attention of researchers worldwide. The objective of this research was to determine the chemical composition of seeds extract from methanol. The phytochemical compound screened by gas chromatography - mass spectrometry (GC-MS) method. Fifty six bioactive phytochemical compounds were identified in the methanolic extract of *Foeniculum vulgare*. The identification of phytochemical compounds is based on the peak area, retention time molecular weight, molecular formula, MS Fragment- ions and Pharmacological actions. The Fourier transform infrared spectroscopy (FTIR) analysis of F. vulgare seeds proved the presence of alkenes, aliphatic fluoro compounds, alcohols, ethers, carboxlic acids, esters, nitro compounds, alkanes, hydrogen bonded alcohols and phenols.

Key words: Gas chromatography - mass spectrometry (GC-MS), bioactive compounds, Fourier transforminfrared spectroscopy (FT-IR), Foeniculum vulgare.

INTRODUCTION

Bitter Fennel (*Foeniculum vulgare* Mill.) is one of the oldest herbs and possesses beneficial medicinal effects, belongs to the Apiaceae family and native to Mediterranean regions (Hornok, 1992). In botany the Umbllifererae (apiaceae) family is widespread and includes 300 genus and 3000 aromatic herbaceous species (Hay et al., 1993). *F. vulgare* is a well known aromatic medicinal plant which is used in traditional medicine as spice and substrate for different industrial purpose (Telci et al., 2009). Fennel is used for various purposes in the food, cosmetic, and medical industries.

Fennel essential oil has a valuable antioxidant, and has antibacterial, anticancer and antifungal activity (Lucinewton et al., 2005; El-Awadi and Esmat, 2010; Altameme et al., 2015a). It is cultivated and also widespread in many parts of Mediterranean and midlist countries such as Italy, Turkey and Iran (Marino et al. 2007; Altameme et al., 2015b). The increasing commercial value of fennel necessitates the need to identification, recognizing and conservation the existing diversity. The fruits of sweet fennel contain essential oi which is rich source of anethole, limonene, fenchone

*Corresponding author. E-mail: imad_dna@yahoo.com.

estragole and camphene among them the anethole is the most important constituent with determinant role in quality of the essential oil of seeds (Gross et al., 2002; Hameed et al., 2015a). These depend upon internal and external factors affecting the plant such as genetic structures and ecological conditions (Telci et al., 2009).

MATERIALS AND METHODS

Collection and preparation of plant material

The seeds were dried at room temperature for seven days and when properly dried then powdered using clean pestle and mortar, and the powdered plant was size reduced with a sieve. The fine powder was then packed in airtight container to avoid the effect of humidity and then stored at room temperature (Hameed et al., 2015b).

Preparation of sample

About four grams of the plant sample powdered were soaked in 50 ml methanol individually. It was left for two weeks so that alkaloids, flavonoids and other constituents if present will get dissolved (Hameed et al., 2015c). The methanol extract was filtered using Whatman No.1 filter paper and the residue was removed (Hamza et al., 2015).

Identification of component by gas chromatography - mass spectrum analysis

The physicochemical properties of F. vulgare are presented in Table 1. Interpretation of mass spectroscopy (GC-MS) was conducted using data base of National Institute Standard and Technology (NIST) having more than 62000 patterns. The spectrum of the unknown component was compared with the spectrum of the known component stored in the NIST library (Mohammed and Imad, 2013; Imad et al., 2014a). The identity of the components in the extracts was assigned by the comparison of their retention indices and mass spectra fragmentation patterns with those stored on the computer library and also with published literatures. The GC-MS analysis of the plant extract was made in a Agilent 7890 A instrument under computer control at 70 eV. About 1 µL of the methanol extract was injected into the GC-MS using a micro syringe and the scanning was done for 45 min. As the compounds were separated, they eluted from the column and entered a detector which was capable of creating an electronic signal whenever a compound was detected. The greater the concentration in the sample, bigger was the signal obtained which was then processed by a computer (Imad et al., 2014b; Hameed et al., 2015d). The time from when the injection was made (Initial time) to when elution occurred is referred to as the Retention time (RT). While the instrument was run, the computer generated a graph from the signal called Chromatogram. Each of the peaks in the chromatogram represented the signal created when a compound eluted from the gas chromatography column into the detector. The X-axis showed the RT and the Y-axis measured the intensity of the signal to quantify the component in the sample injected. As individual compounds eluted from the Gas chromatographic column, they entered the electron ionization (mass spectroscopy) detector, where they were bombarded with a stream of electrons causing them to break apart into fragments. The fragments obtained were actually charged ions with a certain mass. The M/Z (Mass / Charge) ratio obtained was calibrated from the graph obtained, which was called as the mass spectrum graph which is the fingerprint of a molecule. Before analyzing the extract using gas

chromatography and mass spectroscopy, the temperature of the oven, the flow rate of the gas used and the electron gun were programmed initially. The temperature of the oven was maintained at 100°C. Helium gas was used as a carrier as well as an eluent. The flow rate of helium was set to 1 ml per minute (Imad et al., 2014c; Kareem et al., 2015). The column employed here for the separation of components was Elite 1(100% dimethyl poly siloxane).

Fourier transform infrared spectrophotometer (FTIR)

The powdered sample of Euphorbia lathyrus specimen was treated for FTIR spectroscopy (Shimadzu, IR Affinity 1, Japan). The sample was run at infrared region between 400 and 4000 nm (Hussein et al., 2015; Jasim et al., 2015).

RESULTS AND DISCUSSION

Gas chromatography and mass spectroscopy analysis of compounds was carried out in methanolic seed extract of F. vulgare, shown in Table 1. The GC-MS chromatogram of the 56 peaks of the compounds detected was shown in Figure 1. Chromatogram GC-MS analysis of the methanol extract of F. vulgare showed the presence of fifty six major peaks and the components corresponding to the peaks were determined as follows. The first set up peak were determined to be Cyclohexene, 4-isopropenyl-1-methoxymethoxymethyl. The second peak indicated to be L-Fenchone. The next peaks considered to be α-D-Glucopyranoside,O-α-D-glucopyranosyl-(1.fwdarw.3)-ß-D-fructo, 2-Propyl-tetrahydropyran-3-ol, Estragole, 6-Methylenebicyclo[3.2.0]hept-3-en-2-one, Benzaldehyde ,4-methoxy, Anethole, 2,5-Octadecadiynoic acid , methylester, 2-Methoxy-4-vinylphenol, Ascaridole epoxide, d-Mannose, Benzenemethanol, 2-(2-aminopropoxy)-3-methyl-, 2-Propanone, 1-(4-methoxyphenyl), Pterin -6-carboxylic acid, Cyclopenta [1,3]cyclopropa[1,2]cyclohepten-3(3aH)-one,1,2,3b,6,7, 4-Methoxybenzoic acid, allyl ester, Arisaldehyde dimethyl acetal, Propiolic acid, 3-(1-hydroxy-2-isopropyl-5-methylcyclohexyl), Benzenemethanol,2-(2-aminopropoxy)-3-methyl, 1-Heptatriacotanol, 1-propyl-3,6-diazahomoadamantan-9-ol, Benzhydrazide , 4-methoxy-N2-(2-trifluoroacetylcyclohepten-1-yl), 4-(2,5-Dihydro-3-methoxyphenyl) butylamine, 2-Hydroxy-2-(4-methoxy-phenyl)-N-methyl – acetamide, Corymbolone, Apiol, Spiro[4.5]decan-7-one,1,8-dimethyl-8,9-epoxy-4-isopropyl, Fenretinide, Dihydroxanthin, 9-Ethoxy-10-oxatricyclo[7.2.1.0(1,6)]dodecan-11-one, Bicyclo[4.3.0]nonan-7-one,1-(2-methoxyvinyl), 1-(4-methoxyphenyl)-1,5-pentanediol, Aceta-mide,N-methyl-N-[4-(3-hydroxypyrrolidinyl)-2-butynyl], Gibberellic acid, 2,3-Dimethoxy-5-methyl-6- decaisoprenyl- chinon, Cyclopropanebutanoic acid, 2-[[2-[[2-[(2-pentylcyclopropyl)methyl]cym, [1,2,4]Triazolo[1,5-a]pyrimidin-7(4H)-one,5-methyl-6-(3-methylbutyl)-, 2-[4-methyl-6-(2,6,6-trimethylcyclohex-1-enyl)hexa-1,3,5 -trienyl]cyclo, Cis-Vaccenic acid, 6,9,12,15-

Table 1. Major phytochemical compounds identified in methanolic extract of *Foeniculum vulgare*.

Serial No.	Phytochemical compound	RT (min)	Molecular weight	Exact mass	Chemical structure	MS fragmentations	Pharmacological actions
1	Cyclohexene, 4-isopropenyl-1-methoxymethoxymethyl-	4.117	196	196.14633		53, 79, 91, 119, 164, 196	Anti periodic *effect*
2	L-Fenchone	4.935	152	152.120115		53, 69, 81, 91, 109, 123, 137, 152	Anti-tumour activity
3	α-D-Glucopyranoside,O-α-D-glucopyranosyl-(1.fwdarw.3)-ß-D-fructo	5330	504	504.169035		60, 69, 73, 81, 85, 97, 113, 126133, 145, 163, 175, 187, 199	Unknown
4	2-Propyl-tetrahydropyran-3-ol	5.936	144	144.115029		55, 73, 87, 101, 116, 144	Anti-angiogenic effect
5	Estragole	6.331	148	148.088815		51, 55, 63, 77, 91, 105, 121, 133, 148	Anti-inflammatory activity

Table 1. Cont'd

#	Name			Structure	Biological activities
6	6-Methylenebicyclo[3.2.0]hept-3-en-2-one	6.806	120	120.0575147		Biological activities, including bacteriostatic, fungistatic, anti-parasitic
					51, 65, 77, 91, 120
7	Benzaldehyde ,4-methoxy-	7.201	136	136.052429		Anti-Toxoplasma gondii activity
					50, 63, 77, 92, 107, 119, 135
8	Anethole	7.619	148	148.088815		Anti-edematogenic effects
					51, 55, 63, 74, 7791, 105, 117, 121, 1333, 148
9	2,5-Octadecadiynoic acid methylester	7.802	290	290.22458		Anti-inflammatory
					55, 67, 79, 91, 105, 117, 131, 145, 159
10	2-Methoxy-4-vinylphenol	7.933	150	150.06808		Antioxidant, anti microbial and anti inflammatory
					51, 63, 77, 89, 107, 118, 135
11	Ascaridole epoxide	8.437	184	184.109944		Anti-carcinogenic effects
					55, 69, 79, 91, 97, 107, 135, 150, 168

Table 1. Cont'd

#	Name				Structure	Fragment ions	Biological activity
12	d-Mannose	8.225	180	180.063388		60, 73, 85, 103, 131, 149, 179	Anti-arrhythmic effect
13	Benzenemethanol, 2-(2-aminopropoxy)-3-methyl-	8.540	195	195.125929		58, 91, 121, 152, 178	Anti-microbial, anti-cancer and anti-malarial
14.	2-Propanone, 1-(4-methoxyphenyl)-	8.912	164	164.08373		51, 65, 78, 91, 106, 121, 135, 164	Antiviral, anti-inflammatory, antimalarial and antibacterial
15	Pterin -6-carboxylic acid	9.038	207	207.039239		57, 69, 105, 149, 163, 177, 207	Unknown
16	Cyclopenta [1,3]cyclopropa[1,2]cyclohepten-3(3aH)-one,1,2,3b,6,7	9.330	190	190.135765		69, 78, 91, 119, 133, 147, 162, 190	Anti-pain effect

Table 1. Cont'd

No.	Name		MW	Exact mass	Structure	m/z	Activity
17	4-Methoxybenzoic acid , allyl ester	9.673	192	192.078644		50, 64, 77, 85, 92, 107, 120, 135, 147, 152, 177	Anti-inflammatory, antiviral, antibacterial
18	Arisaldehyde dimethyl acetal	9.965	182	182.094295		51, 65, 77, 92, 108, 121, 135, 151, 165, 182	Neurotoxicity and anti-inflammatory effects
19	Propiolic acid , 3-(1-hydroxy-2-isopropyl-5-methylcyclohexyl)	10.354	224	224.141245		55, 81, 95, 109, 135, 163, 178, 191, 206	Anti-cancer
20	Benzenemethanol,2-(2-aminopropoxy)-3-methyl-	10.434	195	195.125929		58, 65, 77, 91, 105, 121, 152, 178, 195	Anti-nociceptive effect
21	1-Heptatriacotanol	10.777	536	536.58962		55, 81, 95, 147, 161, 190, 229, 244, 257	Anti-Mycobacterium tuberculosis Activity
22	1-propyl-3,6-diazahomoadamantan-9-ol	10.857	210	210.173213		58, 72, 82136, 181, 210	Unknown

Table 1. Cont'd

No.	Name	RT	MW	Exact mass	Structure	Fragments	Activity
23	Benzhydrazide , 4-methoxy-N2-(2-trifluoroacetylcyclohepten-1-yl)	10.960	356	356.134777		64, 77, 92, 107, 115, 135, 153, 175, 203	Antimalarial, anti-inflammatory
24	4-(2,5-Dihydro-3-methoxyphenyl)butylamine	11.172	181	181.146665		55, 65, 77, 91, 107, 121, 134, 150	Antitumor, antispasmolytic, estrogenic, antiviral and anti-helminthic
25	2-Hydroxy-2-(4-methoxy-phenyl)-N-methyl – acetamide	11.384	195	195.089543		66, 77, 94, 109, 137, 148, 178, 195	Anti-inflammatory and antibacterial
26	Corymbolone	11.618	236	236.17763		55, 69, 93, 109, 135, 175, 203, 218	Anti-fungal agent
27	Apiol	11.727	222	222.089209		53, 65, 77, 91, 106, 121, 149, 161, 177, 191, 207, 222	Phytotoxic activity and antifungal activity
28	Spiro[4.5]decan-7-one,1,8-dimethyl-8,9-epoxy-4-isopropyl	11.910	236	236.17763		55, 69, 81, 95, 109, 123, 137, 151, 165, 193, 208, 236	Anti-inflammatory activity

Table 1. Cont'd

#	Name				Fragments	Activity
29	Fenretinide	12.013	391	391.25113		58, 69, 81, 95, 109, 119, 135, 148, 161, 202, 213, 255, 268	Anti-tumoural activity
30	Dihydroxanthin	12.196	308	308.162374		55, 79, 95, 137, 151, 178, 206, 248	Unknown
31	9-Ethoxy-10-oxatricyclo[7.2.1.0(1,6)]dodecan-11-one	12.357	224	224.141245		55, 67, 79, 93, 109, 124, 137, 151, 168, 180, 196, 225	Anticancer effect
32	Bicyclo[4.3.0]nonan-7-one,1-(2-methoxyvinyl)-	12.591	194	194.13068		67, 79, 91, 138, 151, 163, 179, 194	Unknown
33	1-(4-methoxyphenyl)-1,5-pentanediol	12.723	210	210.125594		59, 71, 77, 94, 109, 121, 137, 147, 192, 210	Antipyretic, anti-inflammatory, hematological effects, antimicrobial, antiviral and antitumor

Table 1. Cont'd

No.	Name			m/z	Biological activity
34	Acetamide,N-methyl-N-[4-(3-hydroxypyrrolidinyl)-2-butynyl]	13.804	308	308.162374	56, 68, 124, 192	Unknown
35	Gibberellic acid	14.353	346	346.141638	55, 77, 91, 121, 136, 152, 203, 239, 300, 328	Significant anti-ageing, anti-carcinogenic, and anti-thrombotic effects
36.	2,3-Dimethoxy-5-methyl-6-decaisoprenyl- chinon	14.514	862	862.68391	55, 69, 81, 95, 135, 149, 197, 235, 250, 313, 340, 384	New chemical compound
37	Cyclopropanebutanoic acid , 2-[[2-[[2-[(2-pentylcyclopropyl)methyl]cy	14.806	374	374.318481	55, 67, 74, 95, 121, 135, 149, 161, 199, 227, 270, 298, 334	Anti-inflammatory, antioxidant, antimalarial, anti-tuberculosis antifungal
38	[1,2,4]Triazolo[1,5-a]pyrimidin-7(4H)-one,5-methyl-6-(3-methylbutyl)-	15.120	220	220.132411	53, 67, 80, 95, 109, 122, 136, 164, 177, 220	Unknown
39	2-[4-methyl-6-(2,6,6-trimethylcyclohex-1-enyl)hexa-1,3,5-trienyl]cyclo	16.916	324	324.245316	55, 69, 79, 91, 105, 135, 173, 187, 255, 324	Antimicrobials and anti-virals

Table 1. Cont'd

No	Name	RT	Mass	Exact Mass	Structure	Fragment ions	Activity
40	Cis-Vaccenic acid	17.621	282	282.25588		55, 69, 83, 97, 111, 125, 165, 193, 222, 246, 264, 282	Anti-carcinogenic effect
41	6,9,12,15-Docosatetraenoic acid , methyl ester	18.382	346	346.28718		55, 67, 93, 107, 121, 149, 164, 177, 209, 235, 264, 346	Anti-carcinogenic and anti-atherosclerotic effects
42.	1H-2,8a-Methanocyclopenta[a]cyclopropa[e]cyclodecen-11-one,1-	18.645	364	364.18859		53, 65, 77, 121, 151, 269, 333, 364	Anti-tumor activity
43	9-Octadecenamide,(Z)-	19.040	281	281.271864		59, 72, 83, 114, 184, 212, 264, 281	Anti-inflammatory activity and antibacterial activity
44	dl-3Beta-hydroxy-d-homo-18-nor-5alpha,8alpha,14beta-androst-13(1)	20.144	288	288.208931		55, 79, 110, 147, 165, 216, 255, 270, 288	Anti-inflammatory
45	9-Octadecenoic acid (Z)-,2-hydroxy-1-(hydroxymethyl)ethyl ester	21.512	356	356.29266		55, 69, 81, 98, 137, 151, 165, 221, 264, 280, 325, 354	Antimicrobial, Anticancer, Diuretic and Anti-inflammatory

Table 1. Cont'd

No.	Name	RT	Mass	Exact mass	Structure	Fragment ions	Activity
46	5aH-3a,12-methano-1H-cyclopropa[5´,6´]cyclodeca[1´,2´:1,5]cyclo	22.433	388	388.224974		55, 77, 91, 122, 149, 177, 213, 299, 330	Anti-inflammatory effect
47	Phthalic acid , decyl oct-3-ylester, 1,2-Benzenedicarboxylic acid , bis(8-methylnonyl)ester	23.434	418	418.30831		57, 104, 149, 167, 193, 251, 307	New chemical compound
48	1,2-Benzenedicarboxylic acid , bis(8-methylnonyl)ester	24.355	446	446.33961		71, 99, 149, 167, 193, 228, 289, 307, 321, 361, 389, 417	Anti-leishmanial activity
49	(22S)-21-Acetoxy-6α,11ß-dihydroxy-16α,17α-propylmethylenedioxyp	25.357	488	488.241018		55, 79, 91, 121, 149, 223, 279, 297, 351, 387, 416, 445, 488	Anti-inflammatory
50	Oxiraneoctanoic acid , 3-octyl-, methyl ester	25.591	312	312.266445		55, 74, 97, 155, 199, 214, 263, 281, 312	Antibacterial activity
51	1,5-Bis(4-methoxyphenyl)bicyclo[3.2.0]heptane	25.723	308	308.17763		57, 71, 91, 148, 174, 249, 280, 308	Anti-HIV agent

Table 1. Cont'd

#	Name	RT	MW	Exact mass	Structure	Fragment ions	Activity
52	Ingol 12-acetate	26.169	408	408.214804		55, 122, 137, 165, 192, 245, 273, 301, 330, 377, 408	Anti-inflammatory activity
53	Isoquinoline, 1-[3-methoxy-5-hydroxybenzyl]-1,2,3,4,5,8-hexahydro-	26.301	301	301.167793		55, 77, 121, 164, 210, 268, 299	Anti-cancer activities
54	Cholestan-3-one , cyclic 1,2-ethanediyl aetal,(5ß)-	26.541	430	430.38108		55, 69, 99, 125, 149, 194, 232, 282, 340, 384, 430	Anti-inflammatory agents
55	2,24a,6a,8a,9,12b,14a-Octamethyl-1,2,3,4,4a,5,6,6a,6b,7,8,8a,9,1	27.279	410	410.391253		55, 69, 81, 95, 109, 136, 191, 205, 218, 257, 287, 342, 367, 395, 410	Anti-diarrhoeal activity
56	Undeca -3,4-diene-2,10-dione,5,6,6-trimethyl-	28.464	222	222.16198		55, 69, 123, 137, 179, 222	New chemical compound

hydrogen bonded alcohols and phenol which shows major peaks at 719.54, 889.18, 1029.99, 1141.86, 1244.09, 1317.38, 1373.32, 1595.13, 2677.20, 2852.72, 2922.16, 3005.10, 3244.27 and 3361.993 (Table 2 and Figure 60).

Conclusion

F. vulgare is native plant of Iraq. It contain chemical constitutions which may be useful for various herbal formulation as anti-inflammatory, analgesic, antipyretic, cardiac tonic and antiasthamatic.

Conflict of Interests

The authors have not declared any conflict of interest.

ACKNOWLEDGMENTS

The authors wish to express their deepest gratitude to Prof. Dr. Adul-Kareem for his valuable contributions and support throughout this study. They would also like to express their gratitude to Dr. Ali for his valuable suggestions and comments.

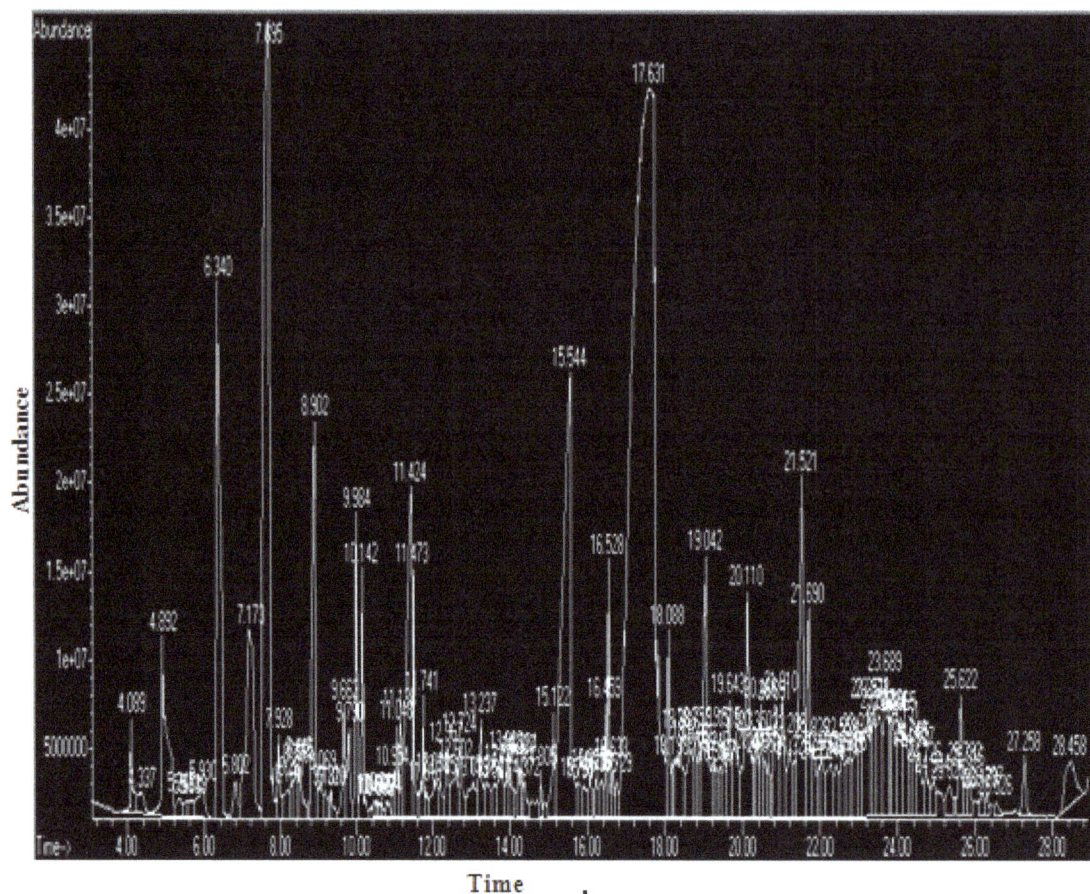

Figure 1. GC-MS chromatogram of methanolic seed extract of *Foeniculum vulgare.*

Table 2. FT-IR peak values of *Foeniculum vulgare.*

No.	Peak (Wave number cm⁻¹)	Intensity	Bond	Functional group assignment	Group frequency
1	665.44	60.383	-	Unknown	-
2	719.54	64.204	C-H	Alkenes	675-995
3	889.18	74.391	C-H	Alkenes	675-995
4	1029.99	53.805	C-F stretch	Aliphatic fluoro compounds	1000-10150
5	1141.86	65.836	C-O	Alcohols, Ethers, Carboxlic acids, Esters	1050-1300
6	1244.09	70.650	C-O	Alcohols, Ethers, Carboxlic acids, Esters	1050-1300
7	1317.38	74.345	NO2	Nitro Compounds	1300-1370
8	1361.74	73.778	NO2	Nitro Compounds	1300-1370
9	1373.32	72.718	-	Unknown	-
10	1417.68	71.920	-	Unknown	-
11	1595.13	72.290	-	Unknown	-
12	1743.65	74.604	-	Unknown	-
13	2677.20	91.620	-	Unknown	-
14	2852.72	77.059	C-H	Alkanes	2850-2970
15	2922.16	70.245	C-H	Alkanes	2850-2970
16	3005.10	86.839	H-O	H-bonded H-X group	2500-3500
17	3066.82	86.670	H-O	H-bonded H-X group	2500-3500
18	3244.27	83.454	O-H	Hydrogen bonded Alcohols, Phenols	3200-3600
19	3275.13	80.640	O-H	Hydrogen bonded Alcohols, Phenols	3200-3600
20	3361.993	81.444	O-H	Hydrogen bonded Alcohols, Phenols	3200-3600

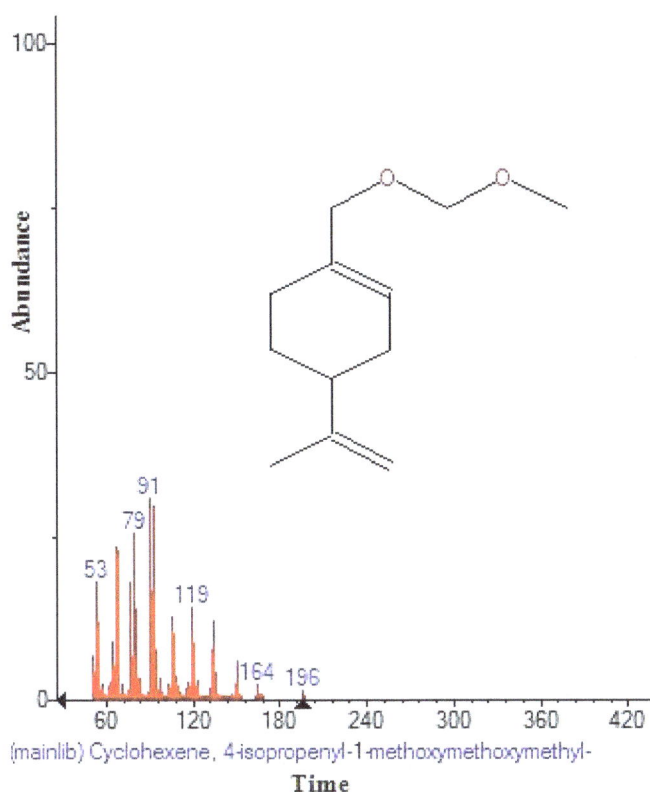

Figure 2. Structure of Cyclohexene, 4-isopropenyl-1-methoxymethoxymethyl present in the methanolic seeds extract of *Foeniculum vulgare* using GC-MS analysis.

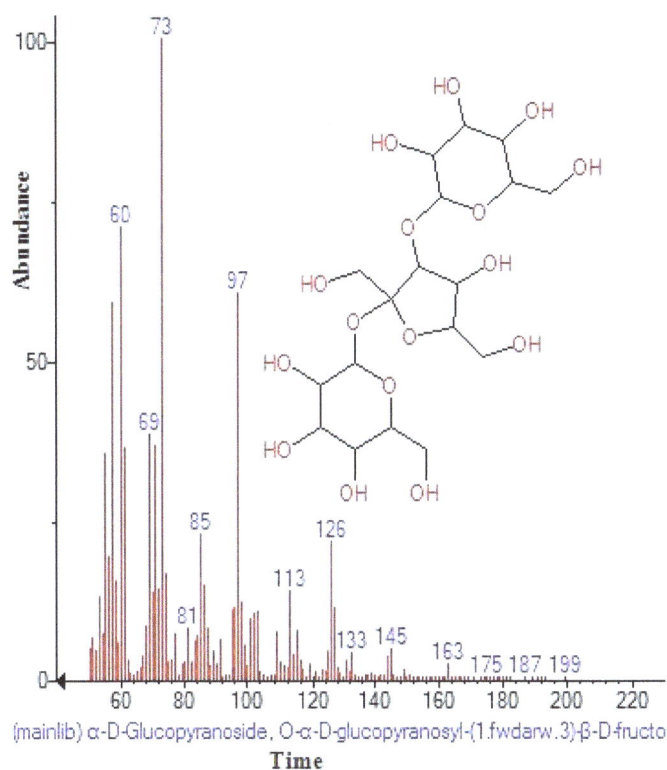

Figure 4. Structure of α-D-Glucopyranoside,O-α-D-glucopyranosyl-(1.fwdarw.3)-ß-D-fructo present in the methanolic seeds extract of *F. vulgare* using GC-MS analysis.

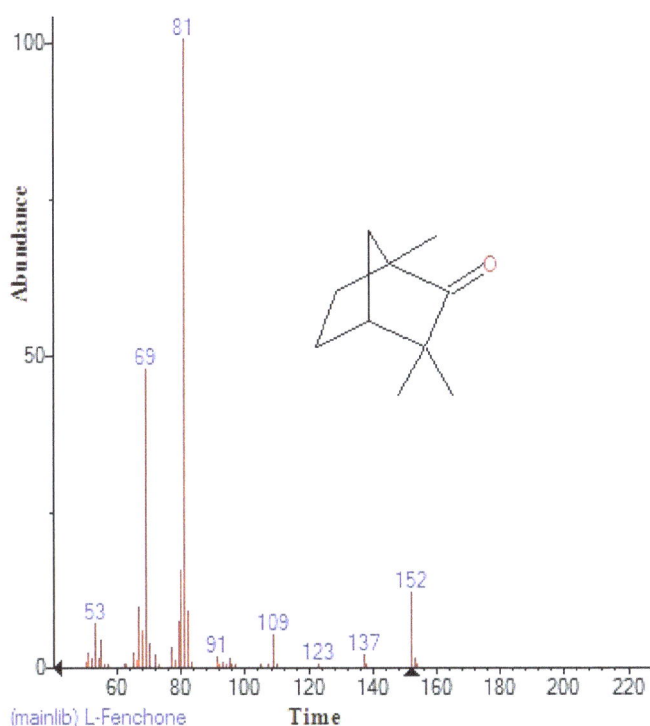

Figure 3. Structure of L-Fenchone present in the methanolic seeds extract of *F. vulgare* using GC-MS analysis.

Docosatetraenoic acid , methyl ester, 1H-2,8a-Methanocyclopenta[a]cyclopropa[e]cyclodecen-11-one,1, 9-Octadecenamide ,(Z), dl-3Beta-hydroxy-d-homo-18-nor-5alpha,8alpha,14beta-androst-13(1), dl-3Beta-hydroxy-d-homo-18-nor-5alpha,8alpha,14beta-androst-13(1), 9-Octadecenoic acid (Z)-,2-hydroxy-1-(hydroxymethyl)ethyl ester, 5aH-3a,12-methano-1H-cyclopropa [5´,6´]cyclodeca[1´,2´:1,5]cyclo, 1,2-Benzenedicarboxylic acid, bis(8-methylnonyl)ester, (22S)-21-Acetoxy-6α,11ß-dihydroxy-16α,17α-propylmethylene-dioxyp, Oxiraneoctanoic acid, 3-octyl-,methyl ester, 1,5-Bis(4-methoxyphenyl)bicyclo[3.2.0]heptane, 1,2-Benzenedicarboxylic acid , bis(8-methylnonyl)ester, (22S)-21-Acetoxy-6α,11ß-dihydroxy-16α,17α-propylmethylene dioxyp, Oxiraneoctanoic acid, 3-octyl-,methyl ester, 1,5-Bis(4-methoxyphenyl)bicyclo[3.2.0]heptane, Ingol 12-acetate, Isoquinoline,1-[3-methoxy-5-hydroxybenzyl]-1,2,3,4,5,8-hexahydro, Cholestan-3-one, cyclic 1,2-ethanediyl aetal,(5ß), 2,24a,6a,8a,9,12b,14a-Octamethyl-1,2,3,4,4a,5,6,6a,6b,7,8,8a,9,1, and Undeca -3,4-diene-2,10-dione,5,6,6-trimethyl (Figures 2 to 59). The FTIR analysis of *F. vulgare* seeds proved the presence of alkenes, aliphatic fluoro compounds, alcohols, ethers, carboxlic acids, esters, nitro compounds, alkanes,

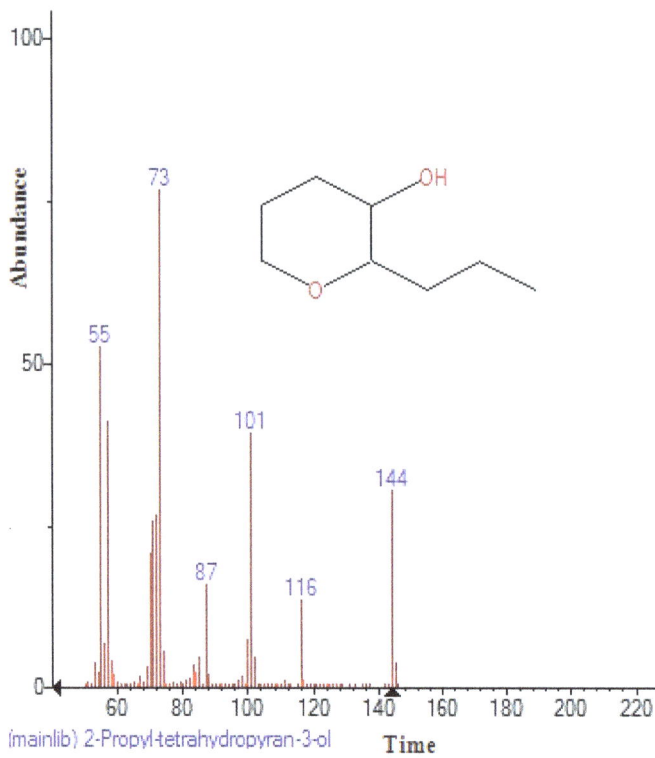

Figure 5. Structure of 2-Propyl-tetrahydropyran-3-ol present in the methanolic seeds extract of *F. vulgare* using GC-MS analysis.

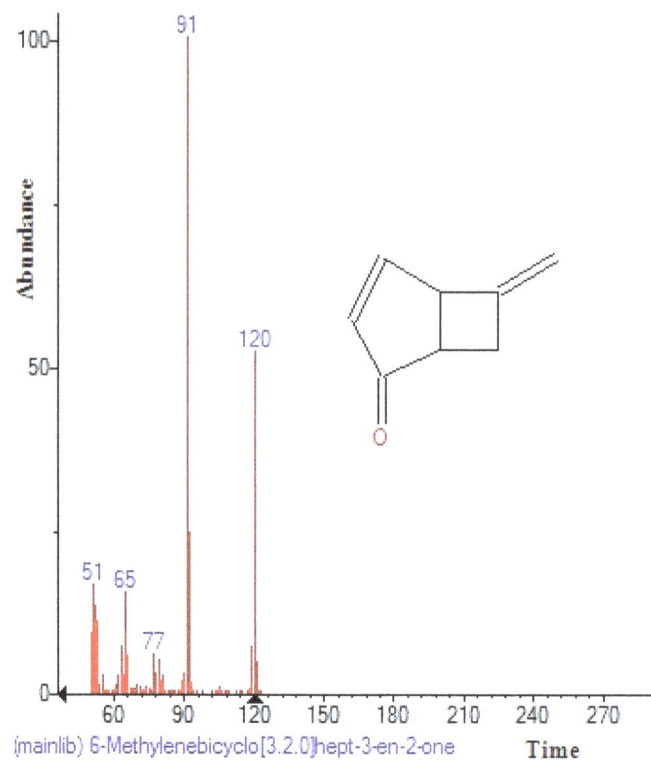

Figure 7. Structure of 6-Methylenebicyclo[3.2.0]hept-3-en-2-one present in the methanolic seeds extract of *F. vulgare* using GC-MS analysis.

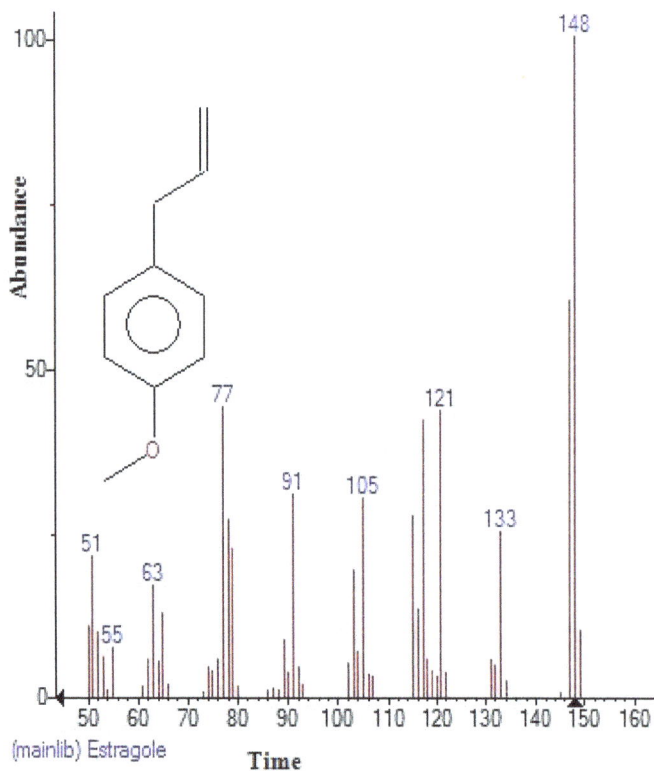

Figure 6. Structure of Estragole present in the methanolic seeds extract of *F. vulgare* using GC-MS analysis.

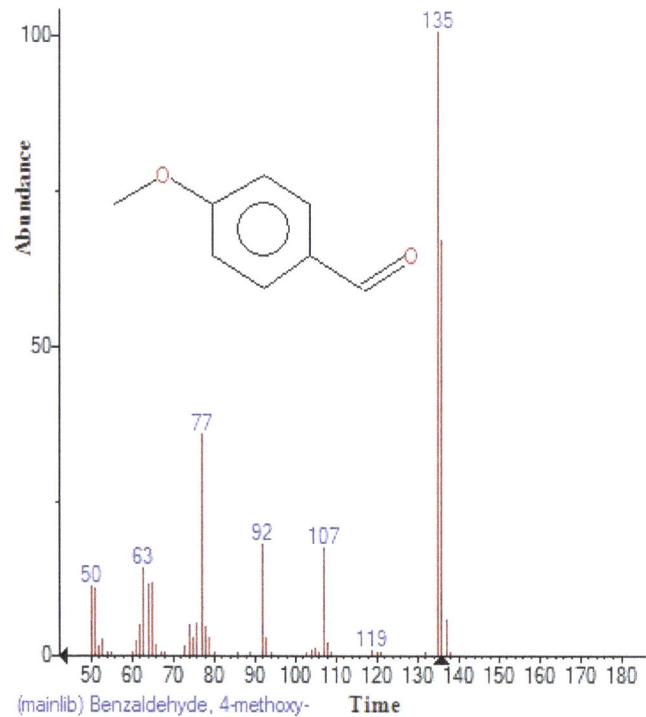

Figure 8. Structure of Benzaldehyde ,4-methoxy present in the methanolic seeds extract of *Foeniculum vulgare* using GC-MS analysis.

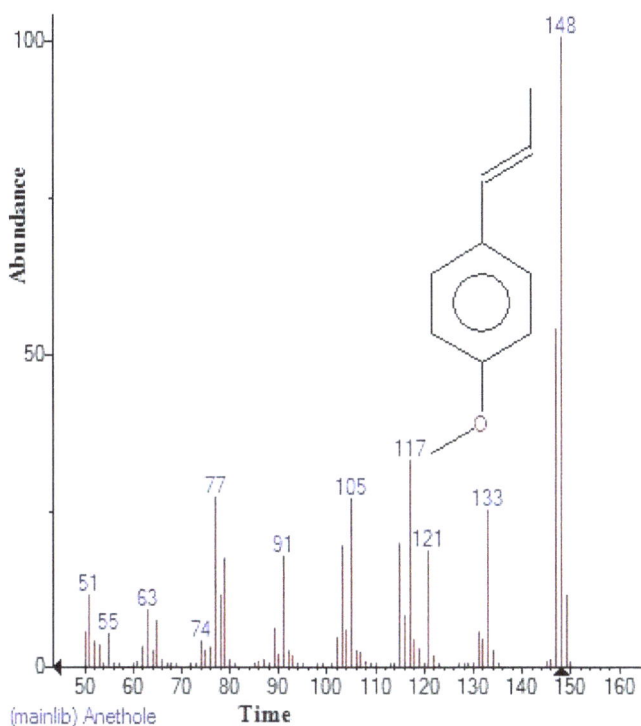

Figure 9. Structure of Anethole present in the methanolic seeds extract of *F. vulgare* using GC-MS analysis.

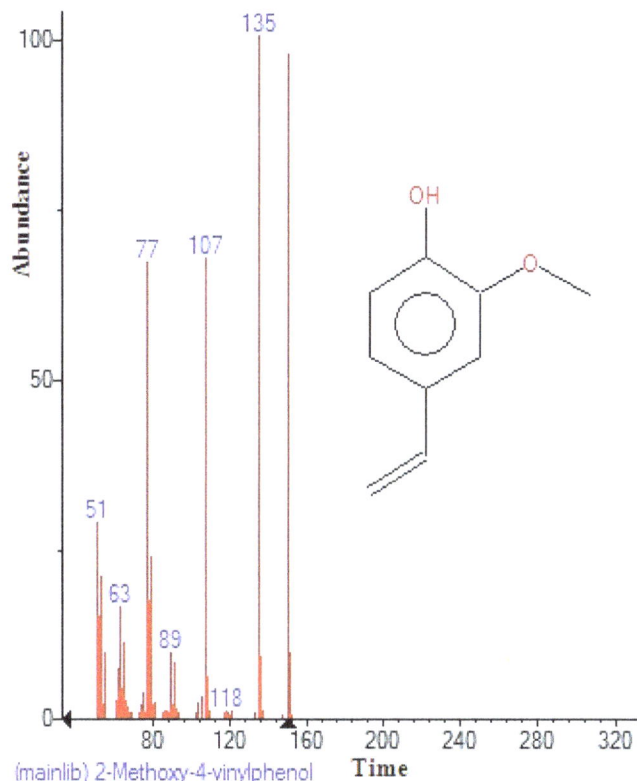

Figure 11. Structure of 2-Methoxy-4-vinylphenol present in the methanolic seeds extract of *F. vulgare* using GC-MS analysis.

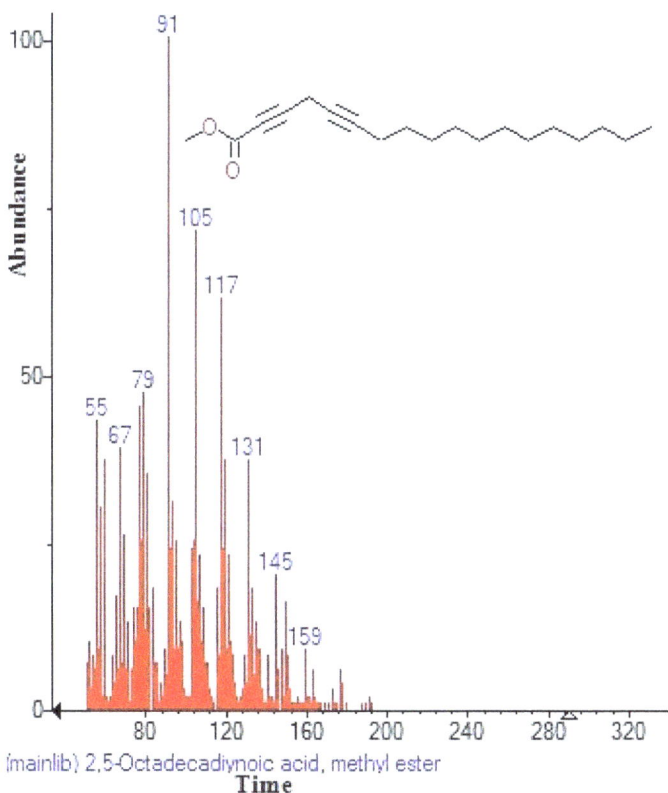

Figure 10. Structure of 2,5-Octadecadiynoic acid , methylester present in the methanolic seeds extract of *F. vulgare* using GC-MS analysis.

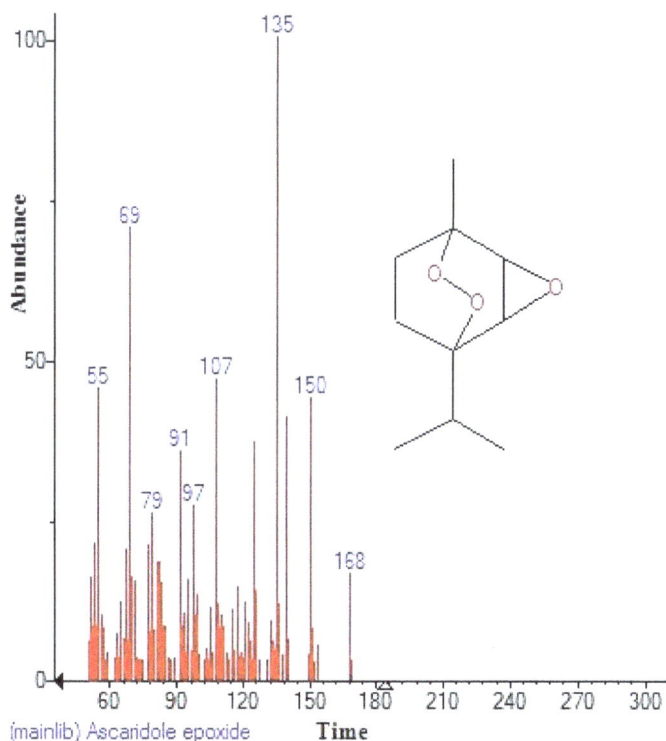

Figure 12. Structure of Ascaridole epoxide present in the methanolic seeds extract of *F. vulgare* using GC-MS analysis.

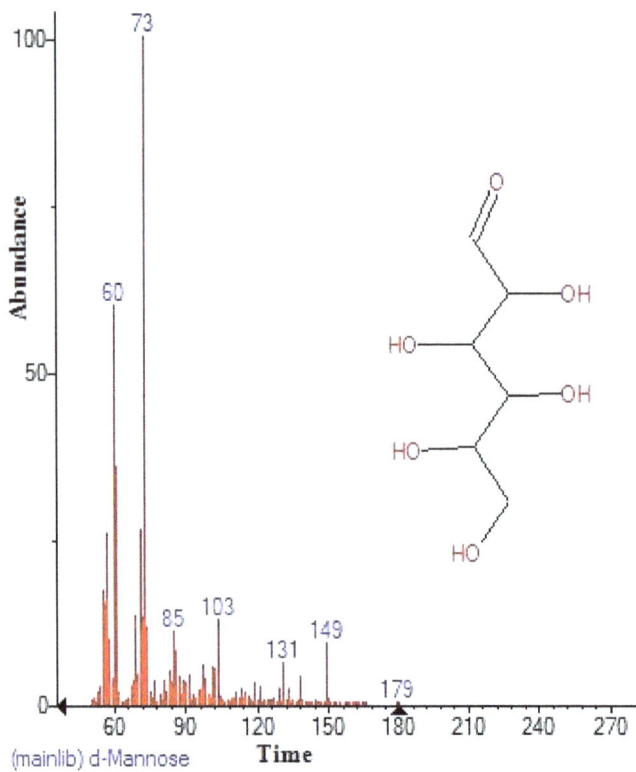

Figure 13. Structure of d-Mannose present in the methanolic seeds extract of *F. vulgare* using GC-MS analysis.

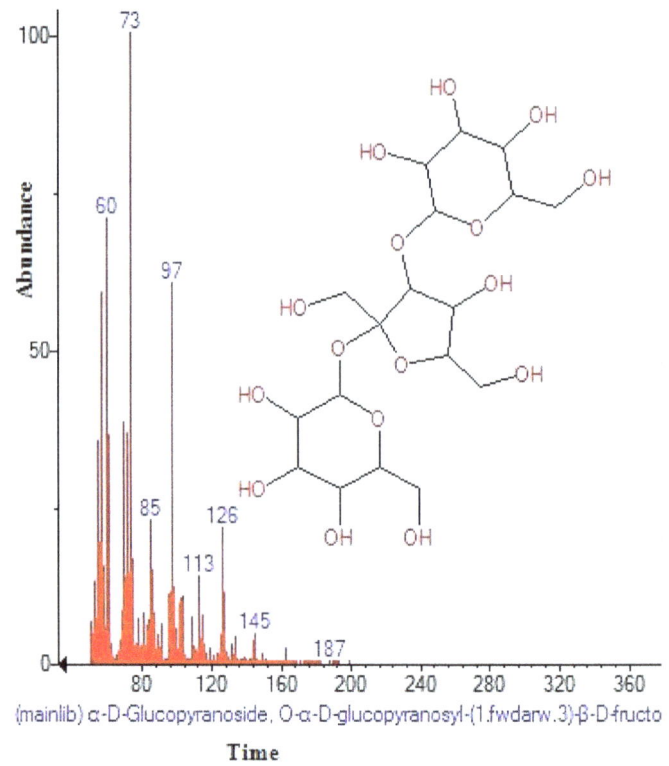

Figure 15. Structure of α-D-Glucopyranoside, O-α-D glucopyranosyl-(1.fwdarw.3)-ß-D-fructo present in the methanolic seeds extract of *Foeniculum vulgare* using GC-MS analysis.

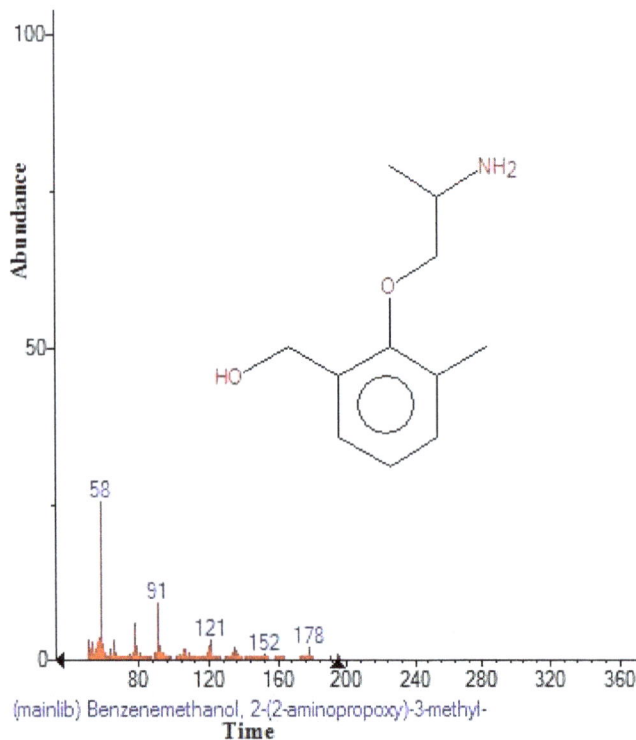

Figure 14. Structure of Benzenemethanol , 2-(2-aminopropoxy)-3-methyl present in the methanolic seeds extract of *F. vulgare* using GC-MS analysis.

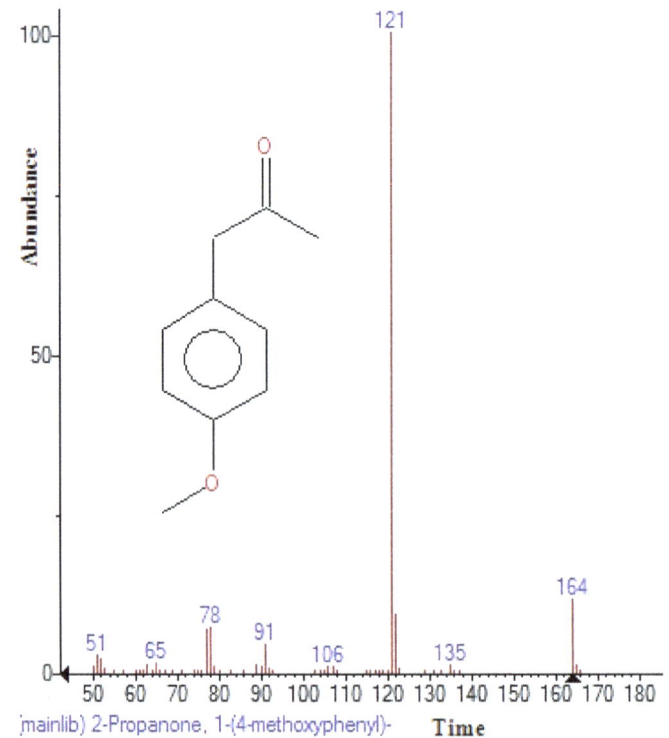

Figure 16. Structure of 2-Propanone, 1-(4-methoxyphenyl) present in the methanolic seeds extract of *Foeniculum vulgare* using GC-MS analysis.

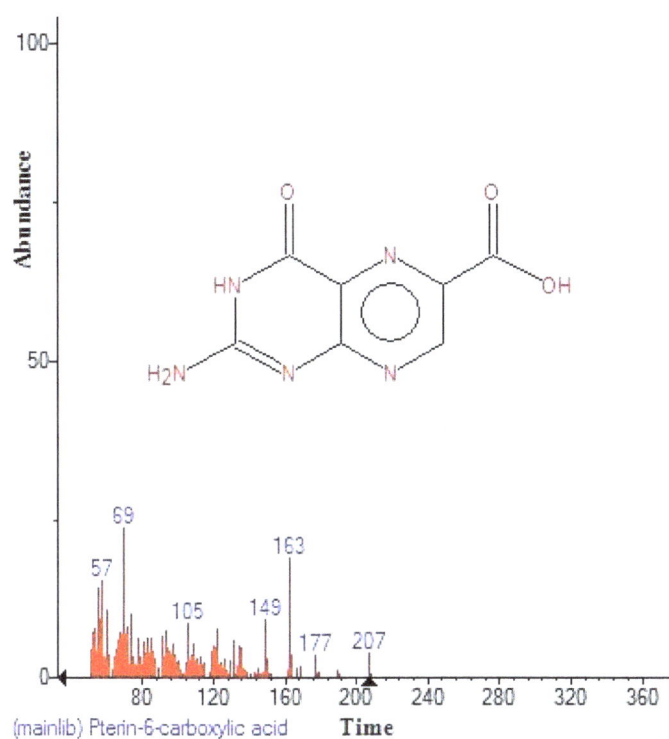

(mainlib) Pterin-6-carboxylic acid   **Time**

Figure 17. Structure of Pterin -6-carboxylic acid present in the methanolic seeds extract of *F. vulgare* using GC-MS analysis.

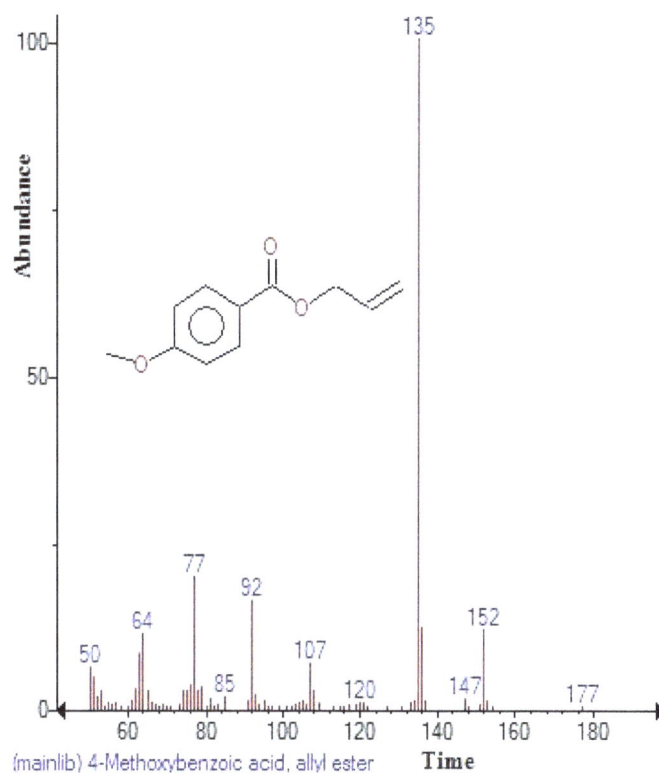

(mainlib) 4-Methoxybenzoic acid, allyl ester   **Time**

Figure 19. Structure of 4-Methoxybenzoic acid, allyl ester present in the methanolic seeds extract of *F. vulgare* using GC-MS analysis.

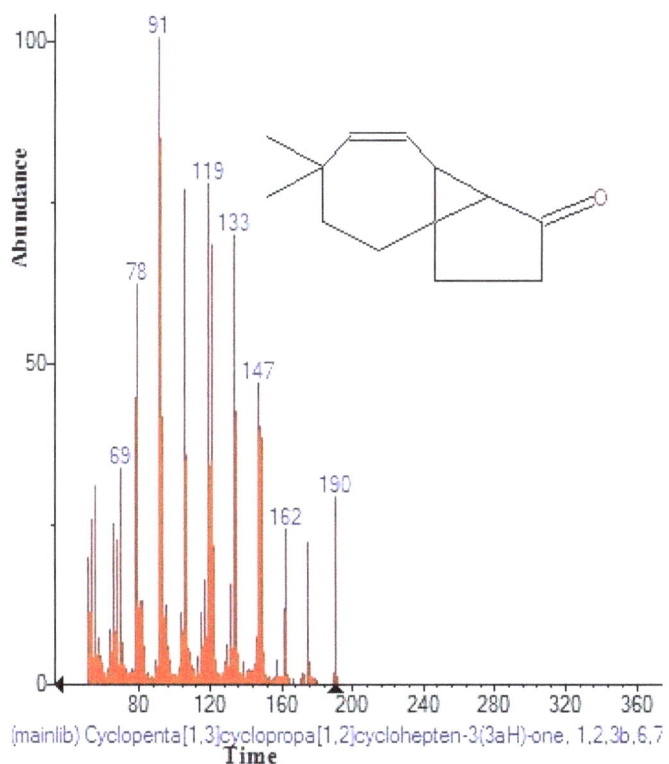

(mainlib) Cyclopenta[1,3]cyclopropa[1,2]cyclohepten-3(3aH)-one, 1,2,3b,6,7   **Time**

Figure 18. Structure of Cyclopenta [1,3]cyclopropa[1,2]cyclohepten-3(3aH)-one,1,2,3b,6,7 present in the methanolic seeds extract of *F. vulgare* using GC-MS analysis.

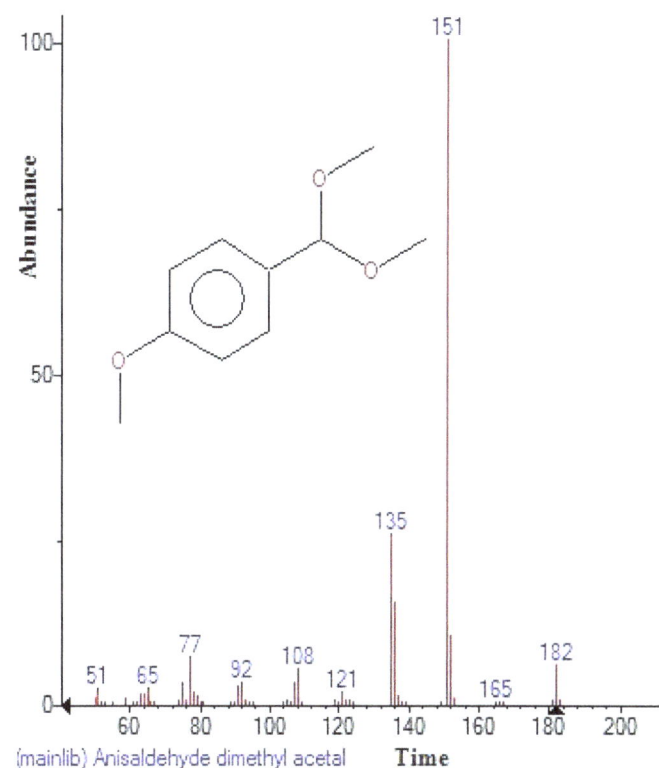

(mainlib) Anisaldehyde dimethyl acetal   **Time**

Figure 20. Structure of Arisaldehyde dimethyl acetal present in the methanolic seeds extract of *F. vulgare* using GC-MS analysis.

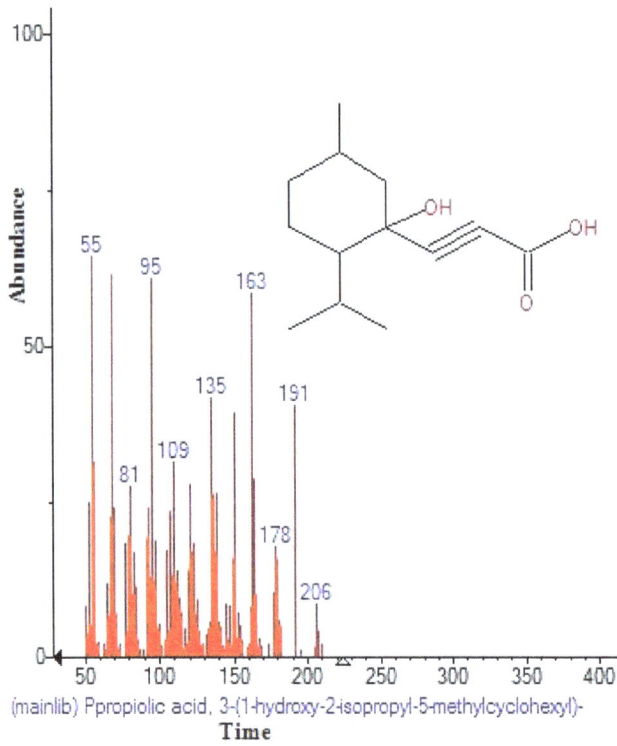

Figure 21. Structure of Propiolic acid, 3-(1-hydroxy-2-isopropyl-5-methylcyclohexyl) present in the methanolic seeds extract of *Foeniculum vulgare* using GC-MS analysis.

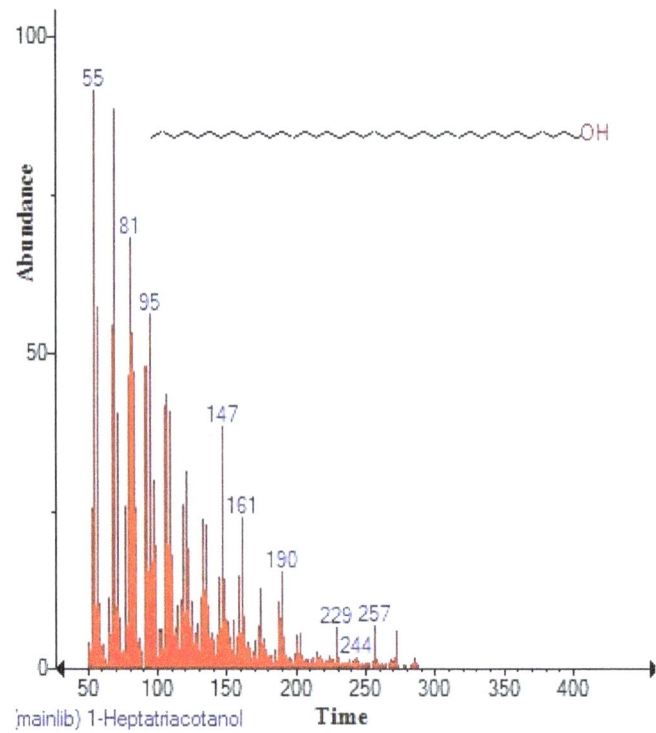

Figure 23. Structure of 1-Heptatriacotanol present in the methanolic seeds extract of *F. vulgare* using GC-MS analysis.

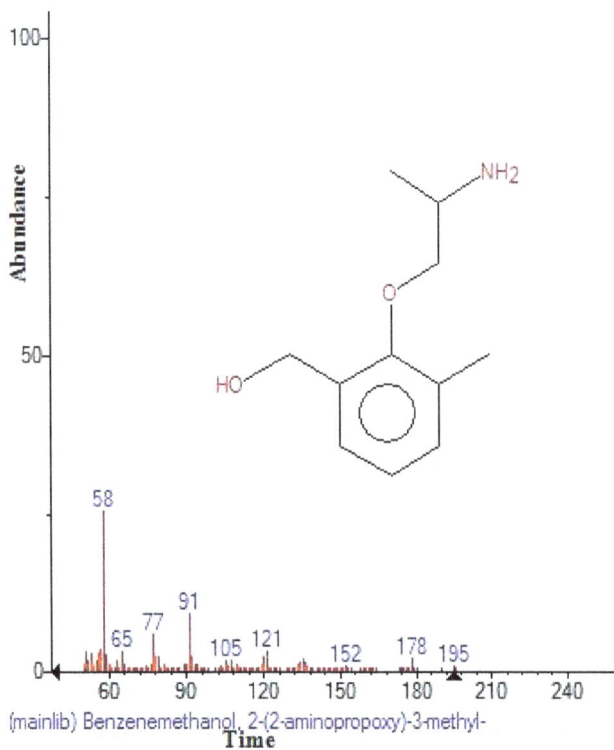

Figure 22. Structure of Benzenemethanol,2-(2-aminopropoxy)-3-methyl present in the methanolic seeds extract of *F. vulgare* using GC-MS analysis.

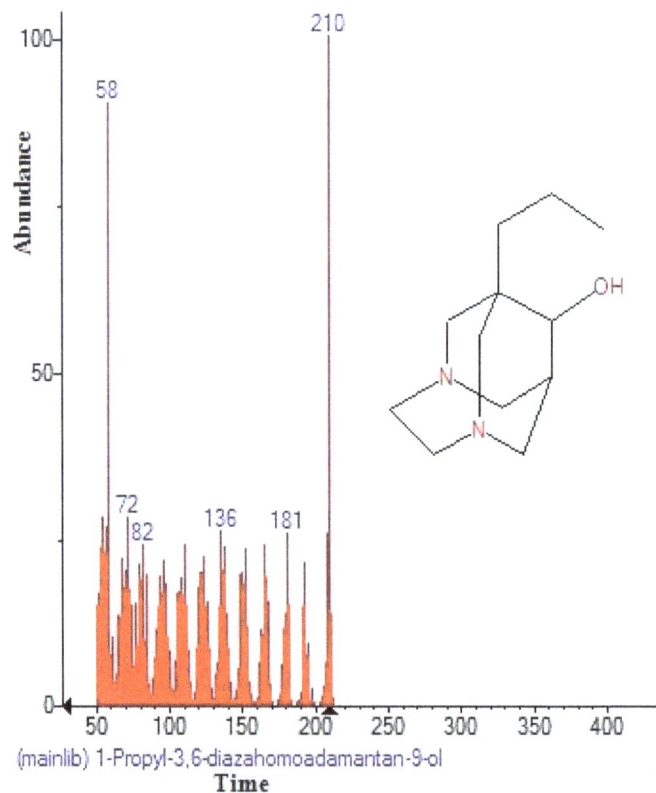

Figure 24. Structure of 1-propyl-3,6-diazahomoadamantan-9-ol present in the methanolic seeds extract of *F. vulgare* using GC-MS analysis.

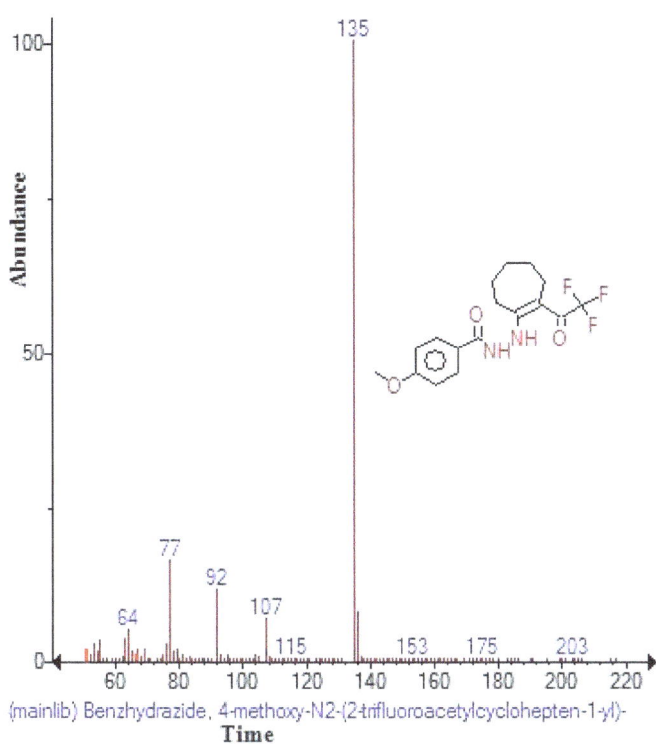

(mainlib) Benzhydrazide, 4-methoxy-N2-(2-trifluoroacetylcyclohepten-1-yl)-

Figure 25. Structure of Benzhydrazide, 4-methoxy-N2-(2-trifluoroacetylcyclohepten-1-yl) present in the methanolic seeds extract of *F. vulgare* using GC-MS analysis.

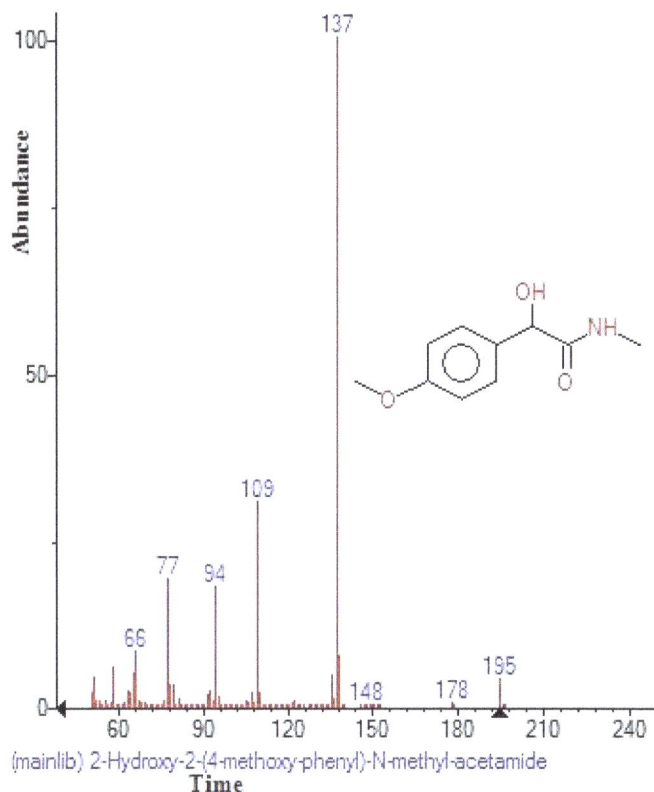

(mainlib) 2-Hydroxy-2-(4-methoxy-phenyl)-N-methyl-acetamide

Figure 27. Structure of 2-Hydroxy-2-(4-methoxy-phenyl)-N-methyl – acetamide present in the methanolic seeds extract of *F. vulgare* using GC-MS analysis.

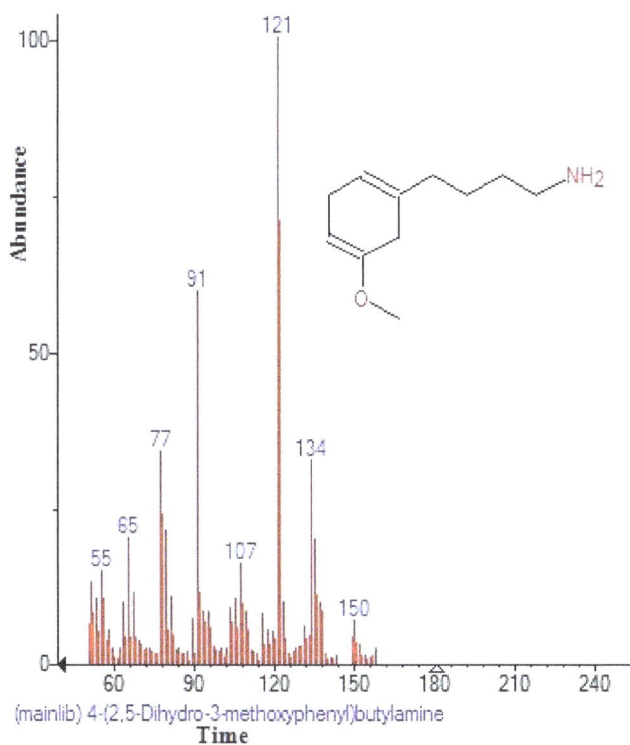

(mainlib) 4-(2,5-Dihydro-3-methoxyphenyl)butylamine

Figure 26. Structure of 4-(2,5-Dihydro-3-methoxyphenyl)butylamine present in the methanolic seeds extract of *F. vulgare* using GC-MS analysis.

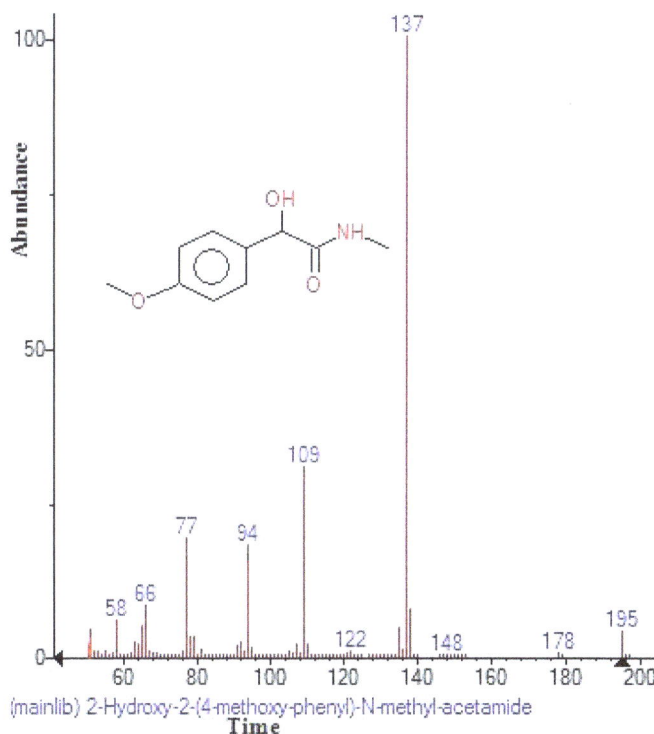

(mainlib) 2-Hydroxy-2-(4-methoxy-phenyl)-N-methyl-acetamide

Figure 28. Structure of 2-Hydroxy-2-(4-methoxy-phenyl)-N-methyl-acetamide present in the methanolic seeds extract of *F. vulgare* using GC-MS analysis.

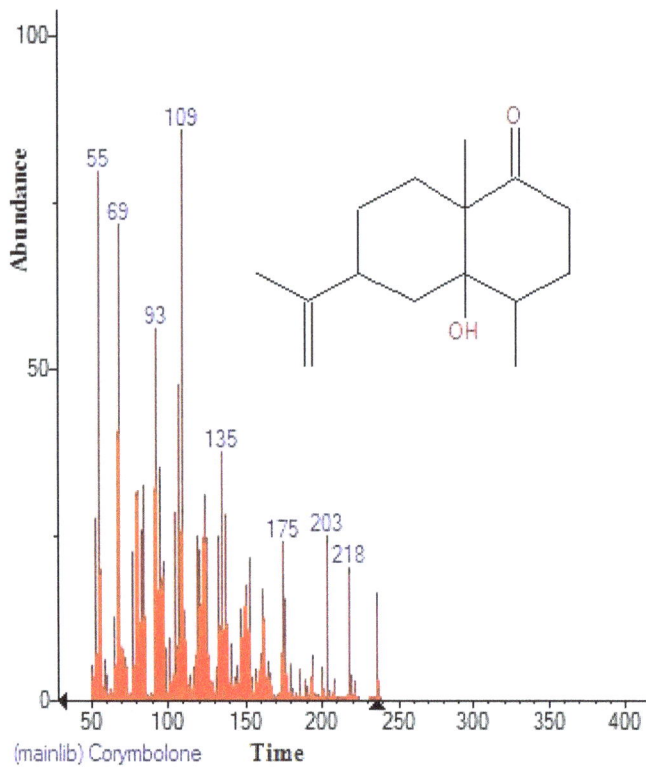

Figure 29. Structure of Corymbolone present in the methanolic seeds extract of *F. vulgare* using GC-MS analysis.

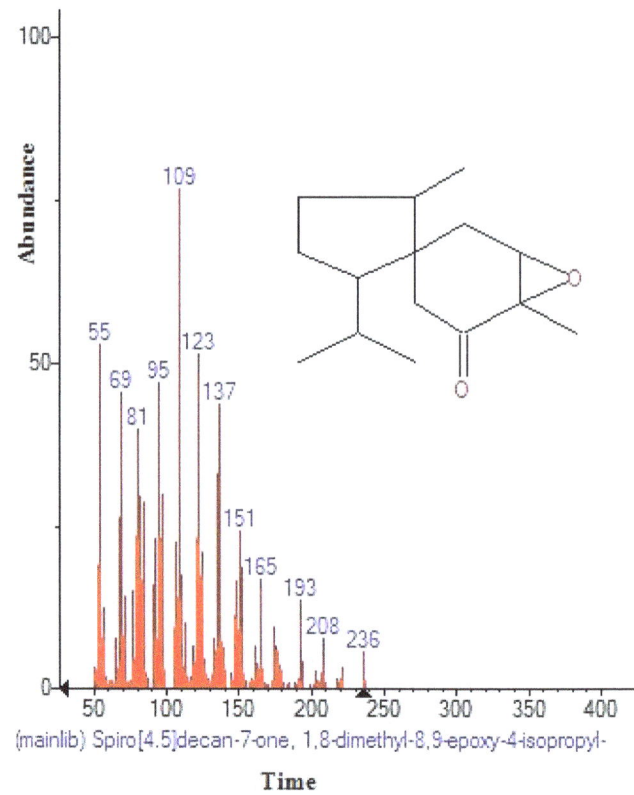

Figure 31. Structure of Spiro[4.5]decan-7-one,1,8-dimethyl-8,9-epoxy-4-isopropyl present in the methanolic seeds extract of *F. vulgare* using GC-MS analysis.

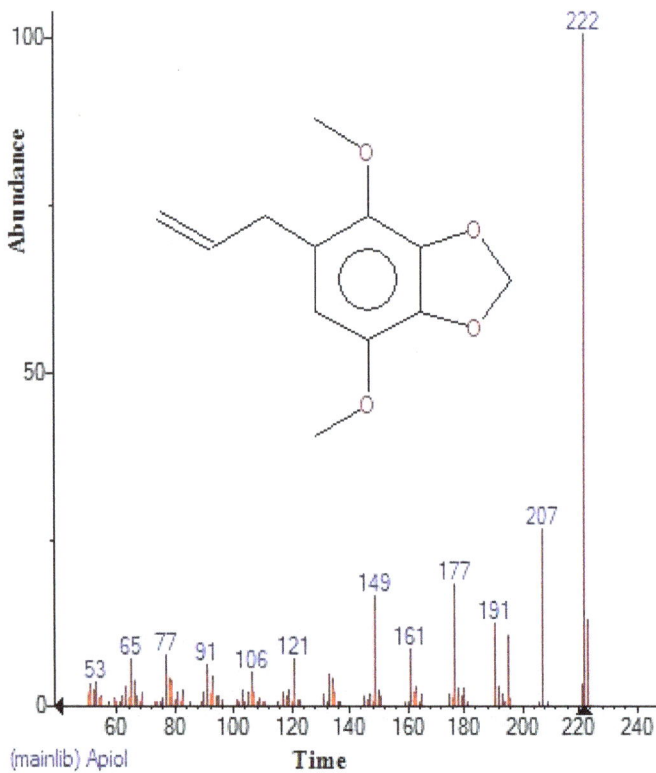

Figure 30. Structure of Apiol present in the methanolic seeds extract of *F. vulgare* using GC-MS analysis.

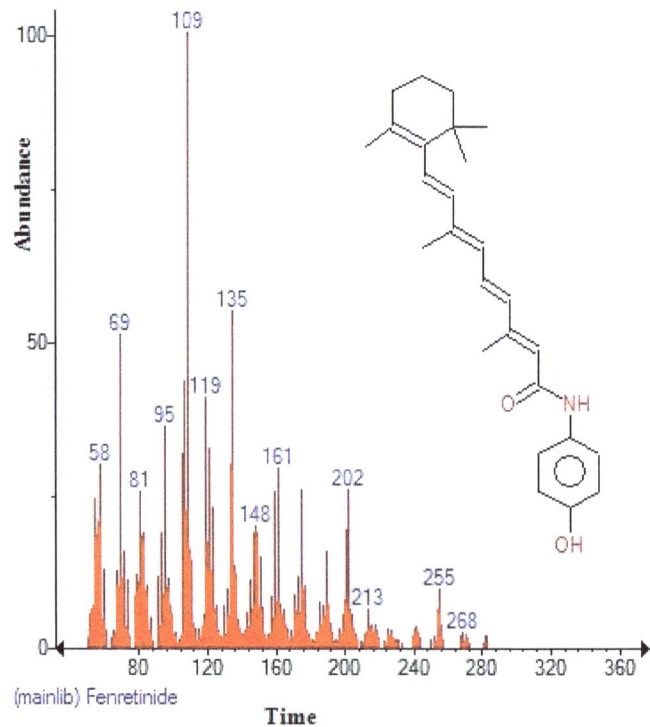

Figure 32. Structure of Fenretinide present in the methanolic seeds extract of *F. vulgare* using GC-MS analysis.

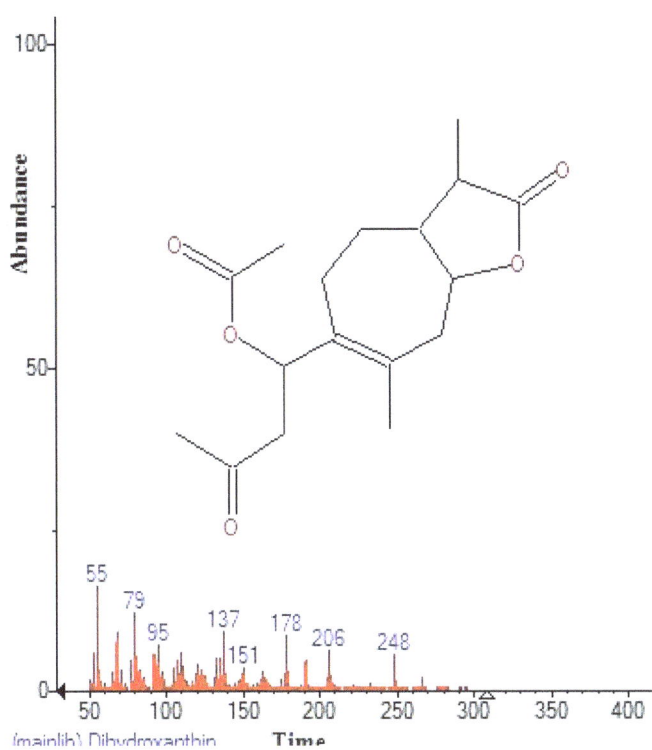

Figure 33. Structure of Dihydroxanthin present in the methanolic seeds extract of *F. vulgare* using GC-MS analysis.

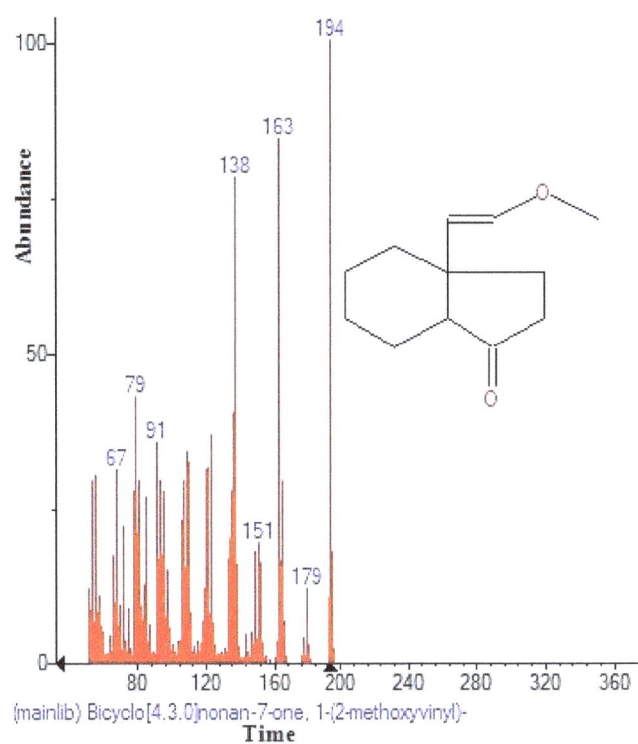

Figure 35. Structure of Bicyclo[4.3.0]nonan-7-one,1-(2-methoxyvinyl) present in the methanolic seeds extract of *F. vulgare* using GC-MS analysis.

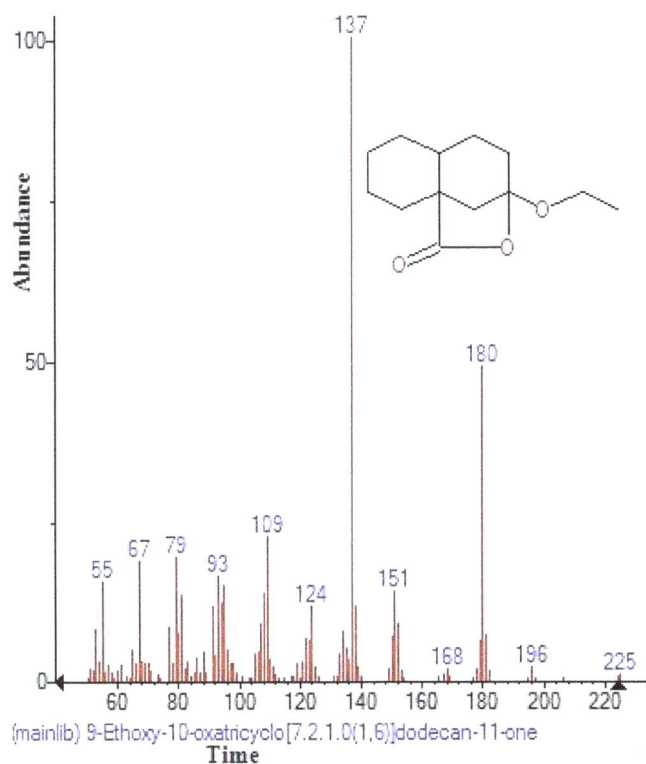

Figure 34. Structure of 9-Ethoxy-10-oxatricyclo[7.2.1.0(1,6)]dodecan-11-one present in the methanolic seeds extract of *F. vulgare* using GC-MS analysis.

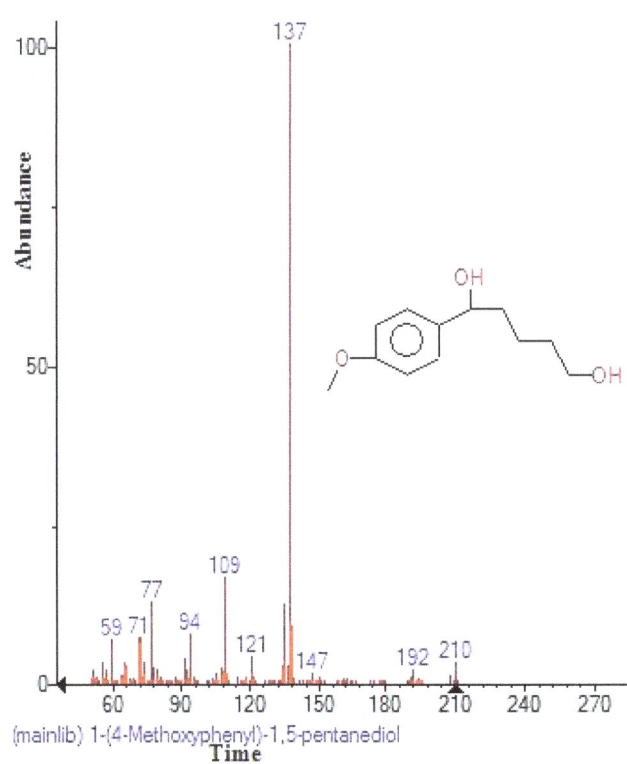

Figure 36. Structure of 1-(4-methoxyphenyl)-1,5-pentanediol present in the methanolic seeds extract of *F. vulgare* using GC-MS analysis.

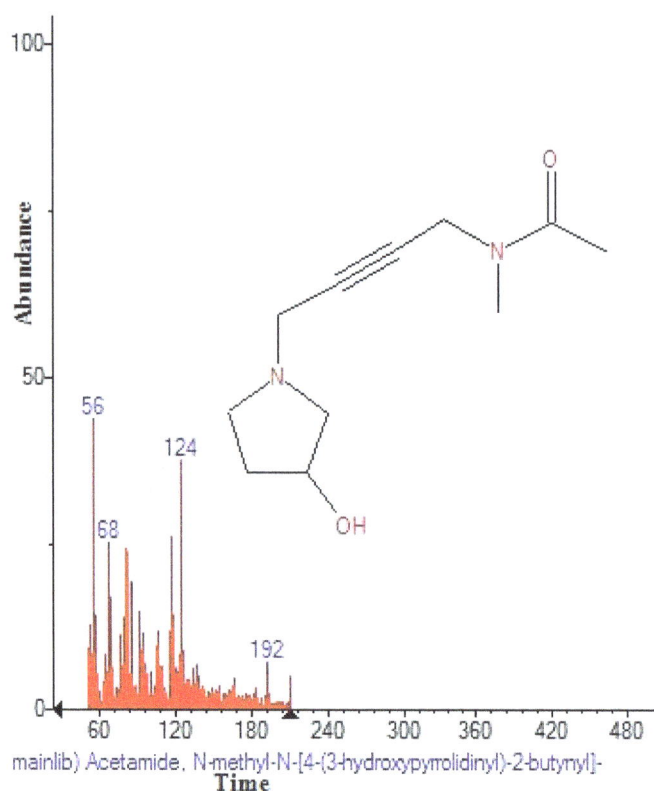

Figure 37. Structure of Acetamide,N-methyl-N-[4-(3-hydroxypyrrolidinyl)-2-butynyl] present in the methanolic seeds extract of *F. vulgare* using GC-MS analysis.

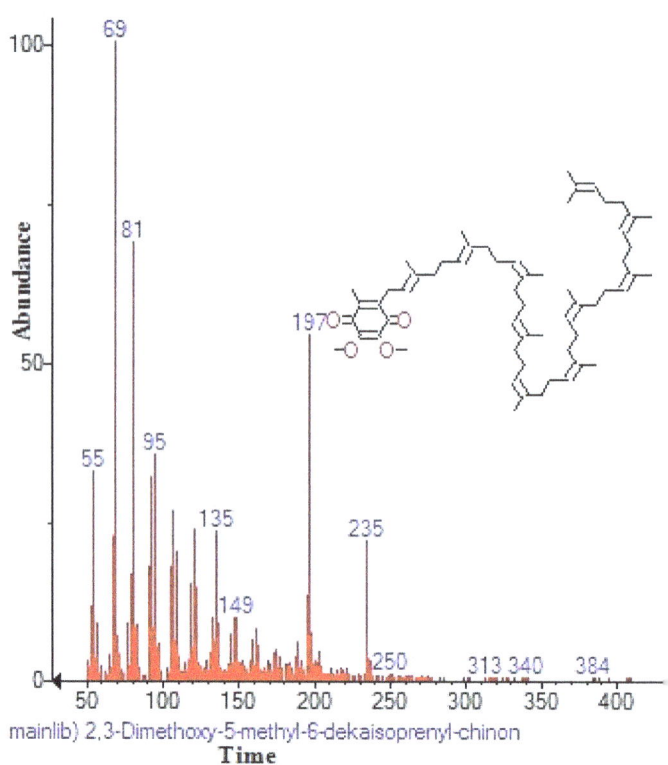

Figure 39. Structure of 2,3-Dimethoxy-5-methyl-6- decaisoprenyl-chinon present in the methanolic seeds extract of *Foeniculum vulgare* using GC-MS analysis.

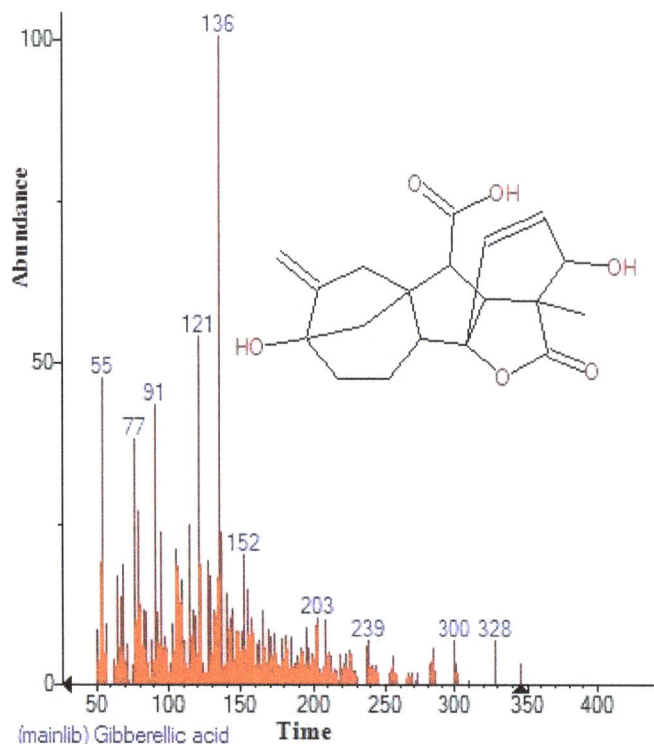

Figure 38. Structure of Gibberellic acid present in the methanolic seeds extract of *F. vulgare* using GC-MS analysis.

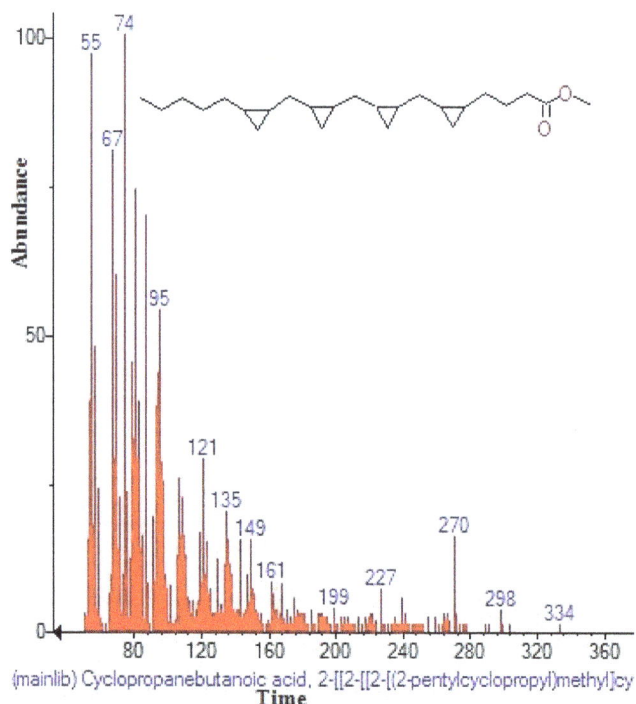

Figure 40. Structure of Cyclopropanebutanoic acid, 2-[[2-[[2-[(2-pentylcyclopropyl)methyl]cy present in the methanolic seeds extract of *F. vulgare* using GC-MS analysis.

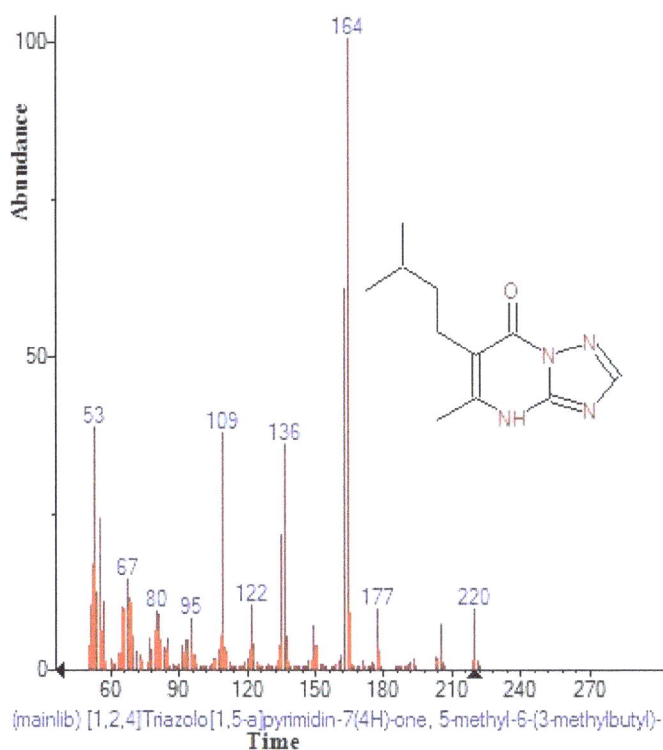

Figure 41. Structure of [1,2,4]Triazolo[1,5-a]pyrimidin-7(4H)-one,5-methyl-6-(3-methylbutyl) present in the methanolic seeds extract of *F. vulgare* using GC-MS analysis.

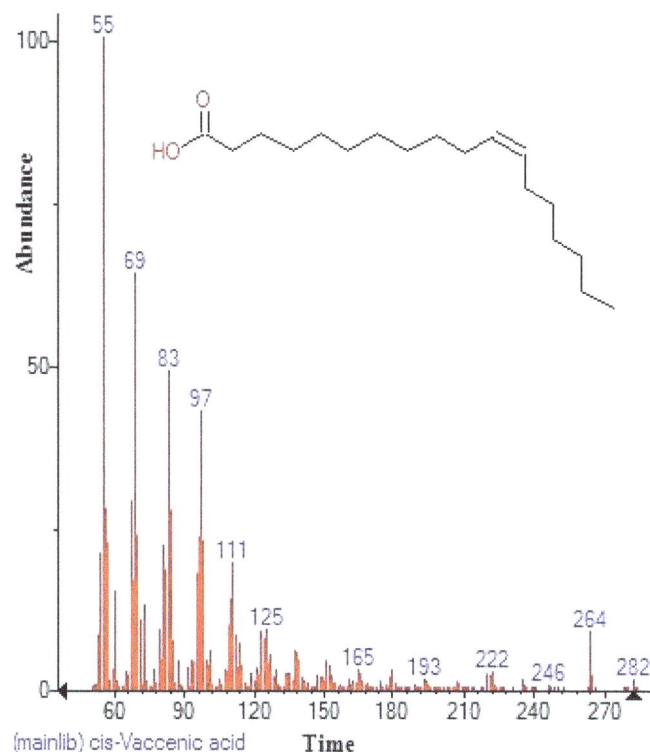

Figure 43. Structure of Cis-Vaccenic acid present in the methanolic seeds extract of *F.vulgare* using GC-MS analysis.

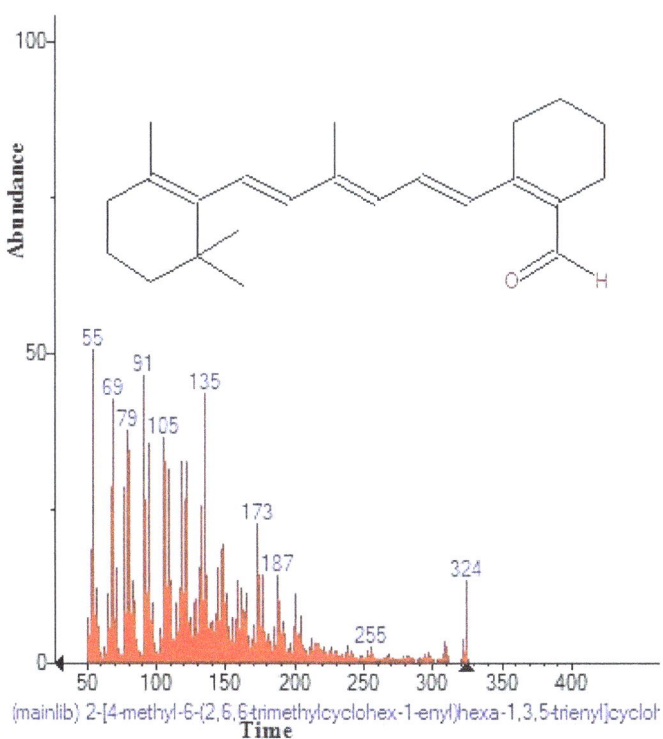

Figure 42. Structure of 2-[4-methyl-6-(2,6,6-trimethylcyclohex-1-enyl)hexa-1,3,5-trienyl]cyclo   present in the methanolic seeds extract of *Foeniculum vulgare* using GC-MS analysis.

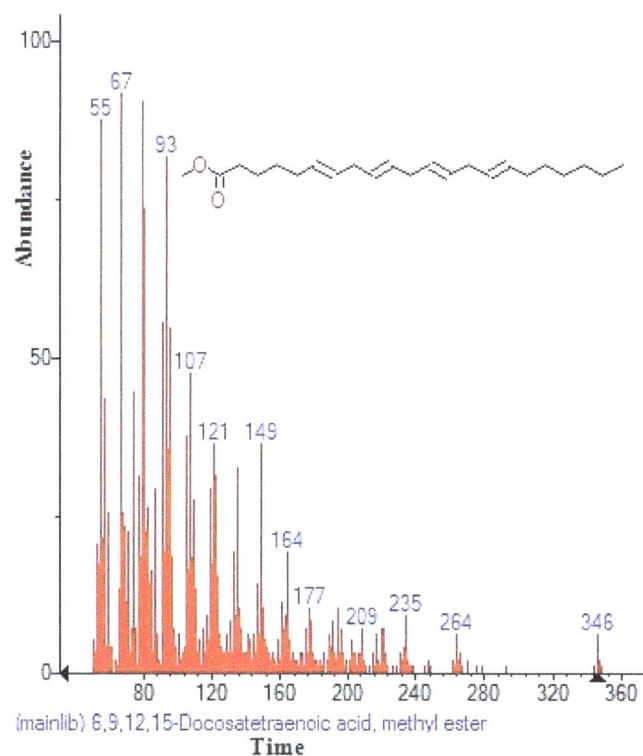

Figure 44. Structure of 6,9,12,15-Docosatetraenoic acid, methyl ester present in the methanolic seeds extract of *F. vulgare* using GC-MS analysis.

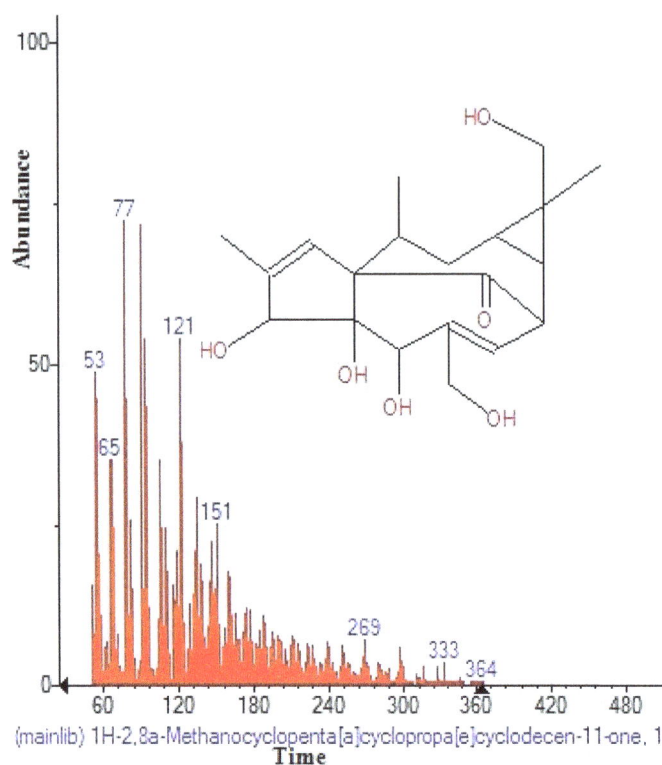

Figure 45. Structure of 1H-2,8a-Methanocyclopenta[a]cyclopropa[e]cyclodecen-11-one,1 present in the methanolic seeds extract of *F. vulgare* using GC-MS analysis.

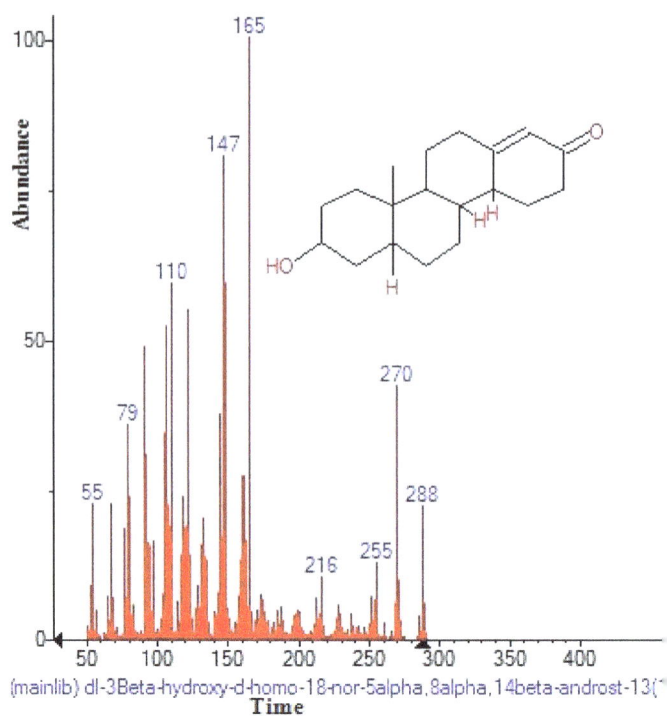

Figure 47. Structure of dl-3Beta-hydroxy-d-homo-18-nor-5alpha,8alpha,14beta-androst-13(1) present in the methanolic seeds extract of *Foeniculum vulgare* using GC-MS analysis.

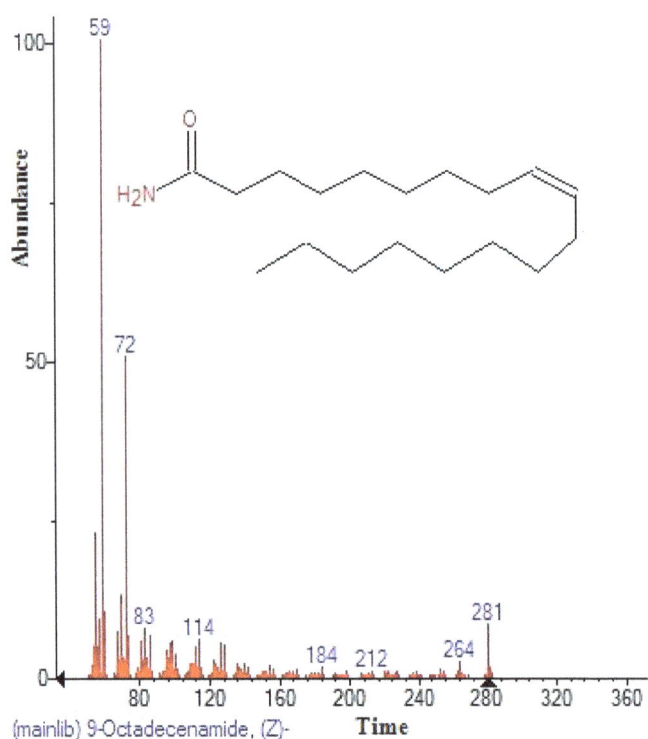

Figure 46. Structure of 9-Octadecenamide, (Z) present in the methanolic seeds extract of *F. vulgare* using GC-MS analysis.

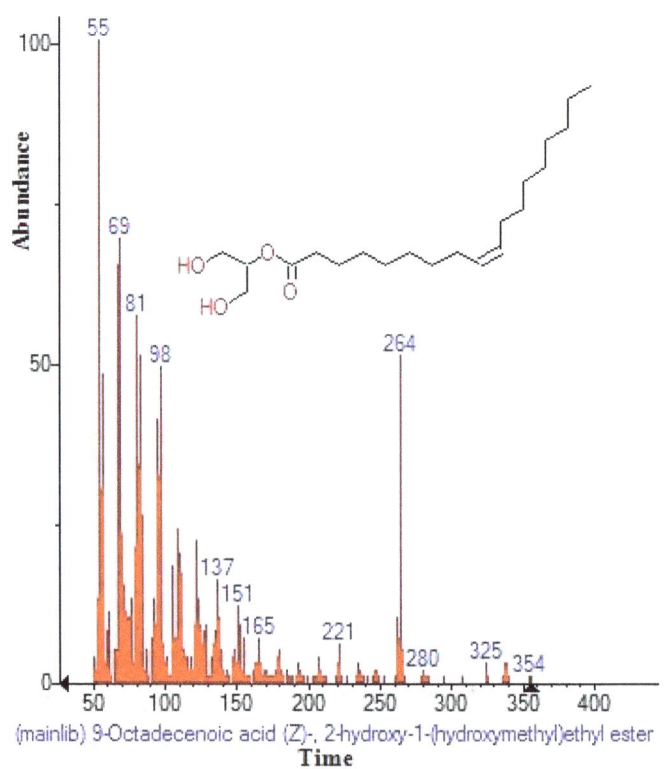

Figure 48. Structure of 9-Octadecenoic acid (Z)-,2-hydroxy-1-(hydroxymethyl)ethyl ester present in the methanolic seeds extract of *F. vulgare* using GC-MS analysis.

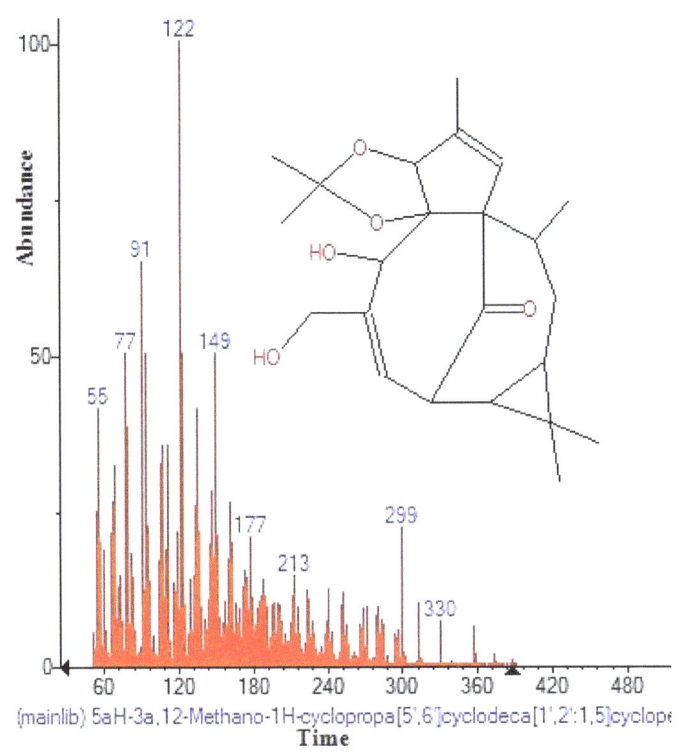

Figure 49. Structure of 5aH-3a,12-methano-1H-cyclopropa[5',6']cyclodeca[1',2':1,5]cyclo present in the methanolic seeds extract of *F. vulgare* using GC-MS analysis.

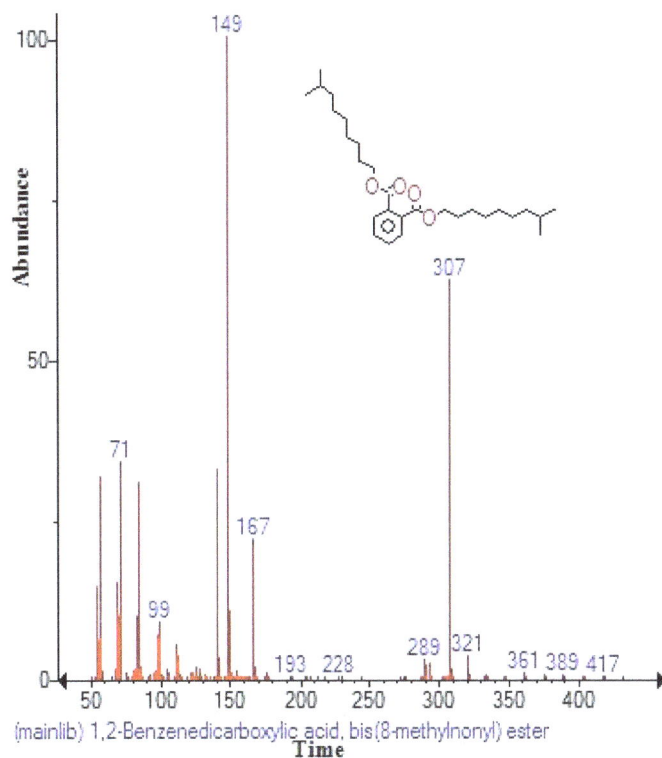

Figure 51. Structure of 1,2-Benzenedicarboxylic acid, bis(8-methylnonyl)ester present in the methanolic seeds extract of *F. vulgare* using GC-MS analysis.

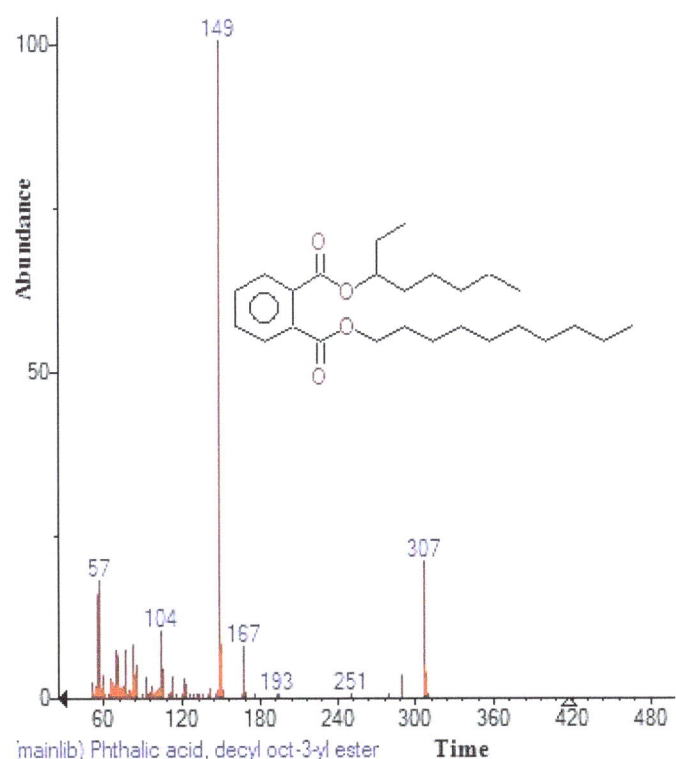

Figure 50. Structure of Phthalic acid, decyl oct-3-ylester present in the methanolic seeds extract of *F. vulgare* using GC-MS analysis.

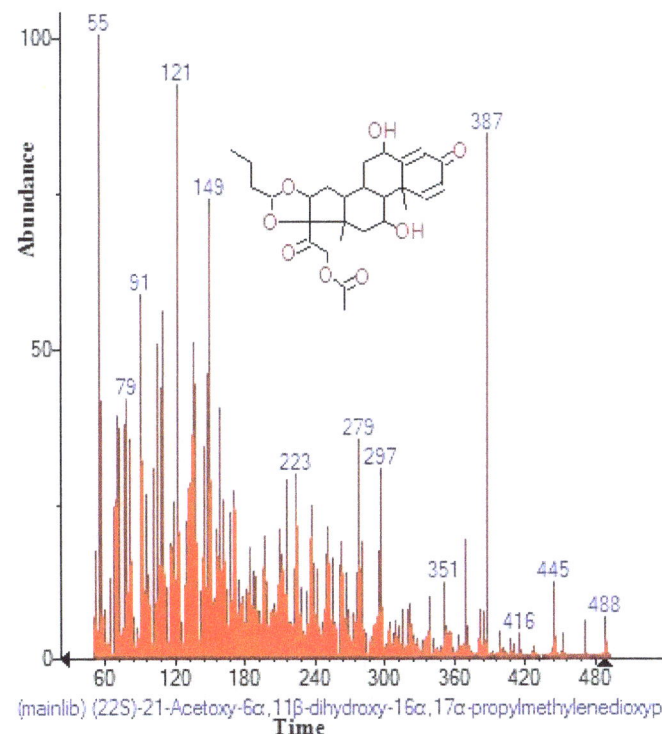

Figure 52. Structure of (22S)-21-Acetoxy-6α,11ß-dihydroxy-16α,17α-propylmethylenedioxyp present in the methanolic seeds extract of *F. vulgare* using GC-MS analysis.

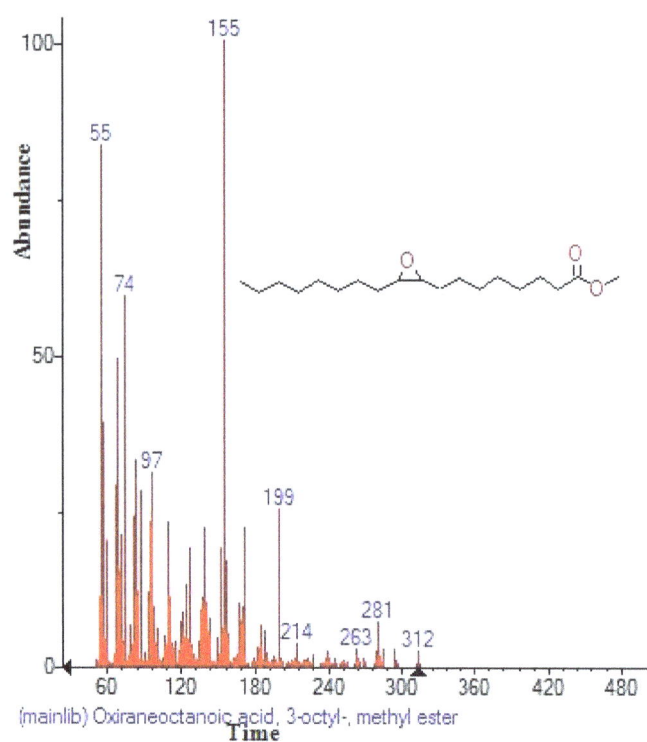

Figure 53. Structure of Oxiraneoctanoic acid, 3-octyl-,methyl ester present in the methanolic seeds extract of *F. vulgare* using GC-MS analysis.

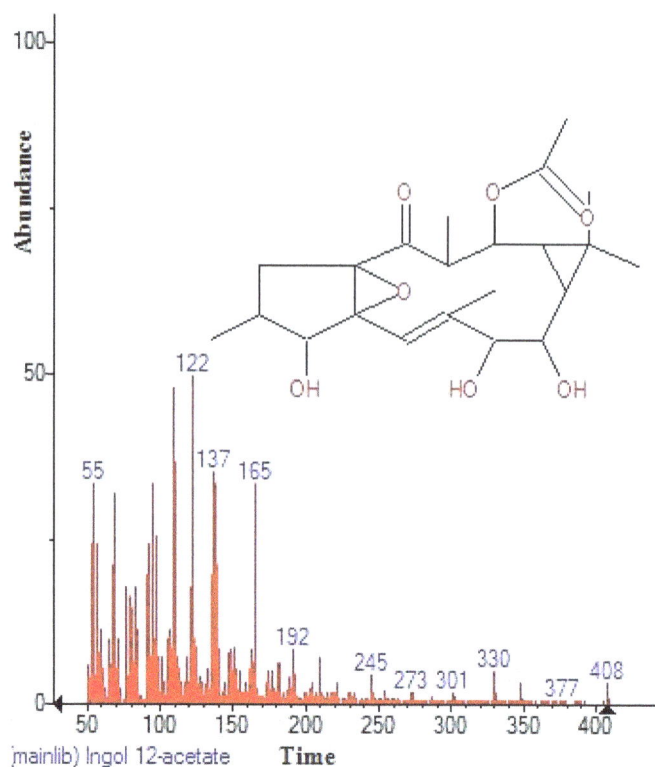

Figure 55. Structure of Ingol 12-acetate present in the methanolic seeds extract of *F. vulgare* using GC-MS analysis.

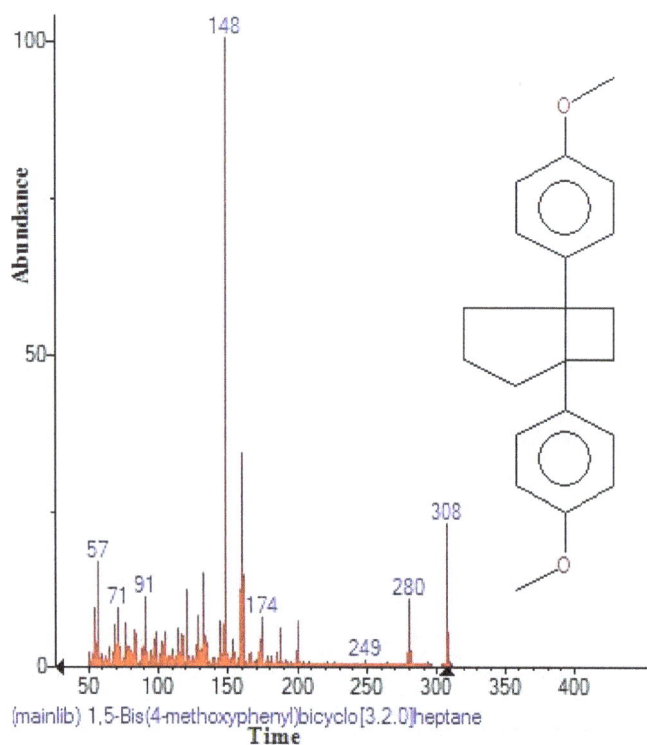

Figure 54. Structure of 1,5-Bis(4-methoxyphenyl)bicyclo[3.2.0]heptane present in the methanolic seeds extract of *F. vulgare* using GC-MS analysis.

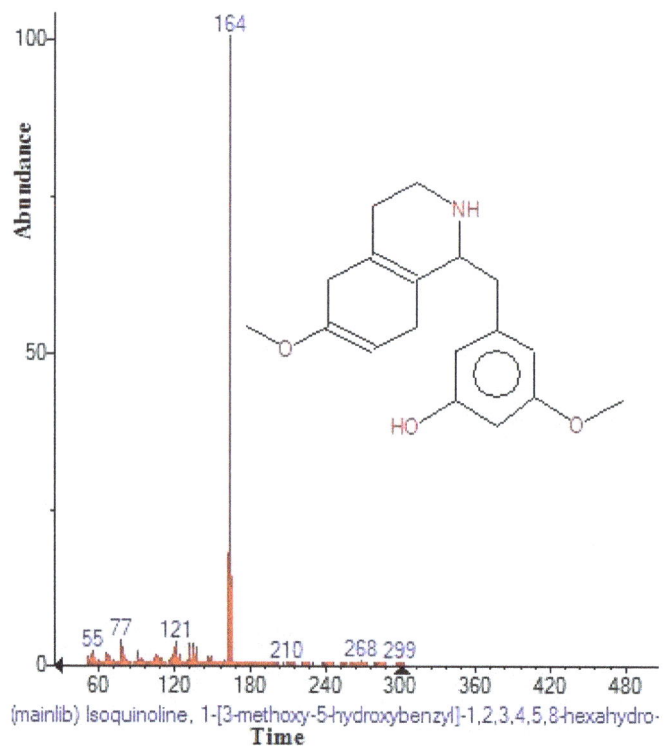

Figure 56. Structure of Isoquinoline,1-[3-methoxy-5-hydroxybenzyl]-1,2,3,4,5,8-hexahydro present in the methanolic seeds extract of *F. vulgare* using GC-MS analysis.

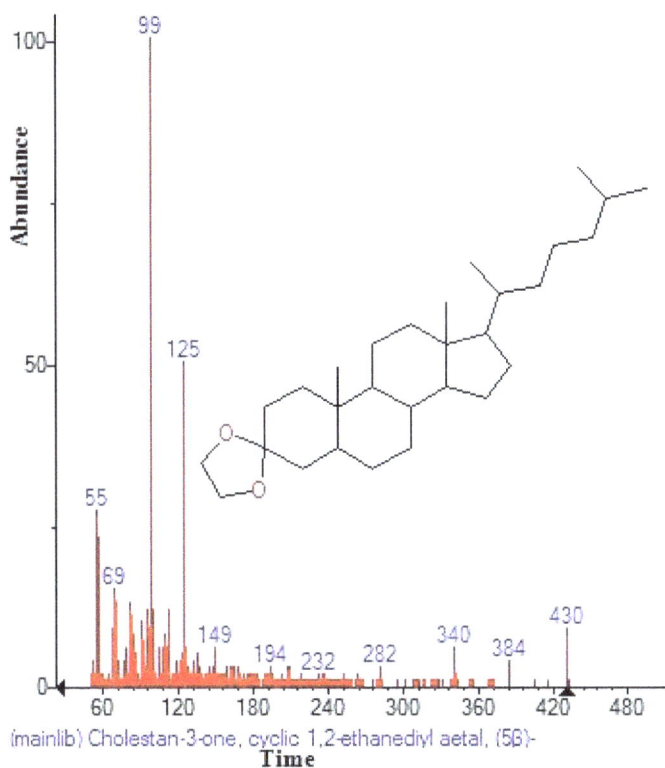

Figure 57. Structure of Cholestan-3-one , cyclic 1,2-ethanediyl aetal,(5ß) present in the methanolic seeds extract of *F. vulgare* using GC-MS analysis.

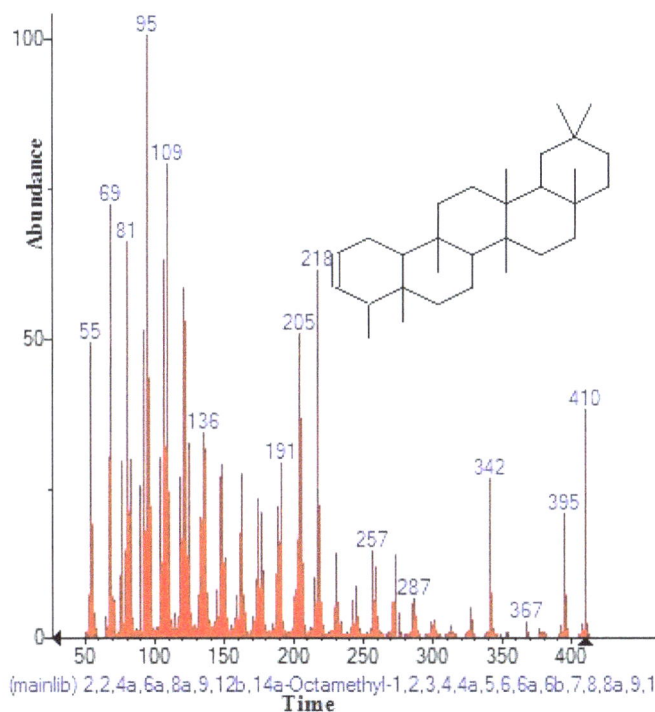

Figure 58. Structure of 2,24a,6a,8a,9,12b,14a-Octamethyl-1,2,3,4,4a,5,6,6a,6b,7,8,8a,9,1 present in the methanolic seeds extract of *F. vulgare* using GC-MS analysis.

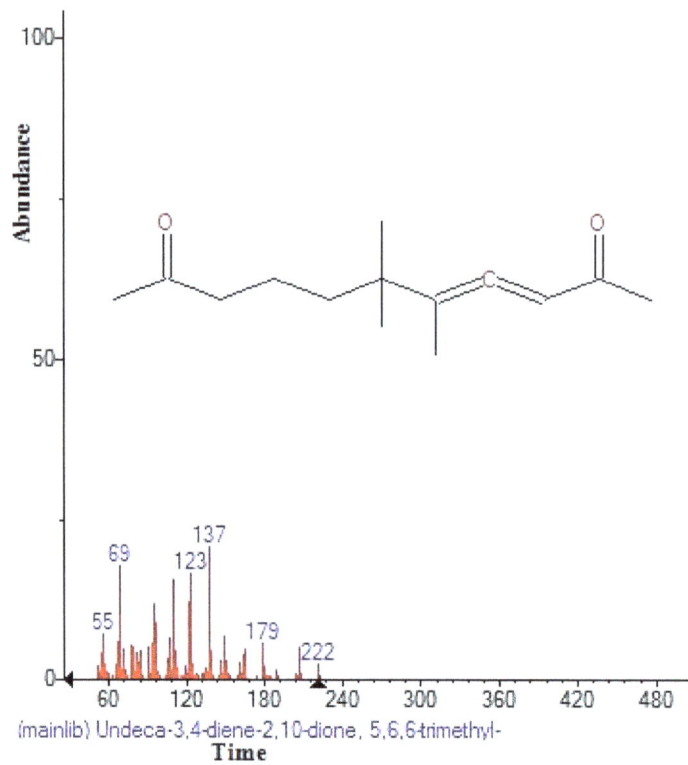

Figure 59. Structure of Undeca -3,4-diene-2,10-dione,5,6,6-trimethyl present in the methanolic seeds extract of *F. vulgare* using GC-MS analysis.

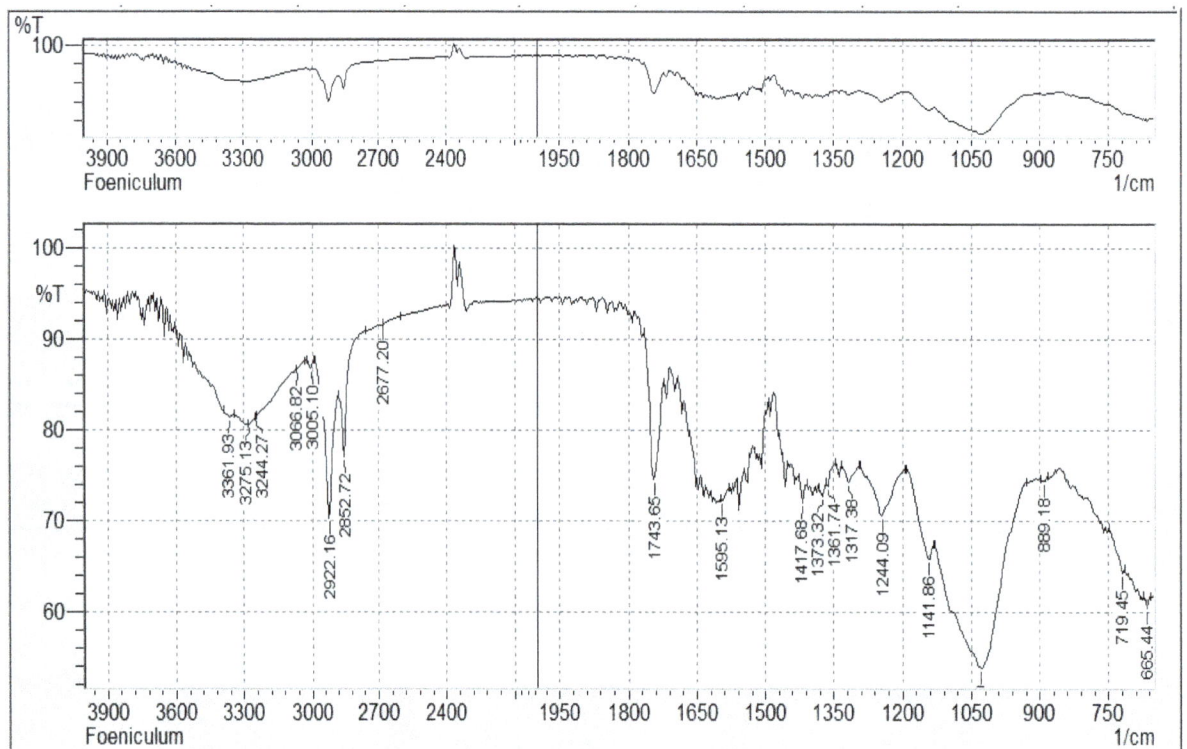

Figure 60. FT-IR profile of *F. vulgare*.

REFERENCES

Altameme HJ, Hameed IH, Idan SA, Hadi MY (2015a). Biochemical analysis of *Origanum vulgare* seeds by Fourier-transform infrared (FT-IR) spectroscopy and gas chromatography-mass spectrometry (GC-MS). J. Pharmacogn. Phytother. 7(9):221-237.

Altameme HJ, Hameed IH, Kareem MA (2015b). Analysis of alkaloid phytochemical compounds in the ethanolic extract of *Datura stramonium* and evaluation of antimicrobial activity Afr. J. Biotechnol. 14(19):1668-1674.

El-Awadi ME, Esmat AH (2010). Physiological Responses of Fennel (*Foeniculum Vulgare* Mill) Plants to Some Growth Substances. J. Am. Sci. 6:985-991.

Gross M, Friedman J., Dudia N, Larkov O, Cohen Y, Bare E (2002). Biosynthesis of estragole and t-anethole in bitter fennel (*Foeniculum vulgare* Mill. var. vulgare) chemotypes. Changes in SAM, phenylpropene o-methyltranferase activities during development. Plant Sci. 163:1047-1053.

Hameed IH, Hussein HJ, Kareem MA, Hamad NS (2015a). Identification of five newly described bioactive chemical compounds in methanolic extract of *Mentha viridis* by using gas chromatography-mass spectrometry (GC-MS). J. Pharmacogn. Phytother. 7(7):107-125.

Hameed IH, Ibraheam IA, Kadhim HJ (2015b). Gas chromatography mass spectrum and Fourier-transform infrared spectroscopy analysis of methanolic extract of *Rosmarinus oficinalis* leaves. J. Pharmacogn. Phytother. 7(6):90-106.

Hameed IH, Jasim H, Kareem MA, Hussein AO (2015c). Alkaloid constitution of *Nerium oleander* using gas chromatography-mass spectroscopy (GC-MS). J. Med. Plants Res. 9 (9):326-334.

Hameed IH, Hamza LF, Kamal SA (2015d). Analysis of bioactive chemical compounds of *Aspergillus niger* by using gas chromatography-mass spectrometry and Fourier-transform infrared spectroscopy. J. Pharmacogn. Phytother. 7(8):132-163.

Hamza LF, Kamal SA, Hameed IH (2015). Determination of metabolites products by *Penicillium expansum* and evaluating antimicobial activity. J. Pharmacogn. Phytother. 7(9):194-220.

Hay RK, Waterman PG (1993). Volatile Oil Crops: Their Biology, Biochemistry and Production, Longman Scientific and Technical, Essex, England,.

Hornok L (1992). The cultivating and Processing of Medicinal Plants. John Wiley, New York. P 338.

Hussein AO, Hameed IH, Jasim H, Kareem MA (2015). Determination of alkaloid compounds of *Ricinus communis* by using gas chromatography-mass spectroscopy (GC-MS). J. Med. Plants Res. 9(10):349-359.

Imad H, Mohammed A, Aamera J (2014a). Genetic variation and DNA markers in forensic analysis. Afr. J. Biotechnol. 13(31):3122-3136.

Imad H, Mohammed A, Cheah Y, Aamera J (2014b). Genetic variation of twenty autosomal STR loci and evaluate the importance of these loci for forensic genetic purposes. Afr. J. Biotechnol. 13:1-9.

Imad H, Muhanned A, Aamera J, Cheah Y (2014c). Analysis of eleven Y-chromosomal STR markers in middle and south of Iraq. Afr. J. Biotechnol. 13(38):3860-3871.

Jasim H, Hussein AO, Hameed IH, Kareem MA (2015). Characterization of alkaloid constitution and evaluation of antimicrobial activity of *Solanum nigrum* using gas chromatography mass spectrometry (GC-MS). J. Pharmacogn. Phytother. 7(4):56-72.

Kareem MA, Hussein AO, Hameed IH (2015). Y-chromosome short tandem repeat, typing technology, locus information and allele frequency in different population: A review. Afr. J. Biotechnol. 14(27):2175-2178.

Lucinewton S, Raul N, Carvalho J, Mlrlan B, Lln C, Angela A (2005). Supercritical fluid extraction from fennel (*Foeniculum vulgare*) global yield, composition and kinetic data. J. Supercrit. Fluids 35:212-219.

Marino SD, Gala F, Borbone N, Zollo F, Vitalini S, Visioli F, Iorrizi M (2007). Phenolic glycosides from *Foeniculum vulgare* fruit and evaluation of antioxidative activity. Phytochem. 68:1805-1812.

Mohammed A, Imad H (2013). Autosomal STR: From locus information to next generation sequencing technology. Res. J. Biotechnol. 8(10):92-105.

Telci I, Demirtas I, Sahin A (2009). Variation in plant properties and essential oil composition of sweet fennel (*Foeniculum vulgare* Mill.) fruits during stages of maturity. Ind. Crop Prod. 30:126-130.

## 7

Ethnopharmacological survey of plants used for the treatment of diabetes

M. Laadim*, M. L. Ouahidi, L. Zidane, A. El Hessni, A. Ouichou and A. Mesfioui

Laboratory of Genetics, Neuroendocrinology and Biotechnology, Department of Biology, Faculty of Sciences, Ibn Tofail University, Kenitra, Morocco.

The study aimed to screen the antidiabetic plants used by 700 diabetic patients in the town of Sidi Slimane (northwestern Morocco). The results identified 59 species belonging to 28 botanical families, four of which are predominant (*Lamiaceae*: 9 species; *Apiaceae*: 7 species; *Asteraceae*: 5 species; Fabaceae: 4 species). The most used species are: *Trigonella foenum-graecum, Oreganum vulgare, Salvia officinalis, Marrubium vulgare* and *Olea europaea*. Similarly, majority of the anti-diabetic recipes are prepared as infusion and decoction. Further, seeds and leaves are the most used parts and are administered orally. These results constitute a database for subsequent studies to experimentally assess the potential of these plants.

Key words: Ethnopharmacological survey, medicinal plants, town of Sidi Slimane, diabetes mellitus.

INTRODUCTION

Diabetes is a complex disease due to its physiopathological mechanisms, its genetic determinism, as well as the genesis of its complications. It is a heterogeneous group of metabolic diseases whose main feature is a chronic hyperglycemia resulting from a defect in insulin secretion, of its action, or the association of these two anomalies (OMS, 2002). This disease affects more than 285 million people throughout the world, and the number of people provided for diabetic should increase in an outstanding manner to more than 380 million in 2025, thus becoming quickly the epidemic of the 21st century (International Diabetes Federation, 2009).

The OMS estimates that, in 2030, the diabetes will be the seventh leading cause of death in the world (OMS, 2013).

Across all the continents, Africa is the most affected by this disease (Erasto et al., 2005). In Morocco, the diabetes constitutes a major public health problem, indeed, according to a national survey conducted in 2000, the prevalence of this epidemic is located in the vicinity with about 6.6% (Tazi et al., 2000). In addition, according to another study, the number of diabetics exceeds 2.5 million, 7.81% of the Moroccan population, which makes the situation of national public health

*Corresponding author. E-mail: majda3amal-85@hotmail.com.

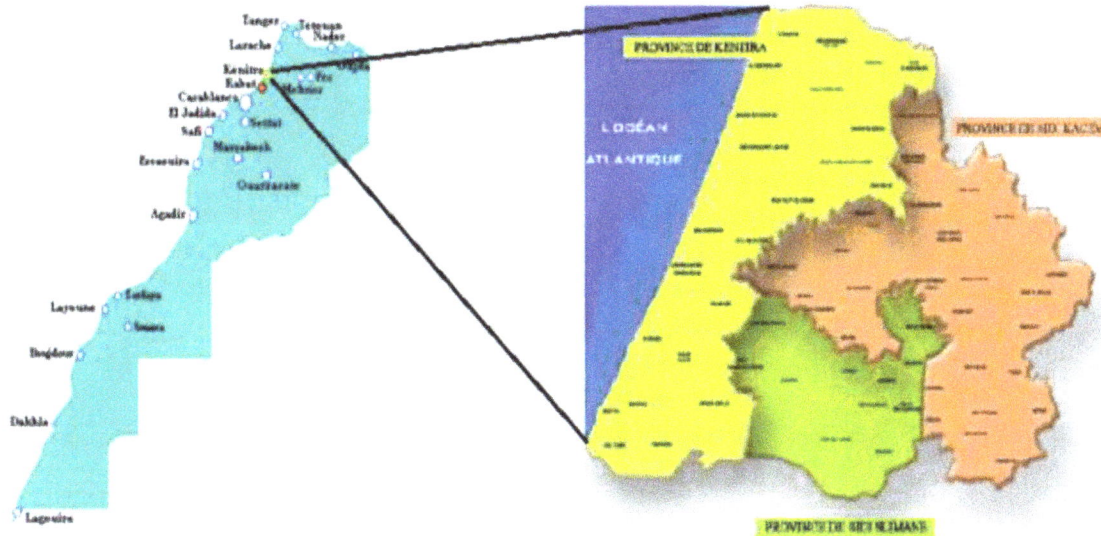

Figure 1. Map of Morocco showing the surveyed city.

eratical in relation to other health and conditions requirements of the population (Ghourri, 2013). More than 1200 species of plants have been used empirically for their presumed glucose lowering activity (Marles and Farnsworth, 1995). The medicinal plants are still a source of medical care in developing countries in the absence of a modern medicinal system (Tabuti et al., 2003).

The objective of this study is to identify the medicinal plants used for the traditional treatment by the diabetic patients in the town of Sidi Slimane which has never been a subject of an ethnobotanical study.

MATERIALS AND METHODS

Description of the studied area

Sidi Slimane is a North West city in Morocco (Figure 1), situated between 34° 15 '36' 'N and 5° 55' 12 '' West with a population of 92,989 people in 2014 (Monography of Sidi Slimane City, 2015). It is centrally located in the region of West by its location in a privileged geo-economic space, and very valued by its demographic weight and the importance of its economic apparatus segment in particular agro-industrial.

The region of Sidi Slimane corresponds to a marked oceanic influence, belonging to the semi-arid bioclimatic stage to temperate winter, the high air humidity, prevailing winds from the west. Hydrologically, Sidi Slimane is part of the Sebou catchment. One of its main tributaries (OuedBeht) passes through the agglomeration. The predominant crop of the area is beets, oranges, cotton, vegetable and grain growing (Monography of Sidi Slimane City, 2015).

Ethnopharmacological survey

The survey was conducted among 700 subjects with diabetes in the province of Sidi Slimane (Rabat- Sale- Kenitra's region). The survey was conducted in three different centers: Laghmariyin, Essalam and Wlad Lghazi, where diabetic patients receive consultations and necessary medicines.

Patients surveyed were of both sexes and aged between 8 and 98 years old.

For the achievement of the survey, a predetermined questionnaire used includes information on the diabetic patients, the disease, the remedy used and the outcome of therapy. The study investigation lasted for 8 months, from September 2013 to April 2014.

The content of the used questionnaire

The study was conducted with the help of a questionnaire which consists of three parts:

1. Identification: information on the diabetic patient (sex, age, weight, level of education, physical activity and socio-economic level)
2. The disease information (type of diabetes, diabetes discovery circumstances, diabetes complications and family history).
3. Traditional remedy: source of supply of medicinal plants, reasons, doses accuracy, plants used, information (parts used, quantity) preparation and cure's dosage, treatment duration and toxic plants knowledge.

RESULTS AND DISCUSSION

Diabetic population's characteristics

The study was carried out on 700 diabetic patients living in the city of Sidi Slimane, the studied population was between 8 and 98 years old, among the two sexes; women were the most affected (72.28%). The results are

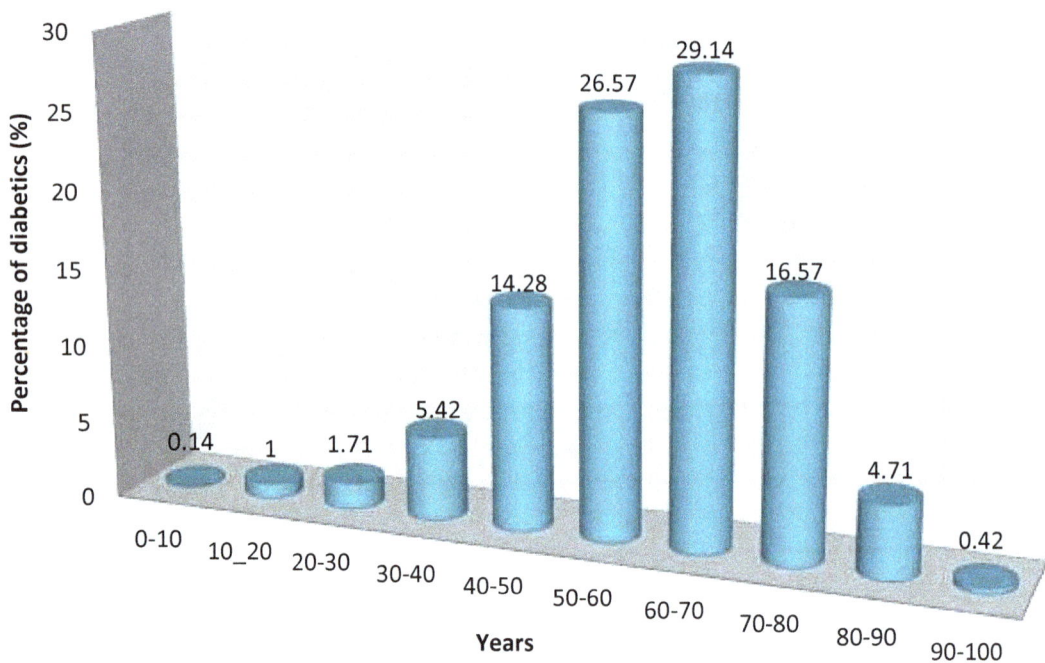

Figure 2. Distribution of diabetics by age.

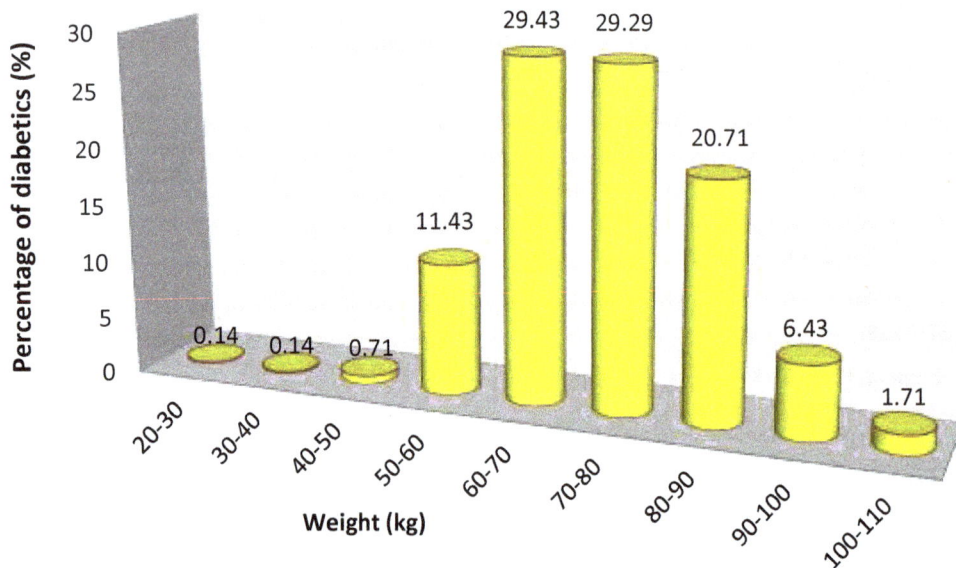

Figure 3. Distribution of diabetics based on weight.

shown in Figure 2. The age group most affected by diabetes is between 60 and 70 years old, concerning the weight, more than 29% have a weight between 60 and 70 kg (Figure 3).

The feeding behavior, physical activity, aging and stress are often considered as factors causing obesity which leads to diabetes (King et al., 1998). This assumes the good control of the food supply, a reasonable level of

physical activity and adapted policies to the populations at risk, particularly for the people older than 60 years (Fagot-Campagna, 2005).

The study has shown that illiteracy is widespread (60% among those with diabetes in Sidi Slimane, while 19.42% have a level of primary schooling, 11% medium (college) 6% secondary and only 3.57% have pursued graduate studies. As regards the socio-economic level, only

Table 1. Percentage of complications associated with diabetes.

Complications associated with diabetes	Number of patients	Percentage
Arterial tension	91	13.43
Cholesterol	10	1.43
Diabetic foot	4	0.57
Heart disease	4	0.57
Eye disease	1	0.14
Kidney disease	1	0.14

15.85% of the patients have a low socio-economic level, 84.14% belong to a medium level, and while only one person lives an easy situation. Sport is neglected by the patients; it was found that only 32.14% part take in sports.

Disease characteristics

The distribution of the studied population according to the type of diabetes is as follows: 1) 72.57% correspond to type 1; 2) 27.42% correspond to type 2.

87.71 %, of diabetics have discovered the disease by suggestive symptoms, 9.28% by a screening test, and 3% of them have discovered it late. Indeed, more than 65% is hereditary, and less than 18% of patients have presented complications associated with diabetes (Table 1).

Characteristics of the diabetic population according to their use of the phytotherapy

More than 61% of people with diabetes have recourse in herbal medicine to treat diabetes and 38.57% use only the conventional treatment. In previous studies, many authors have shown that the percentage of the use of medicinal plants varies between 52 and 90%, depending on the region or where the investigation has been undertaken (Sekkat, 1987; Magoua, 1991; Nabih, 1992; Bellakhdar, 1997; Ziyyat et al., 1997; Eddouks et al., 2007; Benkhnigue et al., 2011). This strong use of medicinal plants is due to the strong belief of diabetic patients in their efficiency (95.86%), accessibility (2.86%) as well as their low cost (1.29%).

This choice of the use of herbal remedies is based on the advice of other diabetics (54.65%) who have already used them (either from media or from other people), and 45.12% have accounted on the advice of the herbalists while only one person was advised by a doctor in herbal medicine.

With regards to the use of these antidiabetic plants, 54.19% of diabetics use them according to a specific doses, 24.42% in non-specific doses and 21.40% of the use by easy acquisition. These patients have shown great satisfaction in relation to the phytotherapy of more than 58%. In addition to these factors, the contribution of

religion in the field of medicinal plants among the plants cited asanti-hyperglycaemic, some are drawn directly from the Koran and religious manuscripts. This is particularly the case of *Lawsonia inermis*, *Trigonella foenum-graecum*, *Ziziphus lotus*, *Punica granatum*, *Myrtus communis*, *Nigella sativa*, *Allium sativum*, *Allium cepa*, *Olea europaea*, *Ficus garcia*, and *Zingiber officinalis* (Eddouks et al., 2007).

The richness of the Moroccan gastronomy in plant species is used both as food ingredients and for their therapeutic properties (Eddouks, 2006), as well as nutritional life style. All these factors are considered as the cornerstone in the treatment and prevention of diabetes (Srivastava and Mehdi, 2005).

The use of the herbal medicine according to sex

Among the 430 (61%) diabetics using the medicinal plants; 76.28% are women, while 23.72% are men, and the study is consistent with other studies which are between 61 and 69 and 31 to 39%, respectively (Eddouks et al., 2002; Jouad et al., 2001; El Beghdadi, 1991; Hamdani, 1984; Jaouad, 1992; Nabih, 1992; Ziyyat et al., 1997). This could be explained by the relative frequency of illiteracy of women in our society, and their commitment to traditional knowledge (Hamdani, 1984; Jaouad, 1992; Nabih, 1992).

Knowledge on toxic plants

In this study, more than 74% of the people with diabetes have no information on the toxicity of medicinal plants and only 26% take into account, the illiteracy of a large number of the patients, and the lack of awareness primarily by the indirect harm. Patients using herbal medicine have reported nine plants that have side effects and they are grouped as shown in Table 2 with their side effects.

Medicinal plants used for the treatment of diabetes in Sidi Slimane

The plants used by the diabetics are divided into 59

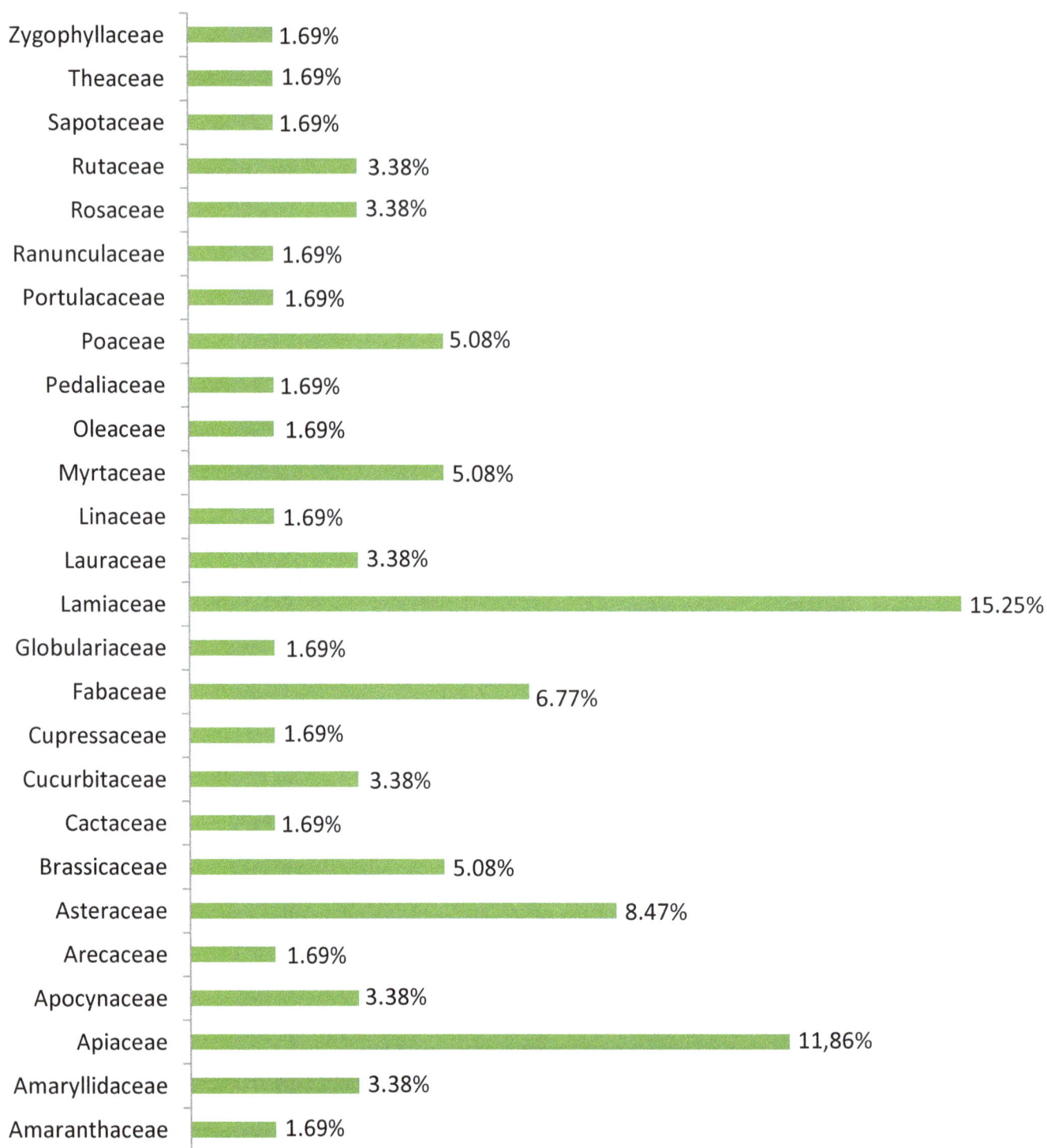

Figure 4. Frequency of botanical families.

species, belonging to 28 botanical families and the most represented are the Lamiaceae: 9 species; Apiaceae: 7 species; Asteraceae: 5 species and Fabaceae: 4 species (Figure 4).

The most used species by diabetic patients are: *T.*

foenum-graecum: 63 persons; *O. vulgare*: 38 persons; *S. officinalis*: 37 persons; *M. vulgare*: 25 persons and *O. europaea*: 24 persons) Also, the most used parts are the seeds and the leaves (Figure 5).

For the mode of preparation, the infusion and decoction

Table 2. List of plants with side effects.

Plant name	Side effects
Lavandula stoeckas	Sore stomach
Rosmarinus officinalis	Generalized pain
Origanum vulgare L.	Abdominal pain
Tetraclinis articulata	Abdominal pain
Olea europaea L.	Vomiting
Artemisia absinthium	Vomiting
Medicago sativa	Sore stomach
Chenopodium ambrosioides L.	Heart ailments
Allium sativum L.	Blood pressure drop

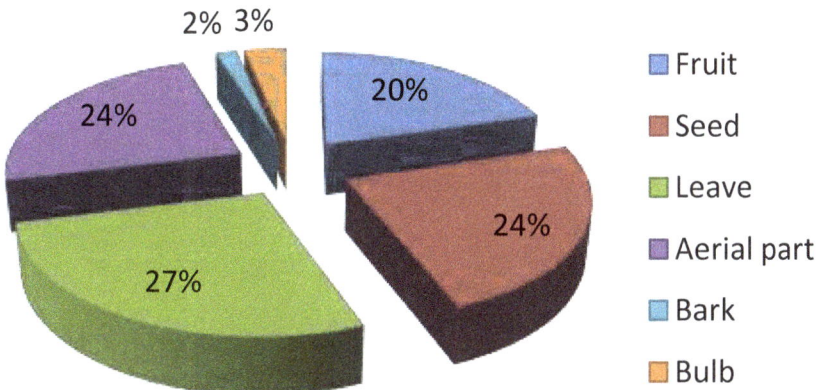

Figure 5. Part of plants used.

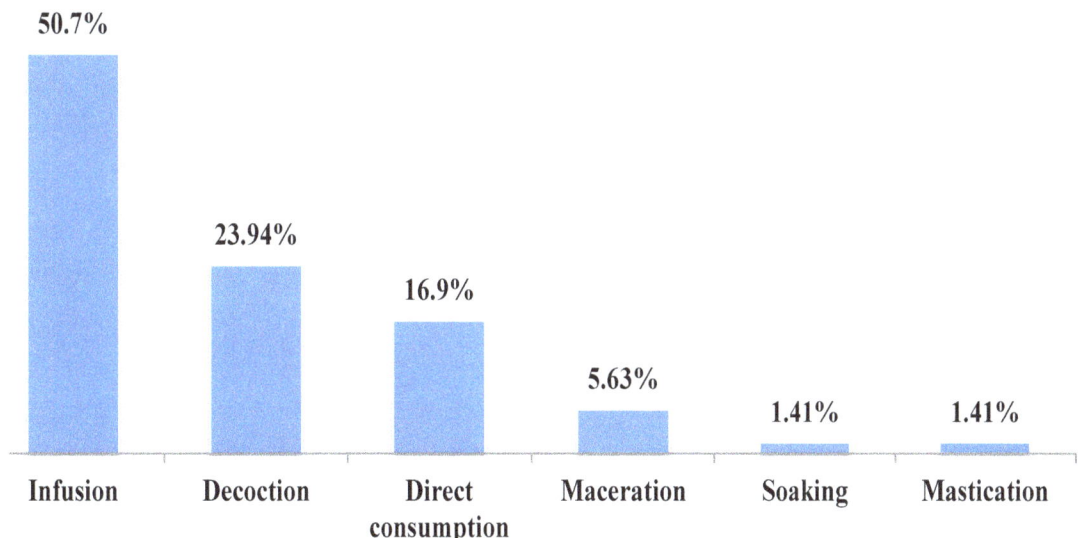

Figure 6. Frequency of form of use of anti-diabetic plants.

are the most used (Figure 6), the bitter taste of plants is widespread, and the remedies are taken orally. Table 3 shows the various plants mentioned, the part used and the method of preparation.

Table 3. Inventory of anti-diabetic plants cited in the survey.

Species	Latin name	Vernacular name	Part of plant used	Method of preparation	Number of citations	Treatment duration	Corresponding References
Amaranthaceae	Chenopodium ambrosioides	Mkhinza	Leaves	Infusion	2	1 Week	Eddouks et al., 2002
Amaryllidaceae	Allium cepa	Basla	Bulbs	Direct consumption	5	6 Month - 1 year	
	Allium sativum	Touma	Bulbs	Decoction	5	3 Year	
	Ammi visnaga	Bachnikha	Fruits	Infusion	9	10 Days	
	Pimpinella anisum	Habathlawa	Seeds	Decoction Direct consumption	8		
Apiaceae	Ammodaucus leucotrichus	Kamounsoufi	Seeds	Infusion	5	2 Month	Eddouks et al., 2002
	Coriandrum sativum L.	Kosbor	Seeds	Infusion	5	3 Month	
	Apium graveolens	Krafess	Seeds	Infusion	8	15 day- 1ans	
	Petroselinum sativum	Maadnouss	Seeds	Infusion	5	1 year	
	Foeniculum vulgare	Basbas	Seeds	Infusion- decoction	7	6 month - 1ans	
Apocynaceae	Nerium oleander	Defla	Leaves	Decoction- infusion	2	ND	Bnouham et al., 2002
	Caralluma europaea	Daghmous	Aerial parts	Maceration	18	1weeks- 4month	
Arecaceae	Phoenix dactylifera	Tmar	Fruits	Direct consumption	3	2 month -6 month	-
	Matricaria nrecutita	Babounj	Aerial parts	Infusion	7		-
	Artemisia absinthium	Chiba	Aerial parts	Infusion	6	1 year -2 year	-
	Artemisia herba-alba	Chih	Aerial parts	Decoction	12		-
Asteraceae	Cynara cardunculus	Kharchouf	Aerial parts	Decoction	8	2 month - 2 year	-
	Lactuca sativa	Khes	Leaves	Direct consumption	4	1 year	-
	Raphanus raphanistrum subsp. sativus	Fjal	Fruits	Direct consumption	1	ND	Ziyyat et al., 1997; Jouad et al., 2001; Jaouhari, 2002
Brassicaceae	Lepidium sativum	Haberrechad	Seeds	Infusion -decoction	8	6 month - 1 year	Eddouks et al., 2002; Merzouki et al., 2003
	Brassica oleracea var. capitata	Krounb-mkaouar	Aerial parts	Maceration	4	6 month -2 year	Jouad et al., 2001

Table 3. Contd.

Family	Scientific name	Local name	Part used	Preparation	No.	Duration	References
Cactaceae	Opuntia ficus-indica	Sabbar-zaaboul-lhendi	Aerial parts	Maceration	12	1 year -2 year	Jouad et al., 2001; Jaouhari, 2002; Merzouki et al., 2003
	Citrullus colocynthis	Hdej	Fruits	Maceration	4	15 year	Bellakhdar et al., 1991; Bellakhdar, 1997; Ziyyat et al., 1997; Merzouki and al., 2000; Jouad et al., 2001;
Cucurbitaceae	Cucumis sativus	Khiar	Fruits	Direct consumption	2	6 month	Eddouks et al., 2002 Jaouhari, 2002; Merzouki et al., 2003); Jouad et al., 2001
Cupressaceae	Tetraclinis articulata	Araar	Leaves	Infusion	9	1week-1month	Eddouks et al., 2002
Fabaceae	Medicago sativa	Fassa	Aerial parts	Infusion	2	1month	-
	Trigonella foenum-graecum	Halba	Seeds	Soaking	63	week -4	Bnouham et al., 2002
	Ceratonia siliqua	Kharoub	Fruits	Direct infusion consumption	4	1month	-
	Glycine max	Soja	Seeds	Decoction	3	1month	Bnouham et al., 2002
Globulariaceae	Globularia repens	Ainlernab	Leaves	Decoction	1	ND	Bellakhdar et al., 1991; Bellakhdar, 1997; Ziyyat et al., 1997; Merzouki et al., 2000; Jouad et al., 2001; Eddouks et al., 2002; Jaouhari, 2002; Merzouki et al., 2003
Lamiaceae	Rosmarinus officinalis	Azir	Leaves	Infusion - decoction	16	3month	
	Mentha pulegium	Fliou	Aerial parts	Infusion-decoction	14	week -3 month	
	Lavandula stoechas	Halhal	Leaves	Infusion-decoction	6	2 month	
	Lavandula dentata	Khzama	Aerial parts	Infusion	7	6 month -1 year	
	Marrubium vulgare	Meriout	Aerial parts	Infusion	25	2 month -1year	
	Salvia officinalis	Salmiya	Leaves	Infusion	37	week -5 year	
	Origanum vulgare	Zaatar	Leaves	Infusion	38	15 day -4 year	Eddouks et al., 2002
	Thymus vulgaris	Zaitra	Leaves	Infusion	6	6 month	
	Ajuga iva	Chandgoura	Aerial parts	Infusion	7	2month	
Lauraceae	Cinnamomum cassia	Karfa	Ecorce	Infusion	8	1 month - 6 month	
	Laurus nobilis	Ouraksidnamoussa	Leaves	Infusion- decoction	3	1 year	
Linaceae	Linum usitatissimum	Zariatelkattan	Seeds	Decoction	8	6 week -2 month	
Myrtaceae	Eugenia caryophyllata	Krantal	Fruits	Infusion	4	6 month	

Table 3. Contd.

Family	Species	Local name	Part used	Preparation		Duration	Reference
Oleaceae	*Eucalyptus globules*	Kritouss	Leaves	Infusion	1	ND	
	Myrtus communis	Rayhan	Leaves	Infusion	2	1month	
	Olea europaea	Zitoun	Leaves	Infusion	24	1 month -5 year	Eddouks et al., 2002
Pedaliaceae	*Sesamum indicum*	Janjlan	Seeds	Infusion-decoction	5	2 month	
	Pennisetum typhoides	Illan	Seeds	Infusion	7	2 month	
Poaceae	*Hordeum vulgare*	Chair	Aerial parts	Infusion	2	1 year	
	Phalaris canariensis	Zouan	Seeds	Infusion	4	2weeks	
Portulacaceae	*Portulaca oleracea*	Rejla	Aerial parts	Decoction	4	ND	
Ranunculaceae	*Nigella sativa*	Sanouj	Seeds	Infusion	17	2 month -1 year	Bnouham et al., 2002
	Prunus amygdalus	Louzalmor	Fruits	Direct consumption	1	ND	
Rosaceae	*Malus communis*	Tofah	Fruits	Direct consumption	1	ND	
	Citrus sinensis	Limoun	Fruits	Direct consomation	3	6 month	Eddouks et al., 2002
Rutaceae	*Citrus bigaradia*	Ranj	Fruits	Direct consommation	3	6 month -1 year	
Sapotaceae	*Argania spinosa*	Argan	Fruits	Direct consumption	5	2 month -1 year	-
Theaceae	*Camellia sinensis*	Atay	Leaves	Decoction- infusion	10	ND	-
Zygophyllaceae	*Zygophyllum gaetulum*	Agaia	Leaves	Infusion	10	1month-1years	Eddouks et al., 2002

REFERENCES

Bellakhdar J, Claisse R, Fleurentin J, Younos C (1991). Repertory of standard herbal drugs in the Moroccan pharmacopoeia. J. Ethnopharmacol. 35:123-143.

Bellakhdar J (1997). La pharmacopéeMarocainetraditionnelle, Médecine arabe ancienne et savoirs populaires. Edition le Fennec et Ibis Press.

Eddouks M (2006). Aspects of food medicine and ethnopharmacology in Morocco, in eating and healing,

traditional food and medicine. Eds Haworth press. New York. pp. 357-82.

Eddouks M, Maghrani, Lemhadri A, Ouahidi ML, Jaouad H (2002). Ethnopharmacological survey of medicinal plants used for the treatment of diabetes mellitus, hypertension and cardiac diseases in the south-east region of Morocco (Tafilalet). J. Ethnopharmacol. 82:97-103.

El Beghdadi M (1991). Pharmacopée traditionnelle du Maroc, Les plantes medicinales et les affections du systéme cardio-vasculaire. Thèse de Pharmacie. Fac. Méd. Pharm. Rabat.

Fagot-Campagna A, Bourdel-Marchasson, Simon D (2005). Burden of diabetes in an aging population: prevalence, incidence, mortality, characteristics and quality of care. Diabet. Metab. 31:5S35-5S52.

Erasto P, Adebola PO, Grierson DS, Afolayan AJ (2005). An ethnobotanical study of plants used for the treatment of diabetes in the Eastern Cape Province South Africa. Afr. J. Biotech. 4:1458-1460.

Hamdani SE (1984). Médecine traditionnelle a Boujaad. Thèse de Pharmacie. Fac. Méd. Pharm. Rabat.

International Diabetes Federation (2009). IDF diabetes atlas, 4th ed., Brussels, Belgium: International Diabetes Federation.

Jaouad L (1992). Enquêteethnobotanique, la part de la médecinetraditionnelledans les différentes couches socio-économiques de la population de Casablanca. Thèse de Pharmacie. Fac. Méd. Pharm. Rabat.

Jouad H, Haloui M, Rhiouani H, El Hilaly J, Eddouks M (2001). Ethnobotanical survey of medicinal plants used for the treatment of diabetes, cardiac and renal diseases in the North centre region of Morocco (Fez-Boulemane). J. Ethnopharmacol. 77:175-182.

Jaouhari JT (2002). Contribution a l'étudephytochimique, pharmacologique et clinique d'une plante réputée hypoglycémiante, Zygophyllumgaetulum EMB. EtMaire. Thèse de doctorat d'état. Université Cady Ayyad, Faculté des Sciences Semlalia, Marrakech.

King H, Aubert R, Herman WH (1998). Global burden of diabetes, 1995-2025. Diabet. Care 21:1414-31.

Magoua N (1991). Les recettes familiales à base de plantes médicinales dans la province de Salé. Thèse de Pharmacie. Fac. Méd. Pharm. Rabat.

Marles RJ, Farnsworth NR (1995). Antidiabetic plants and their active constituents. Phytomedicine 2:13-189.

Eddouks M, Ouahidi ML, Farid O, Moufid A, Khalidi A, Lemhadri A (2007). L'utilisation des plantes médicinales dans le traitement du diabete au Maroc. Phytotherapie 5:194-203.

Merzouki A, Ed-derfouri F, Morelo-Mesa J (2003). Contribution to the knowledge of Rifian traditional medicine. III: Phytotherapy of diabetes in Chefchaouen province (North of Morocco). ArsPharmaceutica 44(1):59-67.

Municipalité de SidiSlimane, Division technique (2015). Monography of Sidi Slimane city. Province de Sidi Slimane, Région Rabat-Salé-Kenitra, Ministère de l'intérieur, Royaume du Maroc.

Nabih M (1992). Secrets et vertus thérapeutiques des plantes médicinales utilisées en médecine traditionnelle dans la province de Settat. PharmD thesis. University of Mohamed IV, Rabat. Morocco.

OMS (Organisation Mondiale de la Santé) (2002). Diabète sucré. Aide mémoire; N°138.

OMS (Organisation Mondiale de la Santé) (2013). Diabète. Aide mémoire ; N°312 Octobre 2013.

Sekkat C (1987). Le diabèteet la phytothérapie. Enquête auprès de100 D.I.D. et 100 D.N.I.D. Thèse de Pharmacie. Fac. Méd. Pharm. Rabat.

Srivastava AK, Mehdi MZ (2005). Insulino-mimetic and anti-diabetic effects of vanadium compounds. Diabet. Med. 22(1): 2-13.

Tabuti JRS, Lye KA, Dhillion SS (2003). Traditional herbal drugs of Bulamogi, Uganda: plants, use and administration. J. Ethnopharmacol. 88:19-44.

Tazi AM, abir-khalil S, chaouki N (2003). Prevalence of the main cardiovascular risk factors in Morocco: results of a National survey 2000. J. Hyperten. 21:897-903.

Ziyyat A, Legssyer A, Mekhfi H, Dassouli A, Serhrouchni M, Benjelloun W (1997). Phytothérapie of hypertension and diabetes in oriental Morocco. J. Ethnopharmacol. 58:45-54.

## 8

Anti-cancer efficacy of ethanolic extracts from various parts of *Annona Squamosa* on MCF-7 cell line

Sneeha Veerakumar[1], Safreen Shaikh Dawood Amanulla[1] and Kumaresan Ramanathan[1,2]*

[1]Department of Biotechnology, Periyar Maniammai University, Vallam, Thanjavur-613 403, India.
[2]Department of Biochemistry, Institute of Biomedical Sciences, College of Health Sciences, Mekelle University (Ayder Campus), Mekelle, Ethiopia.

Medicinal plant extracts are known to possess breast cancer antidote. The present investigation is focused on anticancer efficacy of various parts of *Annona squamosa*. The organic (ethanol) extracts from various parts of *Annona squamosa* were prepared using soxhlet apparatus and tested for *in vitro* anticancer efficacy on Breast cancer cell line MCF-7 by MTT (3-(4, 5-dimethylthiazol-2-yl)-2,5-diphenyltetrazolium bromide) assay. The results obtained from MTT assay showed that the inhibitory concentration values of bark, peel and seed were found to be approximately 20, 30 and 10 µg/ml, respectively The ethanolic seed extract had high anticancer activity with IC50 value of 10 ug/ml, reveals that *A. squamosa* inhibits the proliferation of MCF-7 by inducing apoptosis. The plant investigated has anti-cancer activity; hence further studies should be carried out for the isolation of the lead molecules from the parts of the plant to treat the breast cancer.

Key words: *Annona squamosa*, MCF-7 cell line, 3-(4, 5-dimethylthiazol-2-yl)-2,5-diphenyltetrazolium bromide (MTT) assay, anti-cancer activity.

INTRODUCTION

Breast cancer remains pre-eminent in the scientific, clinical and societal challenge, frequently diagnosed in omen, with an estimated 1.38 million new cases per year. There were 458,000 deaths per year from breast cancer worldwide being leading cause in female mortality in both developed and developing world (Suzanne et al., 2013; Ferlay et al., 2010). Even though great advancement has been made in treatment and control, still there is a scope for improvement, due to the toxicity of chemotherapy drugs and the side effect of current treatment that ultimately necessitates the need for alternative therapeutic strategy (Avni et al., 2008). Medicinal plants have been gaining popularity as natural therapies from plant-derived products in cancer treatment may reduce the risk of side effects. Botanical extracts from plants like *Abrus precatorius L, Allium sativum L, Alstonia scholaris*

*Corresponding author. E-mail: kumaresanramanatha@gmail.com.

L and Annona reticulate L exhibit shown anticancer property (Sumitra and Krunal, 2013). Annonaceae, the custard apple family is a family of flowering plants consisting of trees and shrubs. There are about 2300 to 2500 species and more than 130 genera in the Annonaceae family. The genus name, 'Annona' is from the Latin word 'anon', meaning 'yearly produce', referring to the production of fruits of the various species in this genus seasonally. The family is concentrated in the tropics, with few species found in temperate regions (iba et al., 2014; Rajsekhar, 2011).

The taxonomical classification of Annona squamosa is:

Kingdom: Plantae
Order: Magnoliales
Family: Annonaceae
Genus: Annona
Species: squamosa

A. squamosa is a small well-branched tree or shrub that bears edible fruits which are commonly called custard apple or sugar apple. The tree is more willing to grow at lower altitudes. The plant parts are used for treating various diseases. Leaves are used to treat hysteria, fainting spells. Leaf decoction is employed in the treatment of cold, cough, intestinal infections and acidity condition. A bark decoction is used in diarrhoea. Roots are used to treat dysentery. Fruit is used in making of ice creams and milk beverages (Neha and Dushyant, 2011). Some of the novel chemical constituent isolated from A. squamosa showed anti-cancer, anti- HIV and anti-diabetic properties. This medicinal plant exists with diverse pharmacological spectrum (Martino-Roaro et al., 2008; Biba et al., 2014). Few other Annona species (A. triloba) have also showed anti-cancer property (Jerry, 2008). Malignant sores were treated by seeds of A. squamosa as a traditional remedy in the south of china (Guangdong Food and Drug Administration, 2004). Botanical extracts can be easy and effective approach for treating breast cancer. The aim of this study is to determine the anticancer efficacy of A. squamosa and to predict the lead molecule from a natural source with fewer side effects that could be extracted and purified further for the prevention or cure of breast cancer.

MATERIALS AND METHODS

Collection of plant samples

Different plant parts namely bark and leaves were isolated from A. squamosa while its fruits were collected from the local market.

Preparation of sample and extracts

The collected plant parts such as bark, leaves, peel, pulp and seeds were shade dried for ten days. The dried samples were grounded separately into a fine powder and stored at 4°C for further use. The powdered samples (20 g each) were subjected to Soxhlet extraction individually with organic solvent ethanol (200 ml) and the temperature was set at 70°C (boiling point). The extracts of different plant parts were collected and stored in different sterile Petri dish. The excess solvent present in the extracts were removed by oven drying for 10 to 15 min at 50°C.

Different concentrations of plant extracts

The plant extracts were made at different concentrations by dissolving them in any of the following solvents such as water, ethanol or incomplete media. The bark and seed extracts were dissolved in ethanol and the peel extract was dissolved in incomplete media.

Each milligram of the plant extract was dissolved in its respective solvent of 1 ml. Further, the concentrations were taken and added to the 96 well plates.

MTT assay

Collection of MCF-7 cell lines

The breast cancer cell lines, MCF-7 cells were purchased from National Centre for Cell Science (NCCS), Pune. MCF-7 cells were maintained in DMEM medium (Gibco, Gaithersburg, MD) supplemented with 10% of Fetal Bovine Serum (FBS: Gibco) and 2% of Penicillin-Streptomycin Antibiotics (Gibco). The cells along with the medium were maintained in a CO_2 incubator at 37°C at 5% of CO_2. Doubling time of MCF-7 cell line is about 24 h. The cells were quantified using hemocytometer.

Incubation of cells

The purchased cells were sub cultured in a T25 animal tissue culture flask (sigmaaldrich) for further use. Cultures were kept in a CO_2 incubator at 37°C in a 5% CO_2 incubator and cells were harvested by centrifugation.

Cytotoxicity assay

The cytotoxicity assay was performed by the MTT method (Edmondson et al., 1998). MCF-7 ($1 \times 10^{4)}$ cells were seeded into two 96-well plates and incubated overnight. The first plate was divided into two sections; the first section was treated with ethanolic extracts of A. squamosa peel at 5, 10, 20, 30, 40, 50, 100 and 200 µg per well and in the second section the cells were treated with the ethanol extracts of bark at 5, 10, 20, 30, 40, 50 and 100 µg per well. The second plate was treated with the ethanol extract of seed at 5, 10, 20, 30, 40 and 50 µg concentrations. Each concentration of the extract treated 2 plates were incubated at 37°C for 24 h in a CO_2 incubator. An untreated group (without extracts from different parts of A. squamosa) was used as a control in both of the 96-well plates. A vehicles control was added to the plates and ethanol was used as a control for the cells since, the bark, and seed samples were dissolved in ethanol. The cells were incubated for 12 h. Thereafter, 5 mg/ml of the MTT dye (Thiazolyl Blue Tetrazolium Bromide: (3-(4, 5-dimethylthiazol-2-yl)-2, 5-diphenyltetrazolium bromide) was added to each well of the micro-titre plates and the plates were further incubated for 3 h in a dark cupboard. The formazan crystal products were formed. To dissolve the formazan 100 µl of Dimethyl Sulfoxide (DMSO) was added. After 15 min, the amount of purple formazan formed was determined by measuring the optical density (OD) using the ELISA micro plate reader at a wavelength of 595 nm. The amount of formazan formed at each concentration of the extract was measured at 595 nm using a (Thermoscientific) of a

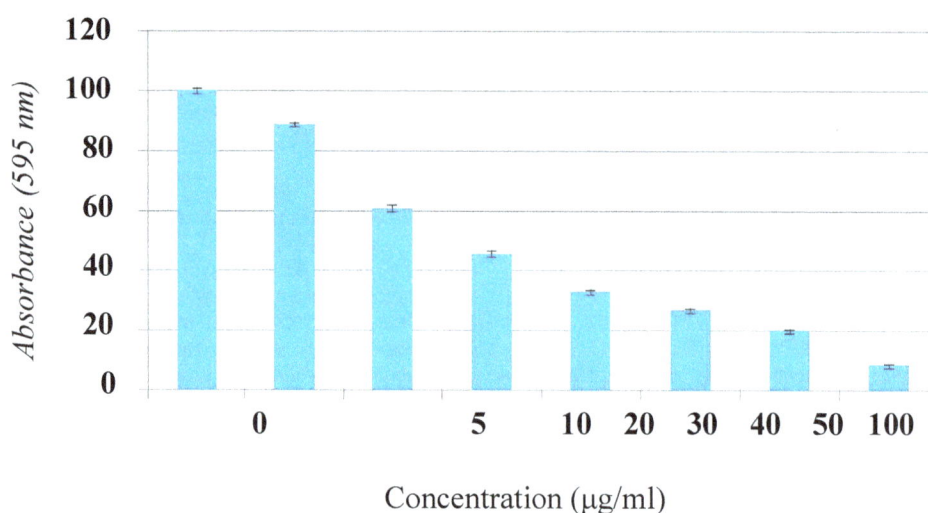

Chart 1. Percentage of cell viability in bark extract treated cells.

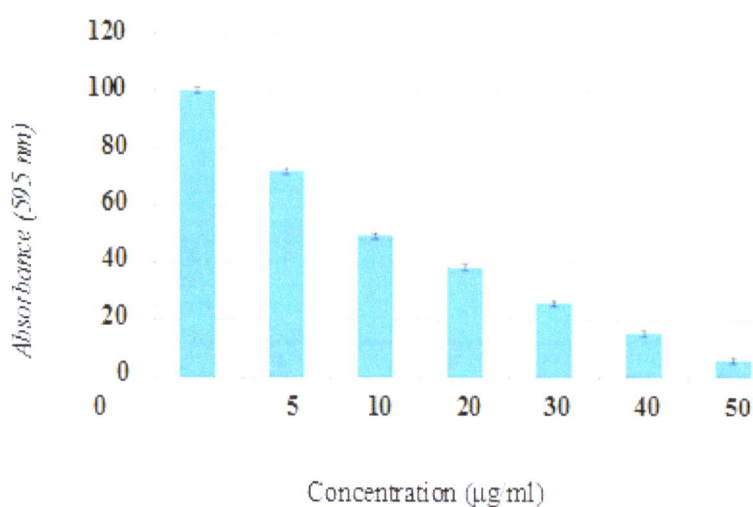

Chart 2. Percentage of cell viability in peel extract treated cells.

spectrophotometer. Each experiment was performed in triplicate. The percentages of viable cells were calculated using the equation:

$$IC_{50} = \frac{\text{Control OD} - \text{Test OD}}{\text{Control OD}} \times 100$$

The viability of the cells was expressed as a percentage of absorbance in cells with treatment to that in cells without treatment. The inhibitory concentration (IC_{50}) was calculated using the formula (Chart 1 to 3).

RESULTS

The percentage of cell viability was found to be gradually decreased from lower concentration to higher concentration. The inhibitory concentration (IC50) of the bark extract was found to be around 20 µg/ml (Table 1).

The percentage of cell viability was found to be gradually decreased from lower concentration to higher concentration. The inhibitory concentration (IC50) of the peel extract was found to be around 30 µg/ml (Table 2).

The percentage of cell viability gradually decreased from lower concentration to higher concentration. The inhibitory concentration (IC50) of the seel extract was found to be around 10 µg/ml (Table 3).

The plant parts were collected, and the extracts were taken with organic solvents using Soxhlet apparatus. The ethanolic extract of the bark, peel and seed extracts were analyzed for their cytotoxic effects. MTT assay was performed to find a percentage of cell viability and inhibitory concentration value (IC50) of the ethanolic

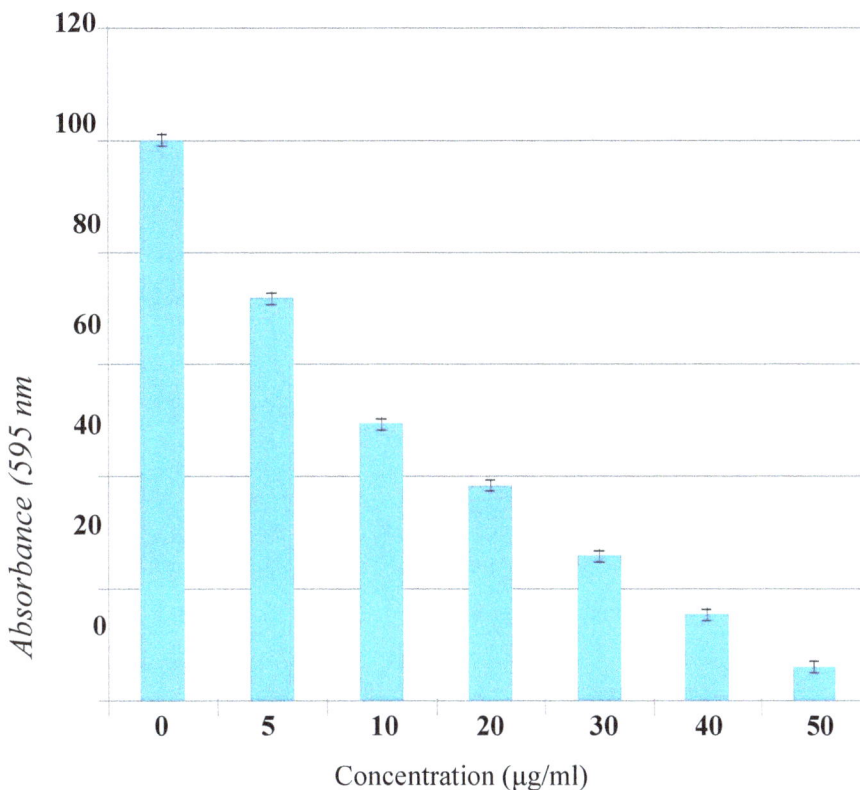

Chart 3. Percentage of cell viability in seed extract treated cells.

Table 1. Various concentrations of bark extract added to the cells.

Concentrations (µg/ml)	Control	5	10	20	30	40	50	100
Row - 1	4.78	3.09	2.89	1.0984	1.243	1.294	0.49	0.602
Row - 2	3.293	3.765	1.081	2.894	1.78	0.454	1.176	0.086
Average	3.958	3.515	2.401	1.800	1.304	1.06	0.791	0.332

Table 2. Various concentrations of peel extract added to the cells.

Concentrations (µg/ml)	Control	5	10	20	30	40	50	100	200
Row - 1	3.8	3.78	3.102	2.9	1.78	1.363	1.094	0.49	0.002
Row - 2	3.789	2.72	2.809	1.231	1.44	1.538	1.454	0.176	0.086
Row - 3	3.003	3.093	2.59	2.8	2.19	1.45	0.432	0.708	0.308
Average	3.530	3.197	2.833	2.310	1.80	1.45	0.993	0.458	0.132

Table 3. Various concentrations of seed extract added to the cells.

Concentrations (µg/ml)	Control	5	10	20	30	40	50
Row - 1	4.76	3.902	1.99	1.79	1.003	1.094	0.034
Row - 2	4.789	2.869	1.781	1.989	1.28	0.094	0.28
Row - 3	4.003	2.949	2.9	1.409	1.205	0.89	0.489
Average	4.51	3.24	2.223	1.729	1.162	0.692	0.267

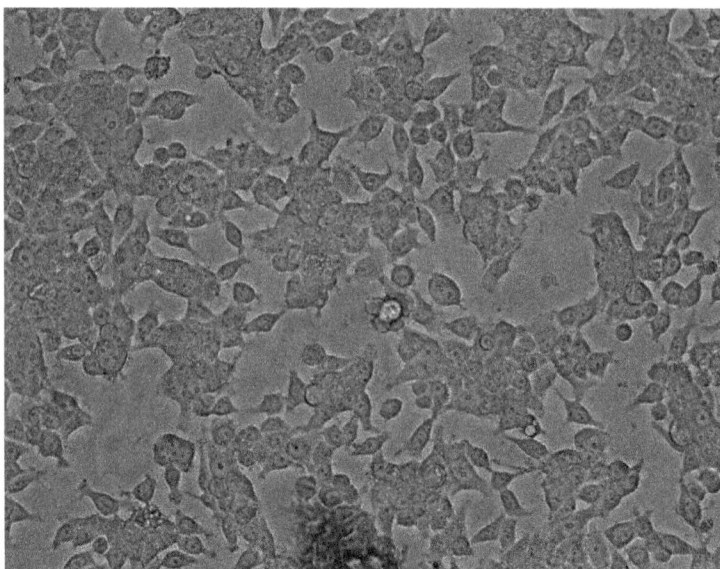

Figure 1. Cells in the control well.

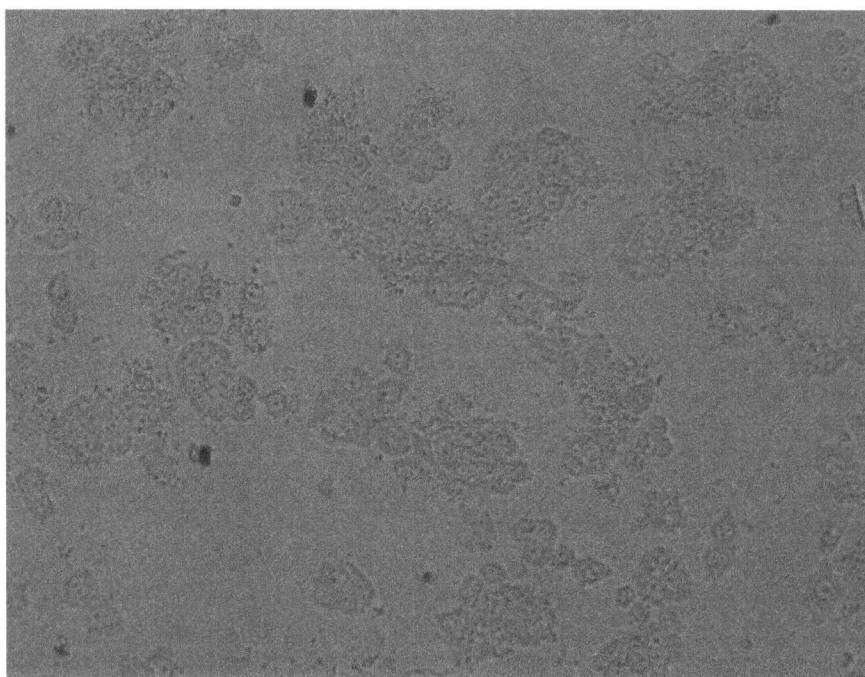

Figure 2. Cells in the bark extract treated well (20 μg).

extracts of bark, peel and seed. The results obtained from MTT assay showed that the inhibitory concentration values of bark, peel and seed were found to be approximately 20, 30 and 10 μg/ml (Figures 1 to 6) respectively. It was observed that the ethanol extracts of the seed had high anticancer activity than bark and peel extract on MCF-7 cell line as they had low IC50 values of 10 μg/ml compared to the latter.

DISCUSSION

Annonaceae species are rich in acetogenin compounds (Craig et al., 1998) exhibit cytotoxic and anti-carcinogenic antioxidant, anti-psoriatic, larvicidal and anthelmintic activities (Martino-Roaro et al., 2008; Jerry, 2008; Feras et al., 1998; Lima et al., 2010; Saelee et al., 2011; Saelee et al., 2011; Kamaraj et al., 2011a,b). Exploration of

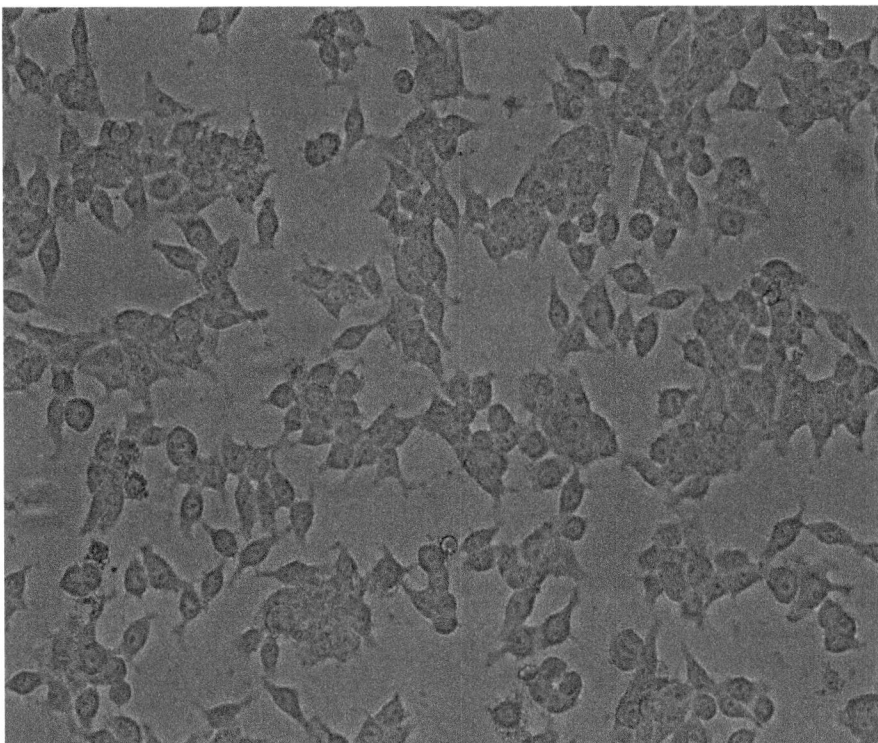

Figure 3. Cells in the control well.

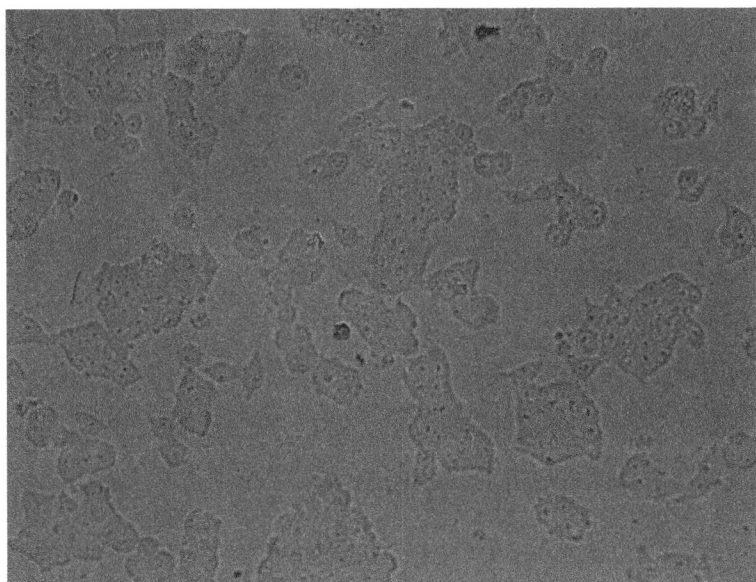

Figure 4. Cells in the peel extract treated well (30 μg).

botanical extract for novel anti-tumor drugs is a significant concern for mankind, as they might prove to be easy and competent approach. Annonaceous acetogenins is the major bioactive compounds from *A. squamosa* seeds that has been identified as well-known inhibitor of multiple drug resistant cancer cells based on phytochemical and pharmacological studies (Jerry, 2008). Previous studies reported identification and quantification of 2 main compounds of annonaceous acetogenins by HPLC analysis: 12, 15-cis-squamostatin-A and bullatacin from

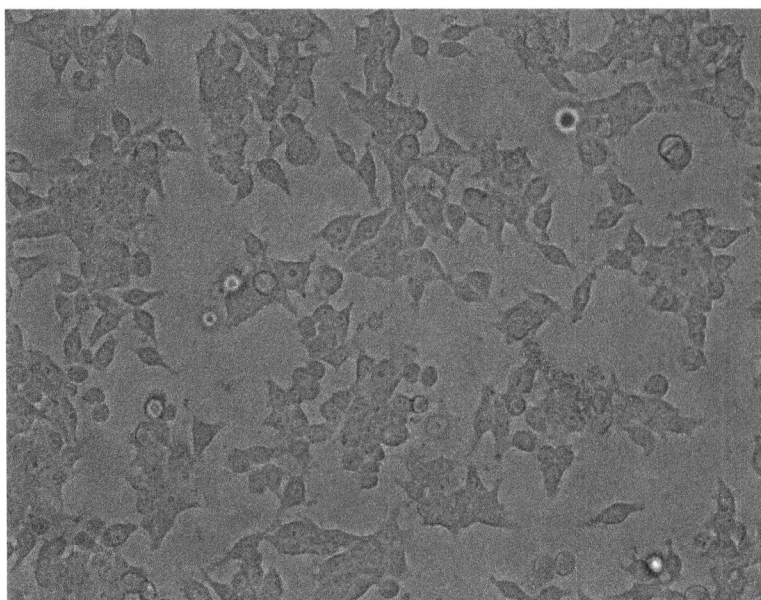

Figure 5. Cells in the control well.

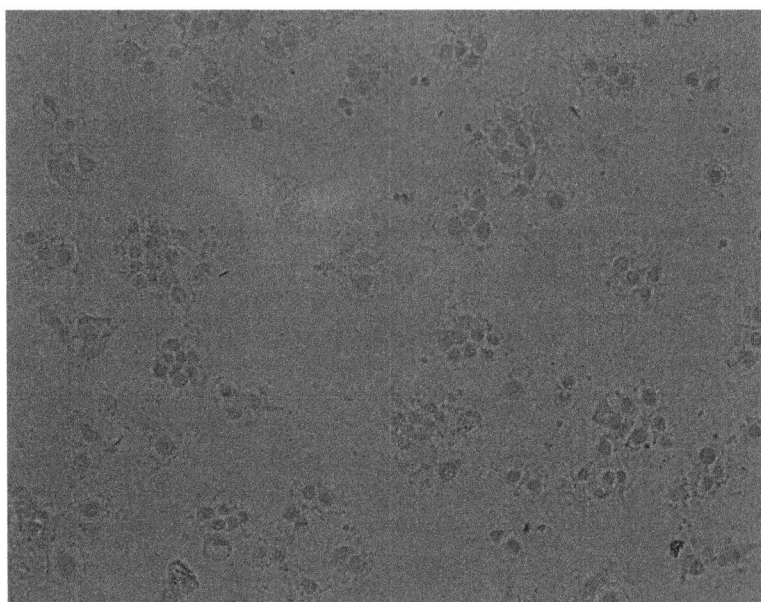

Figure 6. Cells in the seed extract treated well (10 µg).

the extract of A. squamosa seeds. Bullatacin, a bistetrahydrofuran annonaceous acetogenin high degree inhibitory action (300 times more effective than taxol) of the mitochondrial respiratory chain complex I, as tested *in vivo* (Jerry, 2008; Liaw et al., 2010). 12, 15-cis-squamostatin-A and bullatacin also showed anti-cancer property against various tumor cell lines (Yang et al., 2009; Chen et al., 2011). Supplementary assays should be performed to find the accurate inhibitory concentration

values. Thus, it can be concluded that the plant parts of A. squamosa such as bark, peel and seed were found to have anti-cancer activity against the breast cancer cell lines, which is a reliable indication of the presence of drug molecules in the A. squamosa plant that could treat breast cancer. Further studies should be carried out for the isolation of the lead molecules from the parts of the plant to treat the breast cancer. The cell line used has characteristic feature of cancer, hence its cell death contributes directly to the anti-cancer property.

Conclusion

The ethanolic seed extract of the *A. squamosa* is considered to have a high anticancer potential compared to bark and peel. The outcome of the present study encourages future investigation by isolating a lead molecule responsible for anticancer efficacy, so as to design a particular drug for the cancer. Further studies can be performed in the future to predict the underlying mechanism of the anticancer potential of the plant.

ACKNOWLEDGEMENT

The authors express our sincere thanks to Dr. A. Antony Joseph Velanganni, Assistant Professor, Department of Biochemistry, Bharathidasan University for helping us by providing necessary equipment used to carry out cell line studies. They also extend their thanks to the Head of the University for providing the necessary instrumental facilities for Soxhlet extraction to complete the project work. The project is self-funded by the authors.

REFERENCES

Avni GD, Ghulam NQ, Ramesh KG, Mahmoud El-Tamer, Jaswant Singh, Ajit KS, Yashbir SB, Subhash CT, Hari KB (2008). Medicinal Plants and Cancer Chemoprevention. Curr. Drug Metab. 9(7):581-591.

Biba VS, Amily A, Sangeetha S, Remani P (2014). Anticancer, Antioxidant and Antimicrobial activity of Annonaceae family. World J. Pharm. Pharmaceutical Sci. 3(6):1595-1604.

Chen Y, Chen JW, Li X (2011). Cytotoxic bistetrahydrofuran annonaceous acetogenins from the seeds of Annona squamosa. J. Natural Products 74:2477-2481.

Craig Hopp D, Feras QA, Zhe-Ming Gu, McLaughlin JL (1998). Mono-THF ring annonaceous acetogenins from *Annona squamosa*. Int. J. Phytochem. 47(5):803-809.

Edmondson JM, Linda SA, Andrew OM (1998). A rapid and simple MTT-based spectrophotometric assay for determining drug sensitivity in monolayer cultures. J Tissue Cult. Methods 11:15-17.

Feras QA, Xiao-Xi Liu, Jerry LM (1998). Annonaceous Acetogenins: Recent Progress. J. Natural Products 62:504-540.

Ferlay J, Shin HR, Bray F, Forman D, Mathers C, Parkin DM (2010). Estimates of worldwide burden of cancer in 2008: GLOBOCAN 2008. Int. J. Cancer. 127(12):2893-2917.

Guangdong Food and Drug Administration (2004). Guangdong Chinese Materia Medica Standards. Guangdong Science and Technology Press,Guangdong. 1:194.

Jerry LM (2008). Paw Paw and Cancer: Annonaceous Acetogenins from Discovery to Commercial Products. J. Natural Products 71(7):1311-1321.

Kamaraj C, Bagavan A, Elango G, Zahir AA, Rajakumar G, Marimuthu S, Santhoshkumar T, Rahuman AA (2011a). Larvicidal activity of medicinal plant extracts against Anopheles subpictus & Culex tritaeniorhynchus. Indian J. Med. Res. 134:101-106.

Kamaraj C, Rahuman AA, Elango G, Bagavan A, Zahir AA (2011b). Anthelmintic activity of botanical extracts against sheep gastrointestinal nematodes, Haemonchus contortus. Parasitol. Res. 109:37-45.

Liaw CC, Wu TY, Chang FR, Wu YC (2010). Historic perspectives on Annonaceous acetogenins from the chemical bench to preclinical trials. Planta Medica. 76:1390-1404.

Lima LARL, Piment LPS, Boaventura MAD (2010). Acetogenins from Annona cornifolia and their antioxidant capacity. Food Chem. 122:1129-1138.

Martino-Roaro Gerardo Zepeda-Vallejo, Eduardo Madrigal-Bujaidar (2008). Anti carcinogenic and genotoxic effects produced by Acetogenins isolated from *Annona muricata*. Abstracts 180:32-246.

Neha P, Dushyant B (2011). Phytochemical and Pharmacological Review on Annona squamosa Linn. Int. J. Res. Pharmaceutical Biomed. Sci. 2(4):404-1412.

Rajsekhar S (2011). Pharmacognosy and pharmacology of Annona squamosa: A Review. Int. J. Pharm. Life Sci. 2(10):1183-1189.

Saelee C, Thongrakard V, Tencomnao T (2011). Effects of Thai medicinal herb extracts with anti-psoriatic activity on the expression on NF-kB signaling biomarkers in HaCaT keratinocytes. Molecules 16:3908-3932.

Sumitra C, Krunal N (2013). In vitro and in vivo Methods for Anticancer Activity Evaluation and Some Indian Medicinal Plants Possessing Anticancer Properties: An Overview. J. Pharmacogn. Phytochem. 2(1):14-19.

Suzanne AE, Aboagye EO, Ali S, Anderson AS, Armes J, Berditchevski F, Blaydes JP, Brennan K, Brown NJ, Bryant HE, Bundred NJ, Burchell JM, Campbell AM, Carroll JS, Clarke RB, Coles CE, Cook GJ, Cox A, Curtin NJ, Dekker LV, Silva Idos S, Duffy SW, Easton DF, Eccles DM, Edwards DR, Edwards J, Evans D, Fenlon DF, Flanagan JM, Foster C, Gallagher WM, Garcia-Closas M, Gee JM, Gescher AJ, Goh V, Groves AM, Harvey AJ, Harvie M, Hennessy BT, Hiscox S, Holen I, Howell SJ, Howell A, Hubbard G, Hulbert-Williams N, Hunter MS, Jasani B, Jones LJ, Key TJ, Kirwan CC, Kong A, Kunkler IH, Langdon SP, Leach MO, Mann DJ, Marshall JF, Martin L, Martin SG, Macdougall JE, Miles DW, Miller WR, Morris JR, Moss SM, Mullan P, Natrajan R, O'Connor JP, O'Connor R, Palmieri C, Pharoah PD, Rakha EA, Reed E, Robinson SP, Sahai E, Saxton JM, Schmid P, Smalley MJ, Speirs V, Stein R, Stingl J, Streuli CH, Tutt AN, Velikova G, Walker RA, Watson CJ, Williams KJ, Young LS, Thompson AM (2013). Critical research gaps and translational priorities for the successful prevention and treatment of breast cancer. Breast Cancer Res. 15(5):R92.

Yang HJ, Zhang N, Li X, Chen JW, Cai BC (2009). Structure–activity relationships of diverse annonaceous acetogenins against human tumor cells. Bioorganic Medicinal Chem. Lett. 19:2199-2202.

## 9

Antioxidant potential and cytotoxicity of *Randia dumetorum* Lam. leaf extract

Abdullah-Al-Ragib[1], Md. Tanvir Hossain[1], Javed Hossain[2] and Md. Jakaria[2,3*]

[1]Department of Applied Chemistry and Chemical Engineering, Noakhali Science and Technology University, Sonapur, Noakhali-3814, Bangladesh.
[2]Department of Pharmacy, International Islamic University Chittagong, Chittagong-4314, Bangladesh.
[3]Department of Pharmacy, Southern University Bangladesh, Chittagong-4000, Bangladesh.

The aim of the current study was to explore the antioxidant potential and cytotoxicity of different 'fractions from the leaf extract of *Randia dumetorum*. Proximate analysis and phytochemical screening were done with standard protocol. The antioxidant activity was evaluated by using reducing power assay, total antioxidant capacity determination, determination of total phenolic content, determination of total flavonoid content and reduction of ferric ions by ortho-phenanthroline color method. In the antioxidant studies, ascorbic acid, gallic acid and butylated hydroxy toluene (BHT) were used as standard antioxidant compound. The brine shrimp lethality test was used to examine cytotoxicity. In the proximate analysis, moisture content, total ash value, acid insoluble ash and water-soluble ash value were found in the leaf of *R. dumetorum*. Concerning the phytochemical screening, there was the presence of glycosides, flavonoids, reducing sugars, saponins, phenolic compounds, tannins on different fractions, but the absence of gums and mucilage, alkaloid, protein, and amino acid. The results show that all the extracts of *R. dumetorum* leaf possess significant antioxidant activity. 'The methanol and water extracts of the leaves showed significant cytotoxic activity as compared to dimethyl sulfoxide (DMSO) (LC_{50} 1.07 µg/ml). These findings suggest that *R. dumetorum* leaves might be a good antioxidants source and possess mild cytotoxic effect.

Key words: *Randia dumetorum*, proximate analysis, phytochemical screening, antioxidant, lethality bioassay.

INTRODUCTION

Reactive oxygen species (ROS) or free radicals are harmful products or intermediates that may be generated during the processes of biological combustion (Sharma and Vig, 2013; Zaman et al., 2016). The imbalance between oxidants and antioxidants are called oxidative stress, because of the damage in all kinds of biomolecules such as protein, nucleic acid, DNA and RNA (Sharma and Vig, 2013). An excess level of free radicals in living beings causes numerous disorders and diseases including cardiovascular diseases, cancer, asthma, liver diseases, aging, muscular degeneration, neurodegeneration and other inflammatory diseases

*Corresponding author. E-mail: pharmajakaria@rocketmail.com.

(Sharma and Vig, 2013; Saeed et al., 2012; Sen et al., 2010; Kanwar et al., 2009; Chiavaroli et al., 2011).

Antioxidants are known as a reducing agent, free radical scavenger, singlet oxygen molecule quenchers and antioxidative enzyme activators to suppress the damage induced by free radicals in biological system (Sharma and Vig, 2013). The imbalance between ROS and the inherent antioxidant capacity of the body, led to the use of dietary and/or medicinal supplements particularly during the disease attack. Henceforth, the balance between reactive species or free radicals and antioxidants is supposed to be an important concept for maintaining a good biological system. It has been reported that the evidence has brought the attention of scientists to an appreciation of antioxidants for prevention and treatment of diseases and maintenance of human health. Moreover, antioxidants present in plant products support the cellular defense system stimulation and biological system against oxidative damage.

Randia dumetorum Lam. (RD) is an important medicinal plant and it is a big thorny shrub. It belongs to the Rubiaceae family (Jangwan and Singh, 2014; Dharmishtha et al., 2009). This plant is commonly obtainable all over the India and African subcontinent up to 4000 feet elevation. It has been considered that different phytochemicals including iridoid-10-methylixoside, mannitol, triterpenoid glycosides, coumarin glycosides, randianin and saponins named as dumentoronin A, B, C, D, E, F, etc., are available in the RD. In ayurvedic system of medicines, RD has been used because of its potentials for rasa, virya, guna, vipaka, etc. (Patel et al., 2011). Many practitioners believed, the pulp of fruit also have anthelmintic properties and also indicated as an abortifacient. RD fruits are believed to be tonic, demulcent, diuretic and restorative and the drug is claimed as a medical cure for various ailments, such as piles, antidysenteric agent, asthma, jaundice, diarrhea, emetic, and gonorrhea (Satpute et al., 2014). Literature revealed that RD has several pharmacological activities as cytotoxic, immunomodulatory, antifertility, analgesic, anti-inflammatory, antiallergic, antibacterial, insecticidal, and anthalmetics activities (Patel et al., 2011; Satpute et al., 2014). In addition, the methanol extract from the RD leaf and bark shows antioxidant and hepatoprotective activities (Satpute et al., 2014; Kandimalla et al., 2016).

To date, the antioxidant potential and cytotoxicity of different fraction from the leaves of *R. dumetorum* Lam. remain uninvestigated. Therefore, the present study was to explore the antioxidant potentiality and cytotoxicity of fractions from the *R. dumetorum* leaves.

MATERIALS AND METHODS

Plant

Concerning the collection, the leaves of *R. dumetorum* were collected from the Chatkil, Noakhali, Bangladesh on 5th March, 2015. The leaves were washed properly and air dried for several days. The dried leaves were then oven dried for 24 h at a considerably low temperature not exceeding 50°C. The oven dried leaves were then ground into coarse powder using high capacity grinding machine and were used for different investigation.

Proximate analysis

Regarding the proximate analysis, the moisture content, total ash value, acid insoluble ash value and water-soluble ash value of a substance were determined in the samples.

Preparation of plant extracts

The dried leaf powder of *R. dumetorum* (about 190 g) was extracted with n-hexane (600 ml) by using Soxhlet apparatus for 8 h at 60 to 80°C. After n-hexane extraction, the residual dried marc was extracted with chloroform, methanol and water to get chloroform, methanol and water extracts. In the case of aqueous extract preparation, the dried marc was macerated for 3 days with distilled water and the residue was removed by filtration and the filtrate was concentrated to obtain aqueous extract. The extracts of different solvents obtained were concentrated by recovery of the solvent in a rotary evaporator and evaporating them to dryness at low temperature. These concentrated extracts were then weighed and stored for the investigations.

Phytochemical screening

The extracts were exposed to initial phytochemical testing. Small quantity of freshly prepared n-hexane, chloroform, methanol and aqueous extracts of *R. dumetorum* were subjected to preliminary quantitative phytochemical investigation for detection of phytochemicals such as alkaloids, flavonoids, reducing sugars, saponins, phenolic compounds, proteins and amino acids, tannins, gums and mucilage using the standard methods (Mujeeb et al., 2014; Todkar et al., 2010; Thamaraiselvi et al., 2012; Auwal et al., 2014; Mandal et al., 2013; Chinedu et al., 2015; Sumbul et al., 2012).

Antioxidant activity

The antioxidant activity of different extracts of leaf of *R. dumetorum* was evaluated by the following methods: reducing power assay, total antioxidant capacity determination, determination of total phenolic content, total flavonoid content determination and reduction of ferric ions by ortho-phenanthroline color method.

Reducing power assay

The Fe^{3+}-reducing power of the extract was investigated by following the method with a slight modification described by Oyaizu (1986). 2 ml methanol and 2 ml extract of each solvent of different concentrations (31.25, 62.50, 125, 250, and 500 μg/ml) of the extract were mixed with 0.5 ml phosphate buffer (0.2 M, pH 6.6) and 0.5 ml potassium hexacyanoferrate (1%), followed by incubation at 50°C in a water bath for 20 min. For subsequent incubation, 0.5 ml of TCA (10%) was added to terminate the reaction and centrifuged at 3000 rpm for 10 min. 1 ml solution from the upper portion of the solution was mixed with 1 ml distilled water and 0.2 ml $FeCl_3$ solution (0.1%) and the absorbance was measured at 700 nm against an appropriate blank solution. At several concentrations, ascorbic acid was used as standard.

Increased absorbance of the reaction mixture designated increased reducing power.

Total antioxidant capacity

Extracts total antioxidant capacity was assessed by following the method described by Prieto et al. (1999) with slight modification. An aliquot of 0.5 ml of samples solution was combined with 4.5 ml of reagent solution (0.6 M sulfuric acid, 28 mM sodium phosphate, and 4 mM ammonium molybdate). Concerning the blank, 0.5 ml of 45% ethanol was used in place of sample. The tubes were incubated in a boiling water bath at 95°C for 90 min. At room temperature, after cooling the sample, the aqueous solution absorbance of each sample was determined at 695 nm against blank. The total antioxidant activity was shown as the absorbance of the sample at 695 nm. The higher absorbance value specified higher antioxidant activity (Prasad et al., 2009).

Total phenolic content

Folin-Ciocalteu method was used to determine the total phenolic content of all the extracts (Harborne, 1973). Polyphenols containing samples are reduced by the Folin-Ciocalteu reagent, thereby producing blue colored complex. From a gallic acid calibration curve, the phenolic concentration of extracts was estimated. To prepare a calibration curve, 0.5 ml aliquots of 3.9, 7.82, 15.63, 31.25, 62.5, 125, 250 and 500 µg/ml gallic acid solutions were mixed with 2.5 ml Folin-Ciocalteu reagent (diluted ten-fold) and 2.5 ml (75 g/L) sodium carbonate. After incubation at 25°C for 30 min, the quantative phenolic estimation was performed at 765 nm against reagent blank. The calibration curve was constructed by putting the value of absorbance vs. concentration. A similar procedure was adopted for the extracts as described earlier in the preparation of calibration curve. All determinations were performed in triplicate. Total phenolic content was expressed as milligrams of gallic acid equivalent (GAE) per g of the extract.

Determination of total flavonoids

The flavonoids content was determined by aluminium trichloride method using quercetin as a reference compound (Chang et al., 2002). This method is based on the formation of a complex flavonoid-aluminum having the absorptivity maximum at 415 nm, after being left to react at room temperature for 30 min. Briefly, 0.5 ml of each extract (1:10 g/ml) in ethanol was separately mixed with 1.5 ml of ethanol, 0.1 ml of 10% aluminium chloride, 0.1 ml of 1 M potassium acetate and distilled water (2.8 ml). The calibration curve was arranged by preparing quercetin solutions at different concentrations from 0 to 1.00 mg/ml in ethanol.

Reduction of ferric ions by ortho-phenanthroline color method

A reaction mixture containing 0.5 ml o-phenanthroline (5 mg in 10 ml methanol), 2 ml ferric chloride 0.2 µM (3.24 mg in 100 ml distilled water) and 1 ml of numerous concentrations of the extracts was incubated at ambient temperature for 10 min, then the absorbance was determined at 510 nm. In this investigation, ascorbic acid and gallic acid were used as reference standards (Hukkeri and Mruthunjaya, 2008).

Cytotoxicity

The cytotoxicity was conducted by using brine shrimp lethality examination. Concerning the test organism, *Artemia salina* leach

(brine shrimp eggs) collected from pet shops was used. The brine shrimp eggs were placed in 1 L of simulated sea water, aerated for 48 h at 38°C to hatch and become nauplii. After 24 h, ten brine shrimp nauplii were placed in a small container filled with sea water. *R. dumetorum* extract serially diluted with simulated sea water were then added to the container. The lethality of brine shrimp was observed after 24 h of treatment was given. In the present study, positive control group (vincristine sulphate) was not used and the results obtained are only due to the activity of the test agent such as DMSO as the negative control. Following the procedure of Meyer et al. (1982), the lethality of the crude methanol and water extract was determined but n-hexane and chloroform extract was not determined, because of the results of the chemical tests. At different concentrations, each test samples exhibited dissimilar mortality rates; plotting of log of concentration versus percent mortality for all test samples showed an approximate linear correlation. The median lethal concentration (LC_{50}, the concentration at which 50% mortality of brine shrimp nauplii occurred) was determined for the samples by using the graphs. Probity analysis was used to determine lethal concentration (LC_{50}) of *R. dumetorum* extract on nauplii.

RESULTS

Proximate analysis

Proximate analysis of a substance constitutes different classes of nutrients present in the samples such as moisture, ash, carbohydrates, protein, fat and crude fibre. *R. dumetorum* was subjected to evaluate its moisture content, total ash value, acid insoluble ash and water-soluble ash (Figure 1).

Phytochemical screening

In the pharmaceutical screening, it is observed that reducing sugar, flavonoid, phenolic compound and tannins were present in the methanol extract of *R. dumetorum* in addition, except methanol extract saponin was present in all the extracts. On the other hand, no extracts of *R. dumetorum* contains alkaloids, protein, amino acid and gums (Table 1).

Antioxidant activity

Reducing power assay

Figure 2 elucidates the dose response curves for the reducing powers of all extracts (31.25 to 500 µg/ml) from *R. dumetorum*. It shows that the n-hexane and chloroform fraction reduced the Fe^{3+} to ferrous ions (Fe^{2+}) more effectively (2.057 and 2.382) as compared to the methanol and water fraction (1.921 and 1.124), respectively at 500 µg/ml concentration. Ascorbic acid was used as standard antioxidant for comparison.

Total antioxidant capacity determination

Total antioxidant activity (TAC) of the extracts as shown

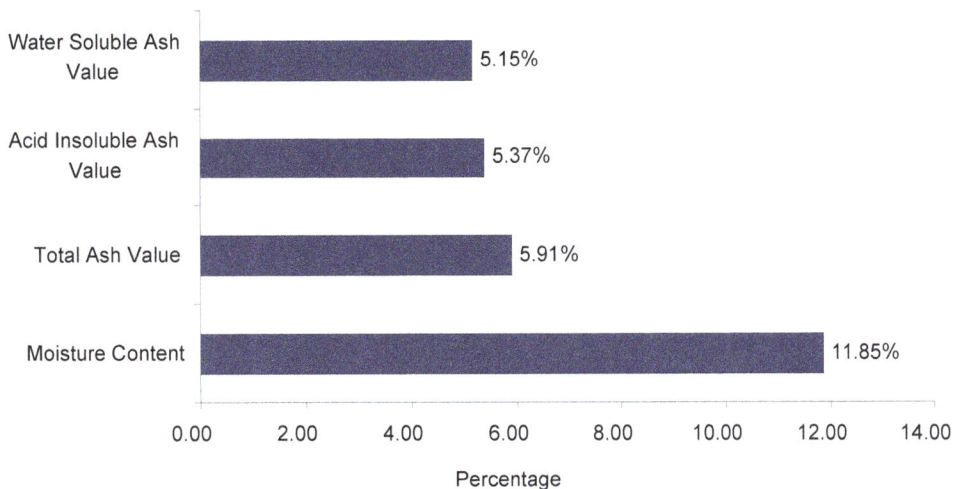

Figure 1. Result of proximate analysis of *R. dumetorum*.

Table 1. Phytochemical compounds in the different fractions of *R. dumetorum*.

Plant name	Phytochemical composition	Results of different extracts			
		n-Hexane	**Chloroform**	**Methanol**	**Water**
	Alkaloid	-	-	-	-
	Reducing sugar	-	-	++	+
	Glycoside	-	-	-	+
	Flavonoid	-	-	++	-
R. dumetorum	Saponin	+	+	-	+
	Phenolic compound	-	-	+	+
	Tannin	-	-	+	+
	Protein and amino acid	-	-	-	-
	Gums	-	-	-	-

+ = Present; - = Absent; ++ = significantly present.

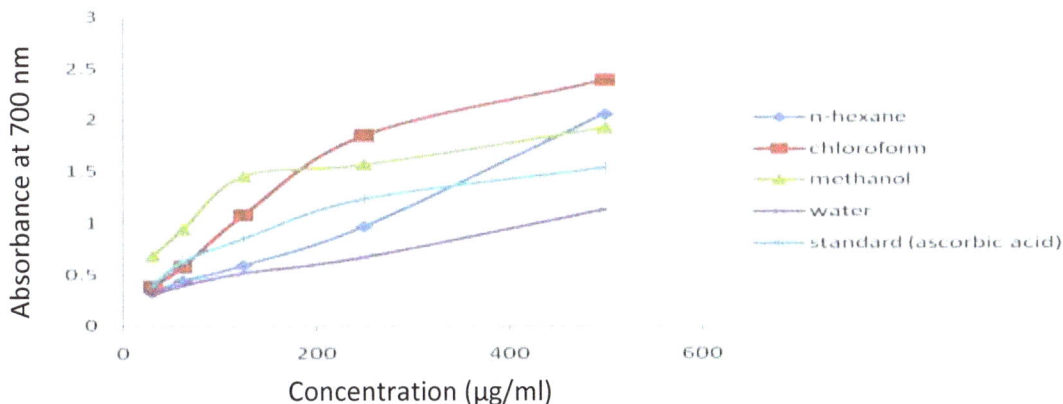

Figure 2. Comparative analysis of different extracts of *R. dumetorum* with standard (ascorbic acid) antioxidant for reducing power assay.

in Figure 3 was based on the reduction of Mo (VI) to Mo (V) by the extract and subsequent formation of green phosphate/Mo (V) complex with a maximum absorbance at 695 nm. The results specify a concentration dependent

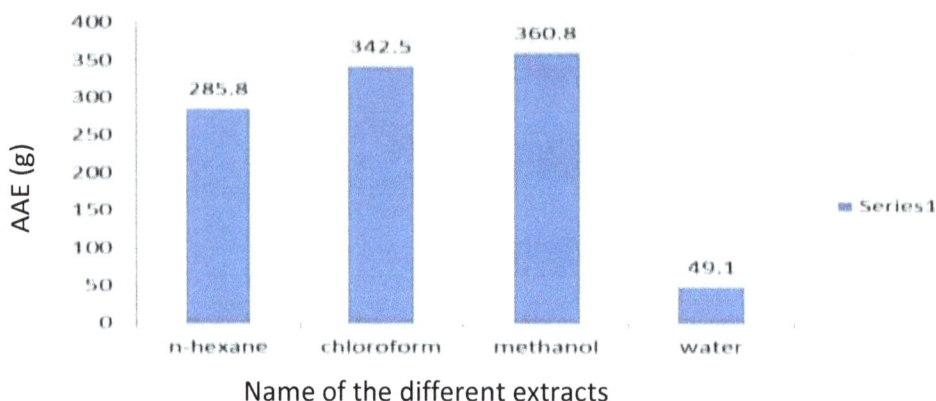

Figure 3. Total antioxidant capacity of different solvent extracts for 500 ppm at 695 nm of *R. dumetorum.*

Table 2. Total phenolic content and total flavonoid content of *R. dumetorum.*

Plant extracts	Total phenolics (mg gallic acid equivalent/g)	Total flavonoid (mg quercetin equivalent/g)
n-Hexane	-	-
Chloroform fraction	-	-
Methanol fraction	131.40	40.71
Water	55.00	-

total antioxidant capacity. The antioxidant activities of the fractions were compared with the standard antioxidant ascorbic acid. The total antioxidant capacity of several solvent fractions of *R. dumetorum* were found to decrease in this order: methanol (360.8 AAE/g) > chloroform (342.5 AAE/g) > n-hexane (285.8 AAE/g) > water (49.1 AAE/g).

Total phenolic content and total flavonoid content

Total phenolic content of the different fractions of *R. dumetorum* was solvent dependent and expressed as milligrams of gallic acid equivalents (GAE). The methanol extracts (131.4 GAE/g) show higher concentration of phenolic content than water extracts (55 GAE/g). The method of aluminium chloride colorimetric is extensively used to detect the total flavonoid. Here, Al^{3+} forms color that give a great absorbance at 415 nm. Flavonoid was found in methanol only in group test results. Methanol extracts of *R. dumetorum* was found to contain the amount of flavonoid content (40.71 mg quercetin equivalent/g of extract) (Table 2).

Reduction of ferric ions by ortho-phenanthroline color method

Figure 4 shows the comparative analysis of different extracts of leaf of *R. dumetorum*. In this figure, the value

of n-hexane and chloroform extract (1.023 and 0.543) is significantly higher than the standard antioxidant gallic acid and ascorbic acid (0.324 and 0.167), respectively tested at 500 µg/ml.

Cytotoxicity

In cytotoxicity study, LC_{50} values of crude methanol and water extract was found to be 0.94 and 0.23 µg/ml respectively. The negative control DMSO showed LC_{50} a a concentration of 1.07 µg/ml (Table 3).

DISCUSSION

As an alternative to clinical therapy, medicine from herbal sources has received enormous attention for different diseases and the demand for these therapies has presently increased speedily. The raise in the number of users as compared to the shortage of scientific evidences on the medicinal plants safety, have raised concerns about the toxicity and detrimental effects of these medications (Saad et al., 2006; Sahgal et al., 2010 Jakaria et al., 2015). Principally, plants are the main source of secondary metabolites apart from their food value, and their plant secondary metabolites prevent diseases in the form of antioxidant, antiviral, antibacterial and anticancer compounds (Makkar et al., 2007). In this study, several *in vitro* tests were used to investigate

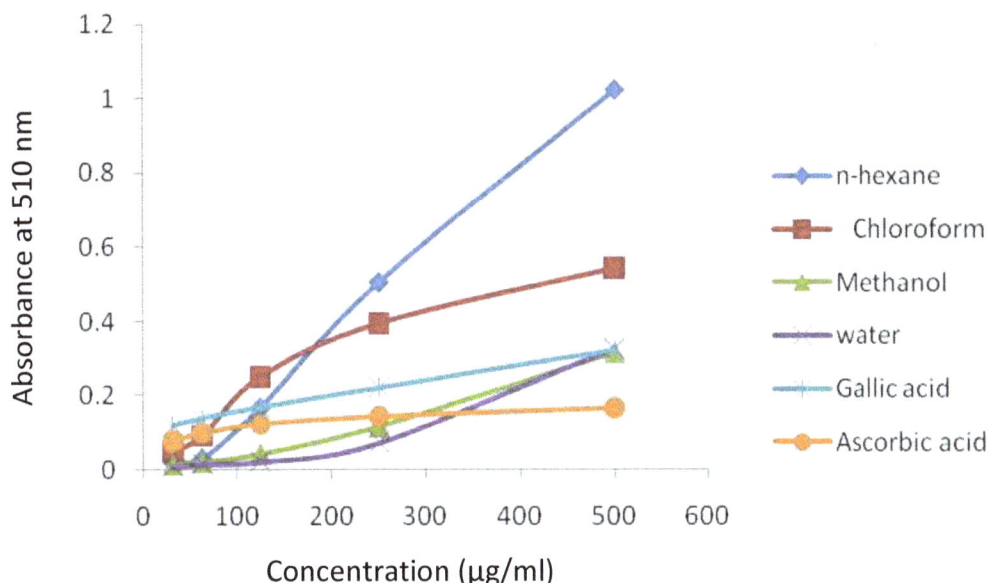

Figure 4. Comparative analysis of different extracts of *R. dumetorum* with standard antioxidants for Reduction of Ferric Ions by Ortho-phenanthroline Color method.

Table 3. Effect of extract of *R. dumetorum* on brine shrimp nauplii.

Sample/Extract	LC_{50} (µg/ml)
DMSO (negative control)	1.07
n-Hexane	-
Chloroform	-
Methanol extract	0.94
Water extract	0.23

antioxidant activity and brine shrimp lethality assay was used to investigate cytotoxic activity.

It has been familiar that free radicals are identified to play a certain role in an extensive variety of pathological manifestations. Antioxidants fight against free radicals and defend the body from several diseases. They show their action either by scavenging the reactive oxygen species or protecting the antioxidant defense mechanisms (Umamaheswari and Chatterjee, 2008).

In the assay of reducing power, depending on the reducing power of the test specimen, the yellow color of the test solution changes to green. The reductants presence in the solution causes the reduction of the Fe^{3+}/ferricyanide complex to the ferrous form. Therefore, Fe^{2+} can be checked by absorbance measurement at 700 nm. According to the previous reports, the reducing properties have been shown to exert antioxidant activity by donating of hydrogen atom to break the free radical chain (Gordon, 1990). At 700 nm, the increasing absorbance indicates an increase in reducing ability. In the fractions of *R. dumetorum*, the presence of the antioxidants caused their reduction of Fe^{3+}/ ferricyanide

complex to the ferrous form, and thus demonstrated the reducing power.

The antioxidant capacity of the fractions was measured spectrophotometrically through phosphomolybdenum method, based on the reduction of Mo (VI) to Mo (V) by the test sample and the consequent formation of green phosphate/Mo (V) compounds. Recent studies have shown that numerous flavonoid and related polyphenols contribute significantly to the phosphomolybdate scavenging activity of medicinal plants (Sharififar et al., 2009; Khan et al., 2012). Regarding the result of total antioxidant activity, the methanol and chloroform fractions of *R. dumetorum* contain antioxidant compounds as equivalents of ascorbic acid to efficiently decrease the oxidant in the reaction matrix.

Phenolic compounds are considered secondary metabolites and these phytochemical compounds derived from phenylalanine and tyrosine occur ubiquitously in plants and are diversified (Naczk and Shahidi, 2004). Plants phenolic compounds are also very important because their hydroxyl groups confer scavenging capability. In the preliminary phytochemical investigation, only methanol and water extract showed the presence of phenol. That is why, only methanol and water extracts are tested for total phenolic content. The other two extracts (n-hexane and chloroform) did not show the presence of phenol in the preliminary phytochemical investigation. Flavonoids are naturally occurring in plants and are believed to have positive effects on human health. Regarding the studies on flavonoidic derivatives, they shown a wide range of antibacterial, antiviral, anti-inflammatory, anti-allergic and anticancer activities (Di Carlo et al., 1999; Montoro et al., 2005).

Flavonoids have been shown to be extremely effective scavengers of most oxidizing molecules, including singlet oxygen and various free radicals (Bravo, 1998) implicated in several diseases. In methanol extract, total phenolic content is significantly higher than total flavonoid content. To estimate antioxidant activity, the ferric ion reduction is expansively used. Gallic and ascorbic acids have been used as standard antioxidant in this method. Fe^{2+} reacts rapidly with 1, 10-o-phenanthroline and forms a red colored complex which is exceptionally stable. The synthesized compounds react with Fe^{3+} to reduce and change it to Fe^{2+}. The degree of coloration designates the reduction potential of the compounds. The methanol and water extract (0.314 and 0.326) also contributed fairly outstanding antioxidant activity at 500 µg/ml. So, n-hexane and chloroform showed appreciable antioxidant activity than methanol and water extract and also standard antioxidants.

As an initial indicator of *in vivo* antitumour activity, the *in vitro* cytotoxicity of the plant extracts were usually tested. Though, an extensive range of phyto compounds are capable of exhibiting nonspecific cytotoxicity, plant extracts with significant cytotoxic activity should be further examined using animal models to confirm antitumor activity, and/or a battery of various cell lines to detect specific cytotoxicity. This step is essential to eliminate cytotoxic compounds with little value for additional investigation as anticancer agents (Ali et al., 1996). From the results of the brine shrimp lethality bioassay, it can be well predicted that both the methanol and water extracts possess less cytotoxic potency. DMSO showed the highest potency than both methanol and water extracts. Besides, cytotoxic potency of methanol extract is higher than water extract of leaves of *R. dumetorum*. When compared with negative control DMSO, it shows that cytotoxicity exhibited by methanol and water extract might have low cytotoxic and anti-tumor activity.

Conclusion

Conclusively, the different leaf extracts of *R. dumetorum* might be potential as antioxidant substances and cytotoxic compounds. Further studies are needed to isolate and reveal the active compounds contained in the different solvent extracts of *R. dumetorum* responsible for

these activities and to establish the mechanism of action.

ACKNOWLEDGEMENT

The authors are grateful to the Department of Applied Chemistry and Chemical Engineering, Noakhali Science and Technology University, for providing the laboratory facilities for the research work.

REFERENCES

Auwal MS, Saka S, Mairiga IA, Sanda KA, Shuaibu A, Ibrahim A (2014). Preliminary phytochemical and elemental analysis of aqueous and fractionated pod extracts of *Acacia nilotica* (Thorn mimosa). Vet. Res. For. 5(2):95-100.

Ali AM, Mackeen MM, Saleh H, Ei-Sharkawy, Hamid JA, Ismail NH, Ahmadi FBH, Lajis NH (1996). Antiviral and cytotoxic activities of some plants used in Malaysian indigenous medicine. Pertanika J. Trop. Agric. Sci. 19(2/3):129-136.

Bravo L (1998). Polyphenols: chemistry, dietary sources, metabolism and nutritional significance. Nutr. Rev. 56:317-333.

Chiavaroli V, Giannini C, De Marco S, Chiarelli F, Mohn A (2011). Unbalanced oxidant-antioxidant status and its effects in pediatric diseases. Redox Rep. 16:101-107.

Chinedu E, David A, Ameh SF (2015). Phytochemical evaluation of the ethanolic extracts of some Nigerian herbal plants. Drug Dev. Ther. 6(1):11-14.

Chang C, Yang M, Wen H, Chern J (2002). Estimation of total flavonoid content in Propolis by two comple mentary colorimetric methods. J. Food Drug Anal. 10(3):178-182.

Dharmishtha AM, Mishra SH, Falguni PG (2009). Antioxidant Studies of Methanolic Extract of *Randia dumetorum* lam. Pharmacologyonline 1:22-34.

Di Carlo G, Mascolo N, Izzo AA, Capasso F (1999). Flavonoids: old and new aspects of a class of natural therapeutic drugs. Life Sci. 65:337-353.

Gordon MH (1990). The mechanism of antioxidant action *in vitro*. In Food antioxidants. Edited by Hudson BJ. London: Elsevier Applied Science Series. pp. 1-18.

Harborne JB (1973). Phytochemical methods. London: Chapman and Hall. pp. 49-188.

Hukkeri VI, Mruthunjaya K (2008). *In vitro* antioxidant and free radical scavenging potential of *Parkinsonia aculeate* Linn, Pharmacog. Mag. 4:42-48.

Jangwan JS, Singh R (2014). *In vitro* cytotoxic activity of triterpene isolated from bark of *Randia Dumetorum* Lamk. J. Curr. Chem. Pharm. Sci. 4(1):1-9.

Jakaria M, Parvez M, Zaman R, Arifujjaman, Hasan MI, Sayeed MA, Ali MH (2015). Investigations of Analgesic Activity of the Methanol Extract of *Haldina cordifolia* (Roxb.) Bark by using *in vivo* Anim. Model Stud. Res. J. Bot. 10:98-103.

Kanwar JR, Kanwar RK, Burrow H, Baratchi S (2009). Recent advances on the roles of NO in cancer and chronic inflammatory disorders. Curr. Med. Chem. 16:2373-2394.

Kandimalla R, Kalita S, Saikia B, Choudhury B, Singh YP, Kalita K, Dash S and Kotoky J (2016). Antioxidant and Hepatoprotective Potentiality of Randia dumetorum Lam. Leaf and Bark via Inhibition of Oxidative Stress and Inflammatory Cytokines. Front. Pharmacol. 7:205.

Khan RA, Khan MR, Sahreen S (2012). Assessment of flavonoids contents and *in vitro* antioxidant activity of *Launaea procumbens*. Chem. Central. J. 6:43.

Mujeeb F, Bajpai P, Pathak N (2014). Phytochemical Evaluation, Antimicrobial Activity, and Determination of Bioactive Components from Leaves of *Aegle marmelos*. BioMed. Res. Intl. ID 497606.

Mandal S, Patra A, Samanta A, Roy S, Mandal A, Mahapatra TD, Pradhan S, Das K, Nandi DK (2013). Analysis of phytochemical profile of *Terminalia arjuna* bark extract with antioxidative and antimicrobial properties. Asian Pac. J. Trop. Biomed. 3(12):960-966.

Meyer BN, Ferrigni NR, Putnam JE, Jacobsen LB, Nichols DJ, McLaughlin JL (1982). Brine shrimp: a convenient general bioassay for active plant constituents. Planta Med. 45(05):31-34.

Makkar HPS, Siddhuraju P, Becker K (2007). Plant Secondary Metabolites, Humana Press, Totowa, NJ, USA.

Montoro P, Braca A, Pizza C, De Tommasi N (2005). Structure-antioxidant activity relationships of flavonoids isolated from different plant species. Food Chem. 92:349-355.

Naczk M, Shahidi F (2004). Extraction and analysis of phenolics in food. J. Chromatogr. A. 1054:95-111.

Oyaizu M (1986). Studies on product of browning reaction prepared from glucose amine. Jap. J. Nutr. 44:307-315.

Patel RG, Pathak NL, Rathod JD, Patel LB, Bhatt NM (2011). Phytopharmacological properties of Randia dumetorumasa potential medicinal tree: an overview. J. Appl. Pharm. Sci. 10:24-26.

Patil MJ, Bafna AR, Bodas K, Shafi S (2014). *In vitro* antioxidant activity of fruits of *Randia dumetorum* Lamk.

Prieto P, Pineda M, Aguilar M (1999). Spectrophotometric quantitation of antioxidant capacity through the formation of a phosphomolybdenum complex: Specific application to the determination of vitamin E. Anal. Biochem. 269:337-341.

Prasad KN, Yang B, Yang SY, Chen YL, Zhao MM, Ashraf M, Jiang Y (2009). Identification of phenolic compounds and appraisal of antioxidant and antityrosinase activities from litchi (*Litchi sinensis* Sonn.) seeds. Food Chem. 116:1-7.

Saeed N, Khan MR, Shabbir M (2012). Antioxidant activity, total phenolic and total flavonoid contents of whole plant extracts *Torilis leptophylla* L. BMC Comp. Altern. Med. 12:221.

Saad B, Azaizeh H, Abu-Hijleh G, Said O (2006). Safety of traditional arab herbal medicine. Evid Based Compl. Altern. Med. 3:433-439.

Sahgal G, Ramanathan S, Sasidharan S, Mordi MN, Ismail S, Mansor SM (2010). Brine shrimp lethality and acute oral toxicity studies on *Swietenia mahagoni* (Linn.) Jacq. seed methanolic extract. Pharmacog. Res. 2(4):215-220.

Sen S, Chakraborty R, Sridhar C, Reddy YSR, De B (2010). Free radicals, antioxidants, diseases and phytomedicines: current status and future prospect. Int. J. Pharm. Sci. Rev. Res. 3(1):91-100.

Sumbul S, Ahmad MA, Asif M, Akhtar M, Saud I (2012). Physicochemical and phytochemical standardization of berries of *Myrtus communis* Linn. J. Pharm. Bioallied Sci. 4(4):322-326.

Sharma S, Vig AD (2013). Evaluation of *In Vitro* Antioxidant Properties of Methanol and Aqueous Extracts of *Parkinsonia aculeata* L. Leaves. The Sci. World J. Article ID 604865.

Sharififar F, Dehghn-Nudeh G, Mirtajaldini M (2009). Major flavonoids with antioxidant activity from *Teucrium polium* L. Food Chem. 112:885-888.

Todkar SS, Chavan VV, Kulkarni AS (2010). Screening of Secondary Metabolites and Anbacterial Activity of Acacia concinna. Res. J. Mcrobiol. 5(10):974-979.

Thamaraiselvi LP, Jayanthi P (2012). Preliminary studies on phytochemicals and antimicrobial activity of solvent extracts of *Eichhornia crassipes* (Mart.) Solms. Asian J. Plant Sci. Res. 2(2):115-122.

Umamaheswari M, Chatterjee TK (2008). *In vitro* antioxidant activities of the fractions of *Coccinnia grandis* L. leaf extract. Afr. J. Trad. Compl. Altern. Med. 5:61-73.

Zaman R, Parvez M, Jakaria M, Islam M, Ali MS, Hossain MA (2016). *In vitro* antibacterial and antioxidant activities of alcoholic extract from the leaves of *Podocarpus neriifolius* D. Don. Afr. J. Pharm. Pharmacol. 10(37):791-795.

## 10

Phytochemical and biological analyses of *Citharexylum spinosum*

Amel M. Kamal[1*], Mohamed I. S. Abdelhady[1#], Heba Tawfeek[1#], Maha G. Haggag[2#] and Eman G. Haggag[1#]

[1]Department of Pharmacognosy, Faculty of Pharmacy, Helwan University, Cairo 11795, Egypt.
[2]Department of Microbiology, Research Institute of Ophthalmology, Giza, Egypt.

The phytochemical screening of *Citharexylum spinosum* L. aerial parts resulted in the presence of flavonoids, tannins, carbohydrates and/or glycosides, triterpenes and/or sterols and saponins. The percentage of hydrocarbons and sterols in *C. spinosum* petroleum ether extract were 99.57 and 0.3%, respectively. In petroleum ether extract, saturated fatty acids (78.76%) and unsaturated fatty acids (9.14%) were found. Chromatographic fractionation of 80% aqueous, methanol and chloroform extracts of *C. spinosum* resulted in isolation of 10 compounds; β-Sitosterol, β-Sitosterol 3-*O*-β-D-glucopyranoside, Oleanolic acid, Gallic acid, Quercetin, 6-Methoxy acacetin 7-*O*-β-D-glucopyranoside, Naringenin, Quercetin 3-*O*-α-L-rhamnopyranoside (Quercetrin), 1, 2, 6-tri-*O*-galloyl-β-D-glucopyranoside and Rutin. The antipyretic activity of aqueous methanolic residue using Brewer's yeast-induced pyrexia in rats was significant at dose 300 mg/kg. All tested samples had no analgesic activity. The major isolated compounds were quercetin and quercetrin, their biological activities, antimicrobial and cytotoxic activities, were determined parallel to the extracts. It was found that the aqueous methanolic residue, chloroform extract, quercetin and quercetrin exerted significant antimicrobial activity. From 3-(4,5-dimethylthiazol-2-yl)-2,5-diphenyltetrazolium bromide (MTT) cell proliferation assay on A2780 human ovarian cell line, quercetrin showed moderate cytotoxic activity, whereas quercetin showed significant cytotoxic activity.

Key words: *Citharexylum spinosum,* lipoidal matter, phenolics, antipyretic, antimicrobial.

INTRODUCTION

Family Verbenaceae includes about 100 genera and more than 3000 species. Among the largest genera of Verbenaceae is *Citharexylum* which comprises 115 species (Dahiya, 1979; Starr et al., 2006; Mohammed et al., 2014). Genus *Citharexylum* was reported to contain triterpenes, sterols, irridoids, lignan glycoside, phenolic and flavonoids.

Different species of genus *Citharexylum* are famous to have antiulcer, antihypertensive, hepatoprotective effects immunomodulatory, antimicrobial, anti-Schistosomal antioxidant, nephroprotective, radical scavenging cytotoxic activities and regulating immediate type o allergic reaction (Khalifa et al., 2002; Ganapaty et al. 2010; Khan and Siddique, 2012; Kadry et al., 2013

*Corresponding author. E-mail: kh.omran@yahoo.com. #Co-authors contributed equally.

Allam, 2014; Mohammed et al., 2016). Among these species is *Citharexylum spinosum* L. which is a popular ornamental tree in many tropical and subtropical regions and are known as fiddlewood. It has been used in folk medicine as diuretic, antipyretic, antiarthritic and in liver disorders (Lawrence, 1951; Turner and Wasson, 1997; Wagner et al., 1999; Starr et al., 2006).

MATERIALS AND METHODS

Plant material

Aerial parts (leaves and stems) of *C. spinosum* L. were collected from Zoo garden, Giza, Egypt in January, 2014. The plant was identified by Mrs. Terase Labib, senior specialist of plant taxonomy, floral and taxonomy department, El-Orman garden, Giza, Egypt. Voucher specimens are kept in the herbarium of Pharmacognosy Department, Faculty of pharmacy, Helwan University, Cairo, Egypt.

Cell line, micro-organisms, animals, chemicals, standard materials, media and drugs

The human ovarian cell line, RPMI-1640 media was supplemented with 10% heat inactivated foetal bovine serum (FBS), L-glutamine and 5% penicillin + streptomycin, MTT: 3-(4,5-Dimethylthiazol-2-yl)-2,5-diphenyltetrazolium bromide, Paracetamol, Saline (0.9%NaCl) and 20% aqueous suspension of Brewer's yeast in normal saline. All chemicals were from Sigma/Aldrich, USA.

Multidrug-resistant strains of *Staphylococcus aureus*, *Escherichia coli* and *Pseudomonas aeuroginosa* were selected among clinical isolates obtained from Outpatient Clinics of the Research Institute of Ophthalmology (RIO) while Imipenem and Ciprofloxacin discs were purchased from Oxoid, England. Adult albino mice weighing 25 to 30 g and rats weighing 120-130 g of either sex were used in the present study. All animals were kept in a controlled environment of air and temperature with access to water and diet *ad libitum*. Anesthetic procedures and animal handling were in compliance with the ethical guidelines of Medical Ethics Committee of the National Research Centre; Polyamide S6 (50-160 μm, Fluka chemie AG, Switzerland) for column chromatography, Microcrystalline cellulose (E. Merck, Darmstadt, Germany) for column chromatography, Sephadex LH-20 (25-100μm, Pharmacia, Uppsala, Sweden) for column chromatography, Silica gel 60 F$_{254,}$ precoated aluminium sheets (20 x 20, 0.2mm thickness), (E. Merck, Darmstadt, Germany) for thin layer chromatography, Silica gel G 60 for column chromatography (70-230 mesh, 60 A°, E. Merck, Germany) and Whatman No.1 for paper chromatography (Whatman Ltd., Maidstone, Kent, England). Spraying reagents were done according to common methods (Smith, 1960; Stahl, 1969; Balbaa et al., 1981; Markham, 1982).

NMR spectrometers

^{1}H and ^{13}C NMR spectra (University of Louisiana at Monroe) were recorded at 400 and 100 MHz, respectively, in appropriate deuterated NMR solvent, on a JEOL Eclipse ECS-400 NMR spectrometer (Boston, MA, USA). For analysis and spectral processing, chemical shifts reported δ ppm values relative to TMS using Detta^{TM} NMR Data Processing Software (JEOL Inc, MA, USA).

HP 5890 series Gas Chromatograph System with an FID/MS detector, Faculty of Agriculture, Cairo University was used for lipoidal matters analysis. We used UV lamp (Marne La Vallee, VL-215 LC, France) for visualization of spots on paper and thin layer chromatograms to follow up the columns fractionation on columns at 254 and/or 365 nm. Hot plate (Harvard Apparatus, Kent, UK), sterile pipettes and 96 well cell culture microplate were used for pharmacological studies.

Preliminary phytochemical screening

Air dried powdered aerial parts (leaves and stems) of *C. Spinosum* L. was subjected to preliminary phytochemical screening for its constituents, according to methods mentioned in the references of Trease and Evans (1989), Evans (1996) and the British Pharmacopea (1993).

Preparation and fractionation of lipoidal matter of *C .spinosum* L. aerial parts

The air-dried powder of *C. spinosum* L. aerial parts (90 g) was extracted with petroleum ether (b.p. 60 to 80°C) and evaporated to give residue (3 g). This residue was kept for the preparation of unsaponifiable matters (USM) and total fatty acids (TFA) according to previous studies (El-Said and Amer, 1965; British Pharmacopea, 1993). TFA and USM of *C. spinosum* L. aerial parts were subjected to methylation followed by GC-MS analysis. Tentative identification was carried out by comparison of their R$_t$-values. The relative concentration of each constituent was calculated based on the peak area integration (Vogel, 1961).

Extraction and purification of active constituents from *C. spinosum* L. aerial parts

The air-dried ground aerial parts (1350 g) of *C. spinosum* L. were subjected to exhaustive extraction with hot 80% aqueous methanol under reflux (50°C). The extract was dried under vacuum (50°C) to give dry total extract (360 g). This dry extract was defatted by petroleum ether which resulted in 20 g of dried petroleum ether residue, and 330 g of the remaining residue was successively extracted with chloroform, under reflux at 50°C to yield 50 g of chloroform extract, 2 g of ethyl acetate extract, 10 g of *n*-butanol extract and 260 g of remaining aqueous methanolic residue.

The 2D-PC and TLC revealed that, ethyl acetate and *n*-butanol extracts had limited constituents, while concentrated in aqueous methanolic residue and chloroform extract. Fractionation, isolation and purification were performed as illustrated in Figure 1. Paper chromatography (PC) according to Mabry et al. (1970), column chromatography and thin layer chromatography (TLC) according to Stahl (1969), GC-MS conditions for unsaponifiable matters analysis and GC - MS conditions for fatty acid methyl esters analysis were performed according to Vogel (1961), mild and complete acid hydrolysis were done according to the methods described by Harborne (1984).

Cell culture and MTT cell proliferation assay

A human ovarian cell line A2780 was incubated at 37°C in an atmosphere of 5% CO$_2$, 95% air and 100% relative humidity, to maintain continuous logarithmic growth. RPMI-1640 media was supplemented with 10% heat inactivated Foetal Bovine Serum (FBS), L-glutamine and 5% penicillin + streptomycin. Cells were checked for Mycoplasma, by measuring the bio-luminescence (Myco Alert sample detection kit; Lonza, Switzerland), using a multiplate reader (Synergy HT, BioTek, USA). The MTT *in vitro* cell viability colorimetric assay was used for measuring cellular proliferation, inhibitory activity and cytotoxicity of the plant samples.

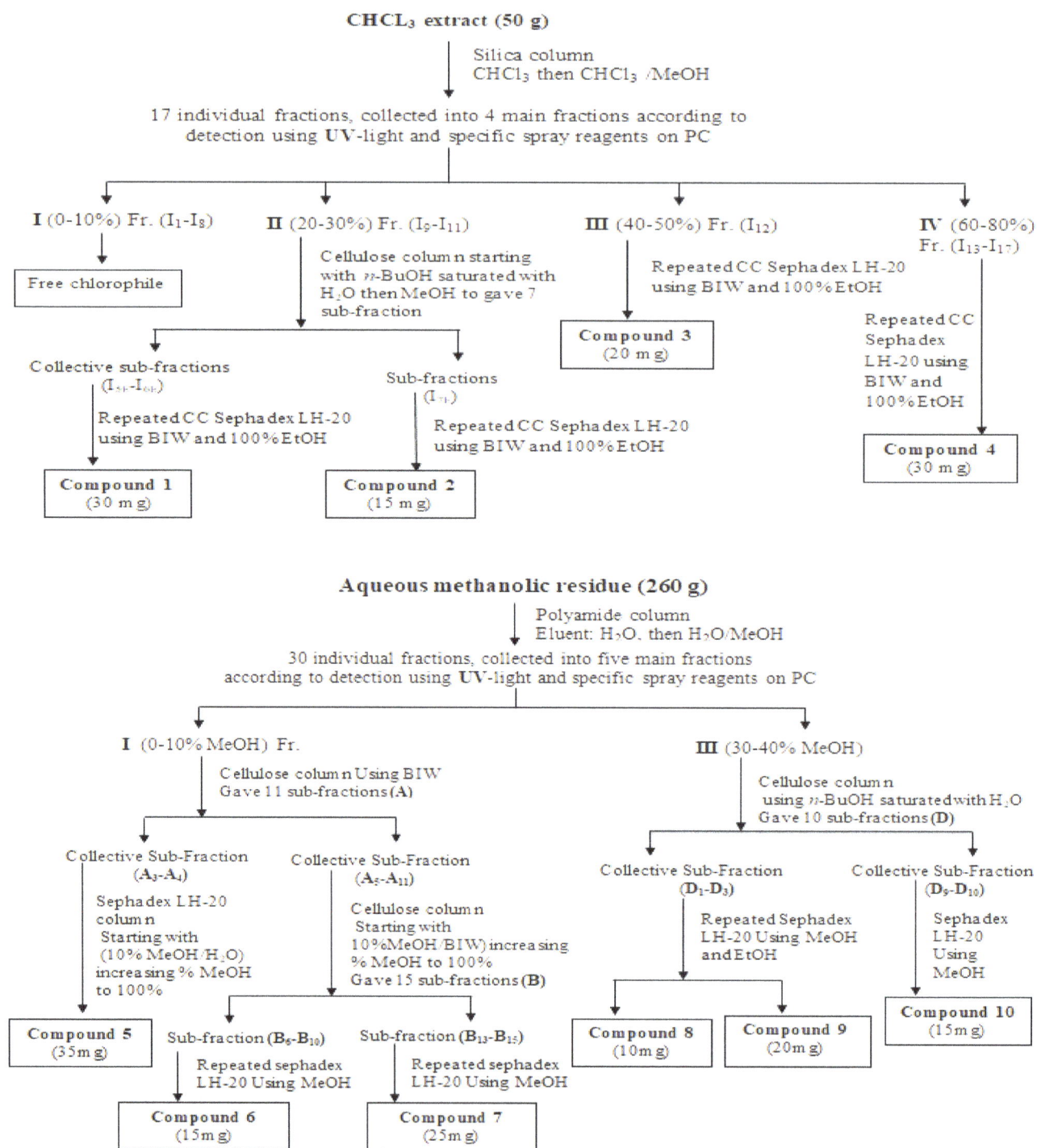

Figure 1. Flow charts of fractionation and purification of compounds isolated from CHCl₃ extract and aqueous methanolic residue of *C. spinosum* aerial parts.

The colour of MTT: 3-(4, 5-Dimethylthiazol-2-yl)-2, 5-diphenyltetrazolium bromide is yellow (tetrazole), which changed to purple (reduced to formazan). When mitochondrial dehydrogenase enzymes are active therefore, reduction indicates cell viability which can be measured as optical density (OD). Cells were incubated at 37°C overnight. Final concentrations of each sample (in DMSO was filtered with Nylon 0.22 µm × 25 mm) in wells were 1, 10, 25, 50 and 100 µg/ml in 200 µl of media (DMSO 0.1%). 20 µl medium was added to each control well, and incubated for 48 h. Each concentration was tested in triplicates (n=3). MTT was added into each well. Plates were incubated for 3 h, supernatant was aspirated, and 100 µl of DMSO was added to each well. Plates were shaken for 5 min at 26°C using STUART scientific orbital shaker (Redhill, Surrey, UK) and absorbance was read on multiplate reader (Synergy HT, BioTek, USA). The OD of the purple formazan A_{570} is proportional to the number of viable cells.

When the amount of formazan produced by treated cells is compared with the amount of formazan produced by untreated control cells, the strength of the drug in causing growth inhibition can be determined. Through plotting growth curves of absorbance against sample(s) concentration, thus formulation concentration causing 50% inhibition (IC_{50}) compared to control cell growth (100%) were determined (Hansen et al., 1989). GraphPad Prism version 5.00 for Windows, GraphPad Software, San Diego California USA (www.graphpad.com) was used for analysis.

Determination of LD_{50}

The alcoholic sample was dissolved in distilled water then given orally to adult albino mice in graded doses up to 4 g/kg (the maximum given dose) and the control group received the same volume of the vehicle. The percentage mortality for samples as well as the general behavior of the animal was recorded 24 h later (Armitage, 1971).

Estimation of analgesic activity using hot Plate Test

Two doses of 100 and 300 mg/kg body weight for chloroform and methanolic extract each and 50 mg/kg paracetamol (as standard) was administered orally to adult albino mice weighing 25 to 30 g of either sex using 25-gauge needle (Farshchi et al., 2009). Tested animal was placed on a hot plate with fixed temperature 55±0.5°C (Harvard Apparatus Ltd., Kent, UK), till the appearance of withdrawal response in terms of hind paw licking, biting or jumped off. A cut-off time to remove mouse from the plate of 30 seconds was used to minimize the tissue damage (Pini et al., 1997; Lavich et al., 2005; National committee for clinical laboratory standard (NCCLS), 1997).

Estimation of antipyretic activity

Aqueous methanolic residue and chloroform extract of C. spinosum L. aerial parts were used to evaluate their antipyretic activity using Brewer's yeast-induced pyrexia in rats as described by, Loux et al. (1972).

Fever was induced by injecting 20 ml/kg of 20% aqueous suspension of Brewer's yeast in normal saline subcutaneously. Temperature across rectum (using thermal probe Eliab thermistor thermometer) was recorded after 18 h and served as base line of elevated body temperature. The extracts samples (100 and 300 mg/kg) was administered orally, using paracetamol (50 mg/kg, orally) as reference. Control group received distilled water. Rectal temperature was determined at 1 and 2 h after test samples/reference drug administration.

Preparation of the plant samples for antimicrobial evaluation

The antimicrobial activity of the aqueous methanolic residue, chloroform extract, compounds 5 and 8 obtained from C. spinosum L. aerial parts were evaluated using the agar well diffusion method as described by Rahbar and Diba (2010). All samples were dissolved in 0.5 ml methanol. A loopful of the tested organisms was inoculated into 5.0 ml of nutrient broth and incubated at 37°C for 24 h.

50 µl of 24 h culture organism was dispensed into 5 ml broth and incubated for 2 h to standardize the culture to 10^6 cfu/ml. Cotton swab was immersed into standardized culture to be spread onto the surface of, the agar plate. Sterilized 6 mm cork borer was used to punch 5 wells for the extracts. From each of the 4 extract samples, 100 µl was dispensed into the corresponding 4 wells while the fifth was used for negative control (methanol). To allow diffusion of the tested extract samples, the plates were left at room temperature for at least 1 h. Two discs of antibiotic (imipenem and ciprofloxacin) were placed as positive control. These plates were incubated at 37°C for 18 to 24 h. Zones of inhibition surrounding the wells and discs were measured to evaluate their antimicrobial activity.

RESULTS

Preliminary phytochemical screening, hydrocarbon, sterol and fatty acid contents in C. spinosum

Phytochemical screening as preliminary tests of aerial parts of C. spinosum revealed the presence of carbohydrate and/or glycosides, tannins, flavonoids, irridoids, unsaturated sterols and/or triterpenes, saponins and the absence of anthraquinones, volatiles, coumarins, and alkaloids or compound containing nitrogenous bases. Identification of hydrocarbons and sterols content of USM fraction was carried out by GC-MS; the conditions were adopted as mentioned. Tentative identification of hydrocarbons and sterols was carried out by, comparison of their retention times.

Quantitation was based on peak area integration. The results of USM analysis for C. spinosum L. are compiled in Table 1 and Figure 2. It was found that, hydrocarbons represented a higher percentage (99.57%) than that of sterols (0.30%). 6-Phenyldodecane (10.03%) and 5-Phenyldodecane (9.96%) represented the major hydrocarbons while β-Sitosterol (0.30%) represented the only sterol identified. It could be concluded that, the saturated fatty acids (78.76%) represented a higher percentage than that of unsaturated ones (9.41%). 14-methyl Pentadecanoic acid (34.8%) and Hexadecanoic acid (25.1 %) represented the major identified saturated fatty acids while 9-Octadecanoic acid (2.62 %) represented the major unsaturated fatty acid, Table 2 and Figure 3.

Characterization and identification of isolated compounds

Air dried powdered aerial parts of the plant under investigation (1350 g) was subjected to exhaustive extraction with 80% MeOH under reflux. After drying the extract under reduced pressure, the residue was defatted by petroleum ether and the remaining residue was fractionated by chloroform, ethyl acetate and n-butanol under reflux (50°C), respectively. The 2D-PC analysis proved that active constituents are concentrated in the chloroform extract and aqueous methanolic residue when compared to ethyl acetate and n-butanol extracts.

Aqueous methanolic residue, and chloroform extract were subjected to fractionation according to the illustrated

Table 1. GC-MS analysis of USM of *C. spinosum* L.

Identified compound	RRT*	Percentage area
5-Phenyl decane	0.8	1.75
4-Phenyl decane	0.814	1.33
3-Phenyl decane	0.834	0.95
2-Phenyl decane	0.872	1.23
6-Phenyl undecane	0.90	3.86
5-Phenyl undecane	0.907	9.78
4-Phenyl undecane	0.917	6.84
3-Phenyl undecane	0.937	4.27
5-Phenyl dodecane	0.966	0.05
2-Phenyl undecane	0.975	7.07
p-Didecyl benzein	0.988	0.07
6-Phenyl dodecane	1	10.03
5-Phenyl dodecane	1.005	9.96
4-Phenyl dodecane	1.02	6.50
3-Phenyl dodecane	1.04	4.54
1-Nonadecene	1.057	0.04
2-Phenyl dodecane	1.07	7.53
6-Phenyl tridecane	1.09	8.57
5-Phenyl tridecane	1.1	5.08
4-Phenyl tridecane	1.11	3.56
3-Phenyl tridecane	1.13	2.47
2-Phenyl tridecane	1.16	4.24
β – Sitosterol	1.19	0.30
Total hydrocarbon		99.57
Total sterols		0.30
Total identified Compounds		99.57
Unidentified compounds		0.13

RRT*: Relative retention time of 6 - Phenyl dodecane with RT = 24.53 min.

Figure 1. Identification of isolated compounds are based on chemical and physical methods including ^{1}H/^{13}C NMR and HMBC. Based on these data and by comparison with reported literature data (Haddock et al., 1982; Barakat et al., 1987; Agrawal and Bansal, 1989; Mahmoud et al., 2001; Seebacher et al., 2003; Shalaby and Bahgat, 2003; Marzouk et al., 2004; Aboutabl et al., 2008; Rahmana et al., 2009; Ahmad et al., 2010; Kamal et al., 2012; Onoja and Ndukwe, 2013; Haggag et al., 2013; Allam, 2014; Khan and Hossain, 2015; Mohammed et al., 2016) and authentic samples, the compounds identified were ten; 1; *β*- Sitosterol, 3; Oleanolic acid and 4; Gallic acid were isolated once before from genus *Citharexylum*, while 2; *β*-Sitosterol 3-*O*- *β* -D-glucopyranoside 5; Quercetin , 6; 6-Methoxy acacetin 7-*O*-β-D-glucopyranoside, 7; Naringenin, 8; Quercetin 3-*O*-α-L-rhamnopyranoside (Quercetrin), 9; 1, 2, 6-tri-*O*-galloyl-β-D-glucopyranoside, 10; Rutin were isolated for the first time from genus *Citharexylum* (Figure 4). Two major compounds (5 and 8) subjected to biological activities, their spectral data are summarized as follow:

Compound 5

Is a yellow amorphous powder (20 mg), with chromatographic properties: R_f values; 0.6 (S_1), 0.4 (S_2); brilliant yellow fluorescent spot by UV- light. It gave pale green color and orange fluorescence with $FeCl_3$ and Naturstoff spray reagents, respectively. ^{1}H-NMR (400 MHz, CD$_3$OD): δ ppm 7.71 (1H, d, *J*=2.0 Hz, H-2`), 7.62 (1H, dd, *J*=8.3, 2.0 Hz, H 6`), 6.86 (1H, d, *J*=8.3 Hz, H-5`), 6.36 (1H, d, *J*=1.8Hz, H-8) 6.15 (1H, d, *J*=1.8Hz, H-6). $^{13}$C-NMR PENDANT (100 MHz CD$_3$OD): δ ppm 175.99 (C-4), 164.23 (C-7), 161.17 (C-5) 156.86 (C-9), 147.34 (C-2), 146.62 (C-4`), 144.88 (C-3`) 135.90 (C-3), 122.79 (C-1`), 120.29 (C-6`), 114.85 (C-2`) 114.48 (C-5`), 103.17 (C-10), 97.85 (C-6), 93.02 (C-8).

Compound 8

Is an orange amorphous powder (16 mg), with chromatographic properties: R_f values; 0.39(S_1), 0.63 (S_2) on PC; dark purple fluorescent spot under long UV-light

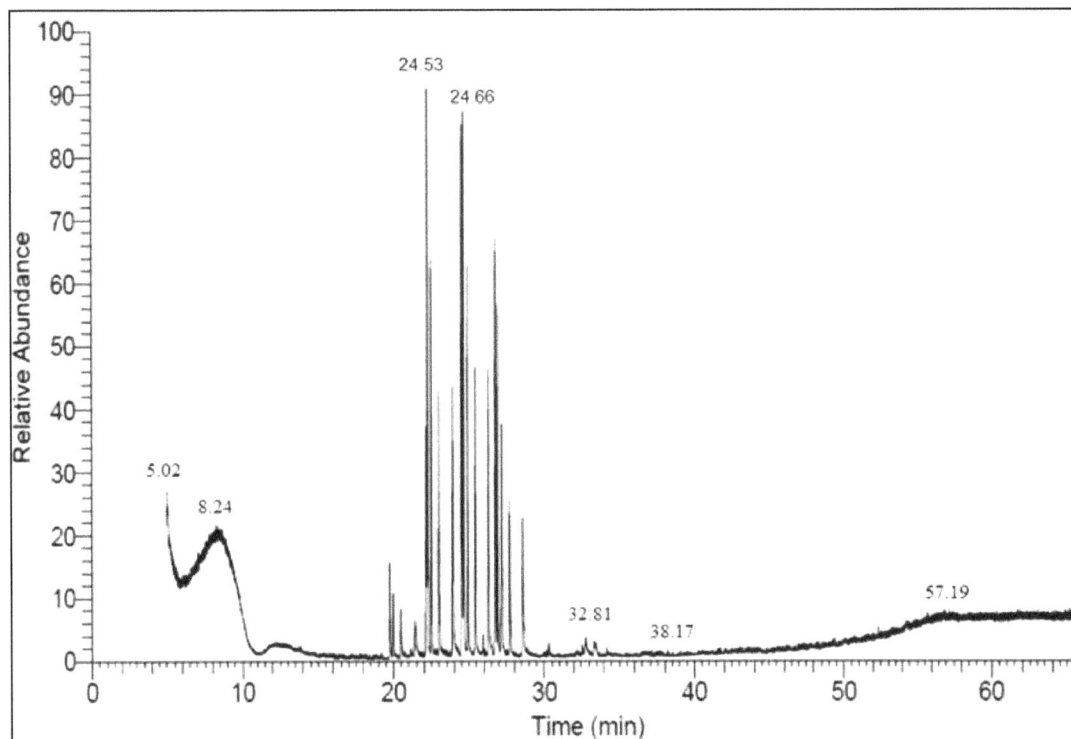

Figure 2. GC-chromatogram of USM of *C. spinosum* L.

Table 2. GC-MS analysis of fatty acids of *C. spinosum* L.

Identified compound		RRT*	Percentage area
Tetradecanoic cid	C(14:0)	0.784	3.38
14-Methyl Pentadecanoic acid	C(16:0)	1	34.8
9-oxo, Nonanoic acid	C(9:0)	1.016	2.64
Hexadecanoic acid	C(16:0)	1.042	25.1
Stearic acid	C(17:0)	1.199	5.22
Octadecanoic acid	C(18:0)	1.237	3.8
10,13-Octadecadienoic acid	C(18:2)	1.278	2.39
18-methyl nonadecanoic acid	C(20:0)	1.38	3.82
Oleic acid	C(18:1)	1.676	1.99
6-Octadecanoic acid	C(18:1)	1.817	2.41
9-Octadecanoic acid	C(18:1)	1.863	2.62
Saturated fatty acid			78.76
Unsaturated fatty acid			9.41
Unidentified compounds			11.83

RRT*: Relative retention time of 14-Methyl Pentadecanoic acid with RT = 23.76 min.

which turned yellow fluorescence on exposure to ammonia vapors and gave a green color and orange fluorescence with $FeCl_3$ and Naturstoff spray reagents, respectively. Complete acid hydrolysis resulted in Quercetin in organic layer and Rhamnose in aqueouslayer (CoPC). ^{1}H-NMR spectrum (400MHz, CD_3OD): δ ppm 7.30 (1H, d, J=2.2 Hz, H-2`), 7.27 (1H, dd, $J$=2.2,8.2 Hz, H-6`), 6.88 (1H, d, J=7.7 Hz, H-5`), 6.32 (1H, d, J=1.8 Hz, H-8), 6.15 (1H, d, J=1.8 Hz, H-6), 5.32 (1H, d, J=1.3 Hz, H- 1``), 4.19 (1H, dd, $J$=1.3, 3.2 Hz, H-2``), 3.71 (1H, dd, J=3.2, 9.6 Hz, H-3``), 3.33 (1H, m, H-5``), 3.32 (1H, m, H-4``), 0.91(3H, d, $J$=5.94 Hz, H-6``). ^{13}C-NMR PENDANT (100 MHz, CD_3OD): δ ppm 178.4 (C-4), 164.8 (C-7), 161.8 (C-5), 157.9 (C-2), 157.2 (C-9), 148.3 (C-4`), 145.1 (C-3`), 134.7 (C-3), 121.6 (C-1`), 121.5 (C-6`), 115.5 (C-2`), 115.0 (C-5`), 104.3 (C-10),

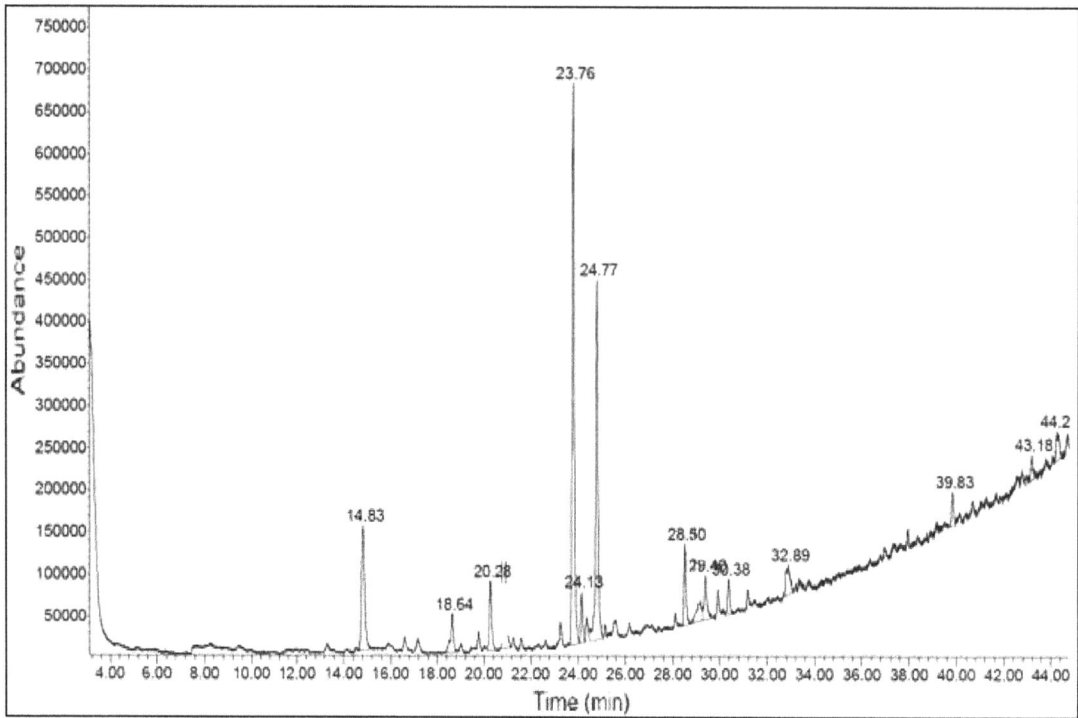

Figure 3. GC-chromatogram of fatty acids of *C. spinosum* L.

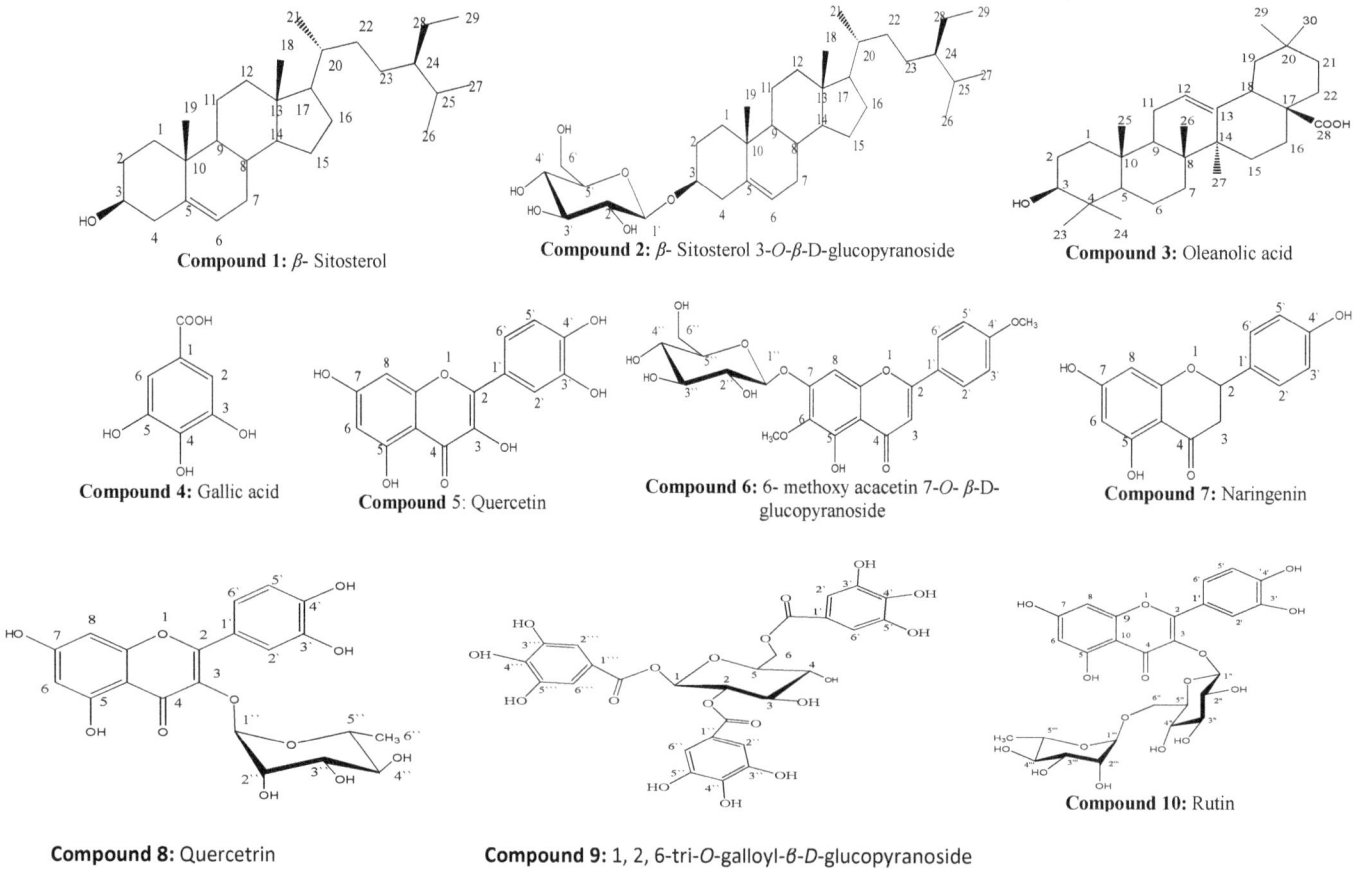

Compound 1: *β*- Sitosterol

Compound 2: *β*- Sitosterol 3-*O*-*β*-D-glucopyranoside

Compound 3: Oleanolic acid

Compound 4: Gallic acid

Compound 5: Quercetin

Compound 6: 6- methoxy acacetin 7-*O*- *β*-D-glucopyranoside

Compound 7: Naringenin

Compound 8: Quercetrin

Compound 9: 1, 2, 6-tri-*O*-galloyl-*β*-D-glucopyranoside

Compound 10: Rutin

Figure 4. Isolated compounds of *C. spinosum*.

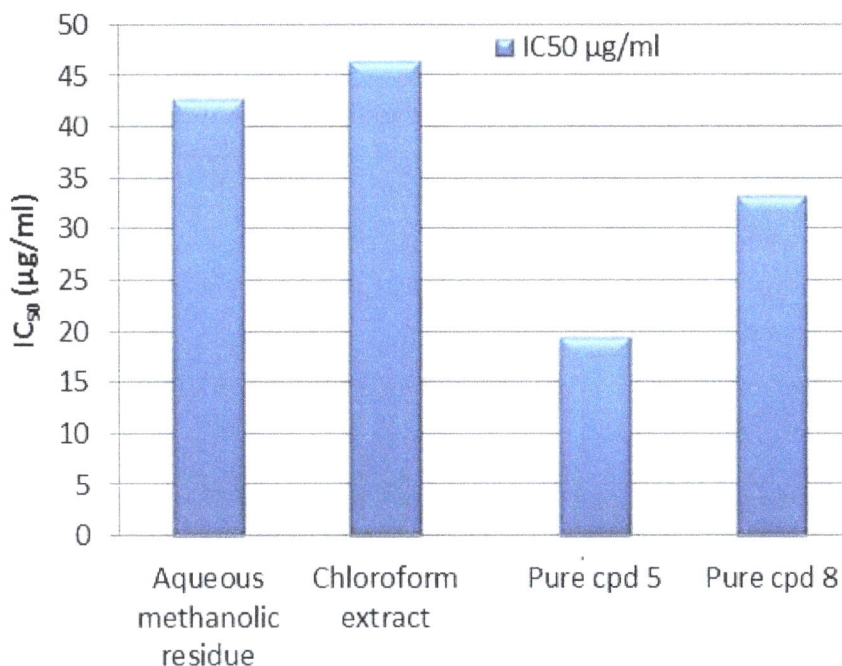

Figure 5. Cytotoxicity of the plant samples against A2780 ovarian cell line.

Table 3. Cytotoxicity of the plant samples against A2780 ovarian cell line.

Sample	IC_{50} µg/ml
Aqueous methanolic residue	42.7
Chloroform extract	46.4
Compound 5 (Quercetin)	19.5
Compound 8 (Quercetrin)	33.2

102.2 (C-1``), 98.5 (C-6), 93.4 (C-8), 71.8 (C-4``), 70.6 (C-3``), 70.5 (C-2``), 70.5 (C-5``), 16.3 ($CH_3$-6``).

Biological study

Cytotoxic activity

Cytotoxic activity of aqueous methanolic residue, chloroform extract, and pure compounds (5 and 8)obtained from the aerial parts of *C. spinosum* were examined against A2780, a human ovarian cell line. Activity was reported in terms of an IC_{50} (concentration in µg/ml necessary to produce 50% inhibition) (Figure 5) and (Table 3). The treatment of A2780 ovarian cell line with an aqueous methanolic residue, chloroform extract showed weak cytotoxic effect as their calculated IC_{50} which were 42.7 µg/ml and 46.4 µg/ml, respectively.

While pure compound 8 (identified later as Quercetrin) showed moderate cytotoxic effect calculated (IC_{50}) as 33.2 µg/ml, pure compound 5 (identified later as Quercetin) showed significant cytotoxic effect as IC_{50} 19.5 µg/ml.

Determination of median lethal dose (LD_{50})

On low doses (less than 2 g/kg of total aqueous methanol extract of *C. spinosum*), it was observed that animals moved and fed normally. The behavior of mice has changed at a dose of 2 g/kg extract. Mice showed abnormal signs like fatigue, loss of appetite and mortality. The 50% of dead animals were estimated at 3 g/kg extract.

In contrast, all animals died at a dose of 4 g/kg. LD_{50} value was calculated by-probit analysis which is 2.86 g/kg body weight.

Analgesic and antipyretic activities

Using hot plate test, the analgesic effect of plant samples

Table 4. Antipyretic activity of aqueous methanolic residue and chloroform extract compared to the effect of paracetamol in yeast suspension-induced hyperthermia in rats

Treatment dose (mg/kg)	Rectal temperature (°C) after yeast injection		
	0 h	1 h	2 h
Distilled water	39.03 ± 0.2	38.95 ±0.16	39.1 ± 0.15
Paracetamol 50	38.95 ±0.25	37.47 ± 0.25**	37.22 ± 0.1**
Aqueous methanolic residue 100	38.88 ± 0.26	38.28 ± 0.15*	38.1 ± 0.26*
Aqueous methanolic residue 300	38.73 ± 0.28	38.07 ± 0.19*	37.87 ± 0.24**
CHCl3 extract 100	38.85 ± 0.29	38.72 ± 0.12	38.87 ± 0.21
CHCl$_3$ extract 300	39.02 ± 0.26	38.32 ± 0.31	38.08 ± 0.31*

Data are represented as mean value ± S.D., n = 6. * Significant difference when compared to untreated group at * $p < 0.05$, ** $p < 0.01$.

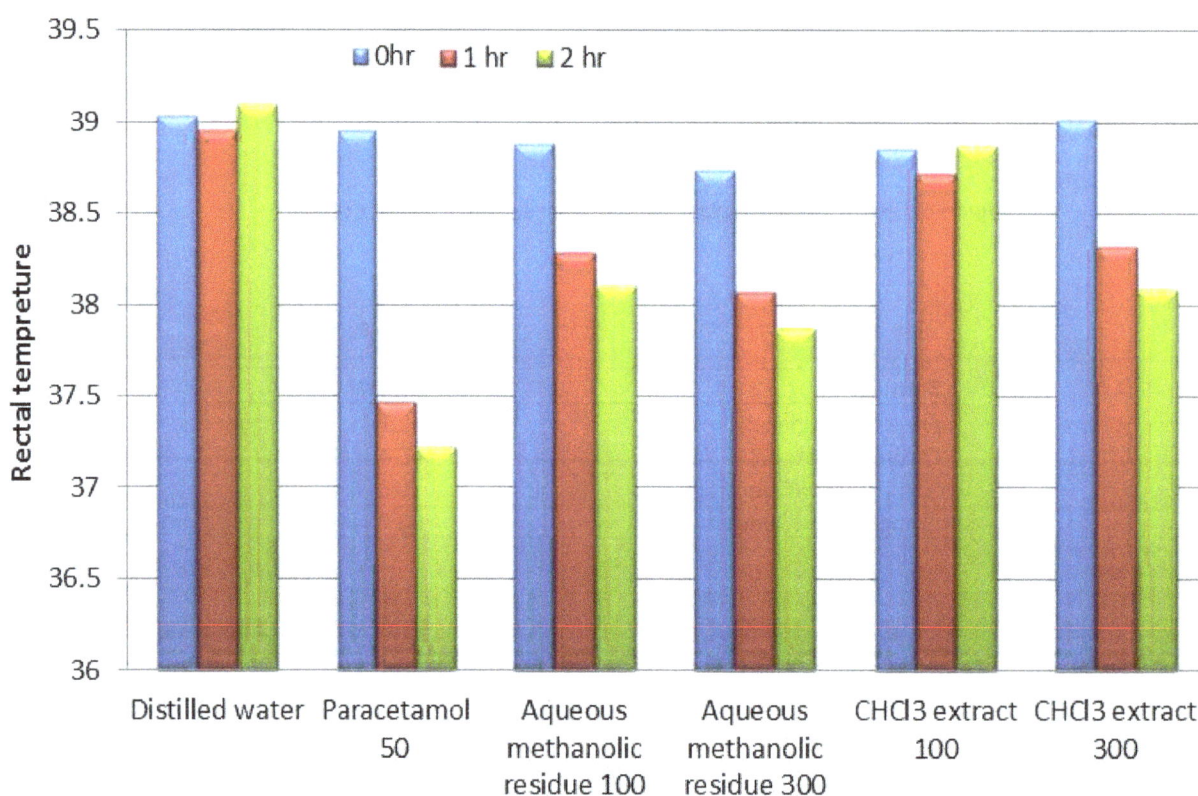

Figure 6. Antipyretic activity of aqueous methanolic residue and chloroform extract compared to the effect of paracetamol and control.

was studied. All tested samples at both concentrations (100 mg/Kg) and (300 mg/Kg) showed non-significant analgesic activity as compared to paracetamol as standard and saline as control. As shown in (Table 4) and (Figure 6), aqueous methanolic residue at concentration 100 mg/kg and chloroform extract at 300 mg/kg showed moderate antipyretic activity while aqueous methanolic residue at 300 mg/kg showed significant antipyretic activity as compared to paracetamol as standard and distilled water as control.

Antimicrobial study

Aqueous methanolic residue of *C. spinosum* exerted marked antimicrobial activity against all tested multidrug resistant Gram +ve and -ve bacteria. Chloroform extrac exerted antimicrobial activity against the tested Gram +ve and -ve bacteria. It showed that, the activity on Gram +ve is higher than Gram -ve bacteria. Pure comound exerted marked activities against the tested Gram +ve S aureus and Gram -ve bacteria E. coli, but showed nc

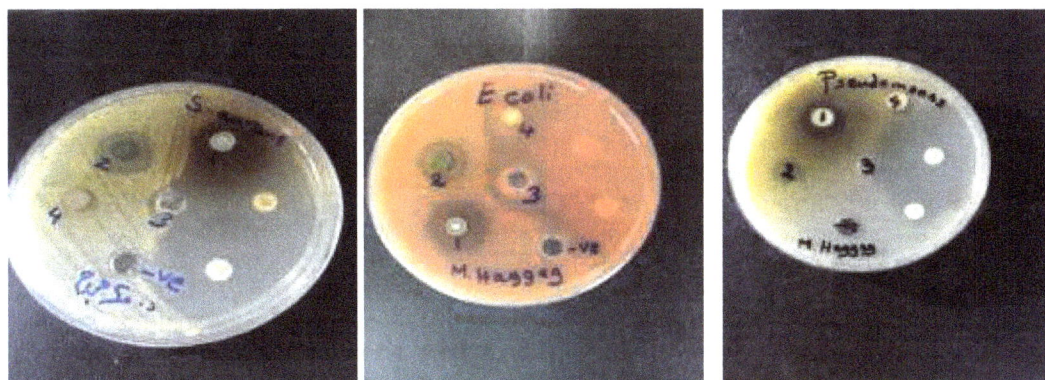

Figure 7. Antimicrobial activity of *C. spinosum* L. against Multidrug-resistant strains of *Staphylococcus aureus, Escherichia coli* and *Pseudomonas aeuroginosa* selected among clinical isolates obtained from Outpatient Clinics of Research Institute of Ophthalmology.

Table 5. Antimicrobial screening.

Sample	*Staphylococcus aureus* (mm)	*Escherichia coli* (mm)	*Pseudomonas aeuroginosa* (mm)
	Mean levels of the inhibition zones		
Aqueous methanolic residue	20	20	15-17
Chloroform extract	20	15	10
Compound 5	17-19	15-17	-
Compound 8	15	10-15	-
Imipenem	25	25	10-15
Ciprofloxacin	25	25	20

antimicrobial activity against *P. aeuroginosa*.

Compound 8 showed moderate antimicrobial activity against the tested Gram +ve *S. aureus* and Gram -ve bacteria *E.coli* but showed no antimicrobial activity against *P. aeuroginosa*. Fortunately, multidrug-resistant *S. aureus* and *E. coli* strains showed sensitivity to all tested samples. The results of agar well diffusion method are shown in (Figure 7 and Table 5).

DISCUSSION

A phytochemical screening of *C. spinosum* aerial parts resulted in the presence of flavonoids, tannins, carbohydrates and/or glycosides, triterpenes and/or sterols and saponins. Also, it revealed the absence of alkaloids, volatiles, anthraquinones and coumarins. The percentages of hydrocarbons and sterols in *C. spinosum* pet-ether extract were 99.57 and 0.3%, respectively. It was found that 6-phenyldodecane (10.03%) and 5-phenyldodecane (9.96%) represented the major hydrocarbons while *β*- Sitosterol (0.30 %) represented only identified sterol.

Concerning the composition of fatty acids content in pet-ether extract, it could be concluded that the percentage of saturated fatty acids (78.76%) represented higher percentage than that of unsaturated fatty acids (9.14%). 14-methyl Pentadecanoic acid (34.8%) and hexadecanoic acid (25.1%) represented the major identified saturated fatty acids while 9-octadecanoic acid (2.62%) represented the major unsaturated fatty acid. These results are in accordance with previous studies of different species of genus *Citharexylum* (Khalifa et al., 2002; Ayers and Sneden, 2002; Shalaby and Bahgat, 2003; Balazs et al., 2006; Ganapaty et al., 2010; Allam, 2014; Mohammad et al., 2016).

Furthermore, the 80% aq. methanolic residue and chloroform extract of *C. spinosum* were purified by employing diversity of chromatographic techniques to afford ten compounds, *β*- Sitosterol Gallic acid and Oleanolic acid were isolated once before from genus *Citharexylum* (Allam, 2014; Khan and Hossain, 2015; Mohammed et al., 2016; Allam, 2017), while *β*- Sitosterol 3-O-*β*-D-glucopyranoside, 6-Methoxy acacetin 7-O-*β*-D-glucopyranoside, Naringenin, 1, 2, 6-tri-O-galloyl-*β*-D-glucopyranoside, Rutin were isolated for the first time from genus *Citharexylum* in addition to two major compounds (5 and 8).

According to chromatographic properties of compound 5 (Rf – value), fluorescent under UV-light and change in color with Fecl3 and Naturstoff reagents compound 5 was expected to be quercetin aglycone (Harborne, 1984). 1H-NMR spectrum showed two characteristic aromatic spin coupling system, the first ABX of three proton resonances at δ 7.71, 7.62, 6.86 were assignable to H-2`,6` and 5` of 3`,4` dihydroxy B-ring. The second coupling system was described as typical AM system of two meta-coupled doublets at δ 6.36 and 6.15 for H-8 and H-6 of 5, 7-dihydroxylated ring- A. The absence of any signals in the aliphatic region proved the aglycone structure. 13C-NMR spectrum exhibited fifteen 13C resonances of the Quercetin moiety with key carbon signals of quercetin nucleus at 175.99 (C-4), 146.62 (C-4`), 144.88 (C-3`), 120.29 (C-6`), 122.79 (C-1`), 114.85 (C-2`) and 114.48 (C-5`) (Agrawal and Bansal, 1989).

Based on the above discussed data and in comparison with previous reported data (Agrawal and Bansal, 1989) and authentic sample, compound 5 was identified as Quercetin which is isolated for the first time from genus *Citharexylum*. The chromatographic properties of compound 8 (R$_f$-values, fluorescence under UV-light and change in color with Fecl$_3$ and natrustoff reagents) and products of acid hydrolysis, was expected to be quercetin rhamnoside (Harborne, 1984).

^{1}H-NMR spectrum showed two characteristic aromatic spin coupling system, the first one ABX of three proton resonances δ7.30, 7.27, 6.88 were assignable to H-2`, 6` and 5` of 3`, 4` dihydroxylated B-ring. The second coupling system was described as typical AM system of two meta-coupled doublets at δ 6.32 and 6.15 for H-8 and H-6, respectively of 5, 7- dihydroxylated ring-A. Concerning the sugar moiety and doublet signal at 5.32 ppm with J=1.3Hz (H-1``), doublet of doublet signal at 4.19 ppm with J=1.4, 3.2 Hz (H-2``) together with a doublet signal at 0.91with J=5.9 Hz (H-6``), were all characteristic for α-L-rhamnopyranoside moiety. In accordance with the earlier discussed data along with a comparison of the previous reported data (Agrawal and Bansal, 1989; Mahmoud et al., 2001), supporting evidence for the structure of glycoside was achieved by ^{13}C-NMR spectrum which showed the characteristic 15 ^{13}C resonance for 3-0-substituted quercetin. The sugar moiety was confirmed as rhamnose from characteristic resonance at δ ppm 102.2 and 16.3 for anomeric carbon and CH$_3$-6``, respectively, together with the rest of carbon resonances for rhamnose carbons. Compound 8 was confirmed as Quercetin 3-O-α-L-rhamnopyranoside (Quercetrin), which is isolated for the first time from genus *Citharexylum*.

Cytotoxic activity of aqueous methanolic residue, chloroform extract and pure compounds (5 and 8) obtained from the aerial parts of *C. spinosum* L. were examined against A2780; a human ovarian cell line using MTT cell prolifiration assay. It was found that, aqueous methanolic residue and chloroform extract had weak cytotoxic activity, pure compound 8 (Quercetrin) had moderate cytotoxic activity, while pure compound 5 (Quercetin) had significant cytotoxic activity. Estimation of analgesic activity done using hot plate test showed that, aqueous methanolic residue and chloroform extract had no analgesic activity. The antipyretic activity of aqueous methanolic residue and chloroform extract were evaluated using Brewer's yeast-induced pyrexia in rats, which found that aqueous methanolic residue at 300 mg/kg had antipyretic activity, while chloroform extract had weak antipyretic activity.

In the present study, the antimicrobial activity was evaluated using agar well diffusion method. For aqueous methanolic residue of *C. spinosum,* results were almost the same against the tested Gram positive and negative bacteria while chloroform extract showed stronger antimicrobial activity against Gram positive than negative bacteria. This is in contrast to the study made by Shalaby and Bahgat (2003), who reported stronger antimicrobial activity against Gram negative bacteria and positive bacteria tested by disc diffusion method. Different species of the genus *Citharexylum* were reported to have antiulcer, antihypertensive and hepatoprotective effects, immunomodulatory, antimicrobial, anti-*Schistosoma mansoni* activities, antioxidant nephroprotective, radical scavenging, cytotoxic activities and regulating immediate type of allergic reaction (Shin et al., 2000; Khalifa et al., 2002; Shalaby and Bahgat, 2003; Bahgat et al., 2005; Khan and Siddique, 2012; Kadry et al., 2013; Allam, 2014).

REFERENCES

Ahmad FB, Sallehuddin NKNM, Assim Z (2010). Chemical constituents and antiviral study of *Goniothalamus velutinus*. J. Fund. Sci. 6(1):72-75.

Aboutabl EA, Hashem FA, Sleem AA, Maamoon AA (2008). Flavonoids, anti-inflammatory activity and cytotoxicity of *Macfadyena unguis-cat* L. Afr. J. Trad. Compl. Alt. Med. 5(1):18-26.

Agrawal PK, Bansal MC (1989). Flavonoid glycosides. Carbon-13 NMR of flavonoids. pp. 283-364.

Allam AE (2014). Stimulation of melanogenisis by polyphenolic compounds from *Citharexylum quadrangular* in B16F1 murine melanoma cells. Bull. Pharm. Sci. Assiut Univ. 37(2):105-115.

Allam AE (2017). Antiallergic polyphenols from *Citharexylum spinosum*. Trends Phytochem. Res. 1(3):129-134.

Armitage P (1971). Statistical methods in medicinal research, 1st Ed. 17.

Ayers S, Sneden AT (2002). Caudatosides AF: New Iridoid Glucosides from *Citharexylum caudatum*. J. Nat. Prod. 65(11):1621-1626.

Bahgat M, Shalaby NM, Ruppel A, Maghraby AS (2005). Humoral and cellular immune responses induced in mice by purified iridoid mixture that inhibits penetration of *Schistosoma mansoni cercariae* upon topical treatment of mice tails. J. Egypt Soc. Parasitol. 35(2):597-613.

Balazs B, Tóth G, Duddeck H, Soliman HS (2006). Iridoid and lignan glycosides from *Citharexylum spinosum* L. Nat. Prod. Res. 20(2):201-205.

Balbaa SI, Hilal SH, Zaki AY (1981). *Medicinal plant constituents. 3rd ed.*, General organization for university and school books, Cairo. P 383.

Barakat HH, Nawwar MA, Buddrus J, Linscheid M (1987). A phenolic glyceride and two phenolic aldehydes from roots of *Tamarix nilotia*. Phytochemistry 26:1837-1838.

British Pharmacopea (1993). Her Majesty's Stationary Office, London.

Dahiya BS (1979). Systematic Botany (Taxonomy of Angiosperms). Kalyani Publishers, Ludhiana, Printed in India. pp. 243-247.

El-Said ME, Amer MM (1965). Oils, fats, waxes and surfactants. Anglo-Egyptian Bookshop, Cairo. pp. 130-132.

Evans WC (1996). Trease and Evan's Pharmacognosy. Edn 14, WB Saunders Company Ltd, London, Philadelphia, Toronto, Sydney, Tokyo. pp. 47-48.

Farshchi A, Ghiasi G, Malek Khatabi P, Farzaee H, Niayesh A (2009). Antinociceptive effect of promethazine in mice. Iran. J. Basic Med. Sci. 12(3):140-145.

Ganapaty S, Rao DV, Pannakal ST (2010). A phenethyl bromo ester from *Citharexylum fruticosum*. Nat. Prod. Commun. 5(3):399-402.

Haddock EA, Gupta RK, Al-Shafi SM, Haslam E (1982). The metabolism of gallic acid and hexahydroxy diphenic acid in plants. Part 1. Introduction of naturally occurring galloyl esters. J. Chem. Soc. Perkin Trans. 1:2515.

Haggag EG, Abdelhady MI, Kamal AM (2013). Phenolic content of Ruprechtia salicifolia leaf and its immunomodulatory, anti-inflammatory, anticancer and antibacterial activity. J. Pharm. Res. 6(7):696-703.

Hansen MB, Nielsen SE and Berg K (1989). Re-examination and further development of a precise and rapid dye method for measuring cell growth/cell kill. J. Immunol. Methods 119:203-210.

Harborne JB (1984). Phytochemical methods: A guide to modern technique of plant analysis, 2nd ed, Champan and Hall Ltd, London, UK. pp. 37-99.

Kadry SM, Mohamed AM, Farrag EM, Fayed DB (2013). Influence of some micronutrients and *Citharexylum quadrangular* extract against liver fibrosis in *Schistosoma mansoni* infected mice. Afr. J. Pharm. Pharmacol. 7(38):2628-2638.

Kamal AM, Abdelhady MIS, Elmorsy EM, Mady MS, Abdel-Khalik SM (2012). Phytochemical and biological investigation of leaf extracts of *Podocarpus polstachya* resulted in isolation of novel polyphenolic compound. Life Sci. J. 9:1126-1135.

Khalifa TI, El-Gindi OD, Ammar HA, El-Naggar DM (2002). Iridoid Glycosides from *Citharexylum quadrangulare*. Asian J. Chem. 14:197-202.

Khan NMU, Hossain MS (2015). Scopoletin and β- sitosterol glucoside from roots of *Ipomoea digitata*. J. Pharmacogn. Phytochem., 4(2), 5-7

Khan MR, Siddique F (2012). Antioxidant effects of *Citharexylum spinosum* in CCl₄ induced nephrotoxicity in rat. Exp. Toxicol. Pathol. 64(4):349-355.

Lavich TR, Cordeiro RSB, Silva PMR, Martins MA (2005). A novel hot-plate test sensitive to hyperalgesic stimuli and non-opioid analgesics. Braz. J. Med. Biol. Res. 38(3):445-451.

Lawrence GHM (1951). Taxonomy of Vascular Plants. Oxford and IBH publishing co. The Macmillan Company, New York. pp. 686-688.

Loux JJ, Depalma PD, Yankell SL (1972). Antipyretic testing of aspirin in rats. Toxicol. Appl. Pharmacol. 22(4):672-675.

Mabry TJ, Markham KR, Thomas MB (1970). The systematic identification of flavonoids, Springer Verlag. New York. pp. 4-35.

Mahmoud II, Marzouk MSA, Moharram FA, El-Gindi MR,Hassan AMK (2001). Acylated flavonol glycosides from *Eugenia jambolana* leaves. Phytochemistry 58:1239-1244.

Markham KR (1982). *Techniques of flavnoids identifaictions*. Academic press, London. P 24.

Marzouk MSA, Soliman FA, Shehta IA, Rabie M, Fawzy GA (2004). Biologically active hydrolysable tannins from *Jassiaea repens* L. Bull. Fac. Pharm. Cairo Uni. 42(3):119-131.

Mohammed MH, Hamed ANE, Khalil HE, Kamel MS (2014). Botanical Studies of the Stem of *Citharexylum quadrangulare* Jacq., cultivated in Egypt. J. Pharmacogn. Phytochem. 3(2):58-62.

Mohammed MHH, Hamed ANE, Khalil HE, Kamel MS (2016). Phytochemical and pharmacological studies of *Citharexylum quadrangulare* Jacq. leaves. J. Med. Plants Res. 10(18):232-241.

National committee for Clinical Laboratory Standard (NCCLS) (1997). Antimicrobial Susceptibility of flavobacteria. P 41.

Onoja E, Ndukwe IG (2013). Isolation of oleanolic acid from chloroform extract of *Borreria stachydea* [(DC) Hutch. and Dalziel]. J. Nat. Prod. Plant Resour. 3(2):57-60.

Pini LA, Vitale G, Ottani A, Sandrini M (1997). Naloxone-reversible antinociception by paracetamol in the rat. J. Pharmacol. Exp. Ther. 280(2):934-940.

Rahbar M, Diba K (2010). *In vitro* activity of cranberry extract against etiological agents of urinary tract infections. Afr. J. Pharm. Pharmacol. 4(5):286-288.

Rahmana SMM, Muktaa ZA, Hossainb MA (2009). Isolation and characterization of β-sitosterol-D-glycoside from petroleum extract of the leaves of *Ocimum sanctum* L. Asian J. Food Agro. Ind. 2(1):39-43.

Seebacher W, Simic N, Weis R, Saf R, Kunert O (2003). Complete assignments of ¹H and ¹³C NMR resonances of oleanolic acid, 18α-oleanolic acid, ursolic acid and their 11-oxo derivatives. Mag. Res. Chem. 41(8):636-638.

Shalaby NMN, Bahgat M (2003). Phytochemical and some biological studies of *Citharexylum quadrangulare* Jacq. Chem. Nat. Microbiol. Prod. 4:219-228.

Shin TY, Kim SH, Lim JP, Suh ES, Jeong HJ, Kim BD, Park EJ, Hwang WJ, Rye DG, Baek SH, An NH, Kim HM (2000). Effect of Vitex *rotundifolia* on immediate-type allergic reaction. J. Ethnopharmacol. 72(3):443.

Smith I (1960). Chromatographic and electrophoretic techniques. Heinman, London. pp. 1-246.

Stahl E (1969). Thin layer chromatography. 2nd ed., Springer Verlag, Berlin, Heidelberg, New York.

Starr FK, Starr, Loope L (2006). *Citharexylum spinosum* (tree). Plants of Hawaii Report. National Biological Information Infrastructure and Invasive Specialist Group.

Trease GE, Evans WC (1989). A text book of Pharmacognsy. 11th ed. Brailliar Tindall Ltd. London. pp. 176-180.

Turner RJ, Wasson E (1997). Botanica. Mynah Publishing, Australia, NSW.

Wagner WL, Herbst DR, Sohmer SH (1999). Manual of the Flowering Plants of Hawaii. University of Hawaii and Bishop Museum Press, Honolulu, HI.

Vogel AI (1961). Practical organic chemistry. 3rd Edition, Longmans pruvate Ltd., Calcutta, Bombay, Madras. pp. 467-468.

Analysis of bioactive chemical compounds of *Nigella sativa* using gas chromatography-mass spectrometry

Mohammed Yahya Hadi[1], Ghaidaa Jihadi Mohammed[2] and Imad Hadi Hameed[3]*

[1]College of Biotechnology, Al-Qasim Green University, Iraq.
[2]College of Science, Al-Qadisia University, Iraq.
[3]Department of Biology, Babylon University, Iraq.

Phytochemicals are chemical compounds often referred to as secondary metabolites. Twenty eight bioactive phytochemical compounds were identified in the methanolic extract of *Nigella sativa*. The identification of phytochemical compounds is based on the peak area, retention time molecular weight, and molecular formula. Gas chromatography-mass spectrometry (GC-MS) analysis of *Nigella sativa* revealed the existence of the ß-Pinene, D-Glucose, 6-O-α-Dgalactopyranosyl, O-Cymene, DL-Arabinose, Trans-4-methoxy thujane, 2-Propyl-tetrahydropyran-3-ol, Terpinen-4-ol, α- D-Glucopyranoside, O-α-D-glucopyranosyl-(1.fwdarw.3)-ß-D-fruc, Thymoquinone, 2-Isopropylidene-5-methylhex-4-enal, Limonen-6-ol, pivalate, Longifolene, 2-(4-Nitrobutyryl)cyclooctanone, ß-Bisabolene, 1,1-Diphenyl-4-phenylthiobut-3-en-1-ol, Phenol, 4-methoxy-2,3,6-trimethyl, Pyrrolidin-2-one-3ß-(propanoic acid, methyl ester),5-methylene-4α, Cholestan-3-ol, 2-methylene-,(3ß,5α), I-(+)-Ascorbic acid 2,6-dihexadecanoate, 9,12-Octadecadienoic acid (Z,Z)-, methyl ester, 1-Heptatriacotanol, 10,13-Eicosadienoic acid, methyl ester, E,E,Z-1,3,12-Nonadecatriene-5,14-diol, 9-Octadecenamide,(Z), 2H-Benzo[f]oxireno[2,3-E]benzofuran-8(9H)-one,9-[2-(dimethylar, Phthalic acid, decyl oct-3-yl ester, 1,2-Benzenedicarboxylic acid, bis(8-methylnonyl) ester and Stiqmasterol.

Key words: Gas chromatography-mass spectrometry, Fourier-transform infrared spectroscopy, *Nigella sativa*, phytochemicals.

INTRODUCTION

Nigella sativa L. (Ranunculaceae) is an annual herbaceous plant native to (and cultivated in) Southwest Asia, and cultivated and naturalized in Europe and North Africa (Al-Johar et al., 2008). The seeds and seed oil have been used as a diuretic, appetizer, hemorrhagic and anti-dandruff therapy in folk medicine (Al-Othman et al., 2006). *N. sativa* L. commonly known as Kalonji in Hindi, a member of Ranunculaceae family, also known as the black cumin seeds is one of the most revered medicinal seeds in history. It is an annual aromatic plant and its cultivation is traced back more than 3000 to the kingdom of the Assyrians and ancient Egyptians (Ashraf et al., 2006; Hameed et al., 2015a). *N. sativa* taxonomic classification (Ashraf, 2011), depicts it is a flowering

*Corresponding author. E-mail: imad_dna@yahoo.com.

dicotyledon plant belonging to family Ranunculaceae under kingdom plantae. Morphology *N. sativa* is an annual medicinal herb, about 30 to 60 cm high (Boskabady et al., 2007; Jasim et al., 2015), with finely divided, linear leaves. The flowers are usually pale blue and white, with 5 to 10 petals. The fruit is a large inflated capsule that composed of 3 to 7 united follicles, each containing numerous black trigonal seeds (Chaudhry and Tariq, 2008; Hameed et al., 2015b).

The black kalonji seeds possess the anthelmintic, insecticidal, antimalarial, antibacterial, antifungal, and antitumor effects. There are also reports that black seeds possess diuretic, carminative, digestive and antiseptic properties (Burits and Burcar, 2000; Ali and Blunden, 2003; Saleh, 2006; Abdulelah and Abidin, 2007; Ali et al., 2008). The seeds have also been used traditionally for centuries in the Middle East, Far East, and some Mediterranean and European countries for the treatment of different ailments, such as diabetes, hypertension, cardiac diseases, hemorrhoids, and sexual diseases and as an abortifacient (Kanter, 2008; Iqbal et al., 2010).

Seeds of *N. sativa* are reported to contain amino acids, carbohydrates, fixed and volatile oils. The yield of black seed fixed oil ranges from 22.0 to 40.35% (Ali and Blunden, 2003; Cheikh-Rouhou et al., 2007; Altameme et al., 2015a). The extracts of *N. sativa* (Black seeds) have been used by patients to suppress coughs, disintegrate renal calculi (Hashem and El-Kiey, 1982), retard the carcinogenic process, treat abdominal pain, diarrhea, flatulence, and polio (Enomoto et al., 2001), exert choleretic and uricosuric activities, anti-inflammatory and antioxidant effects (Mansour et al., 2002; Altameme et al., 2015b). Besides, the essential oil was shown to have antihelminthic, antischistosomal (Mahmoud et al., 2002), antimicrobial (Aboul-Ela et al., 1996), and antiviral.

MATERIALS AND METHODS

Preparation of extract

N. sativa were purchased from local market in Hilla city, middle of Iraq. After thorough cleaning and removal of foreign materials, the seeds were stored in airtight container to avoid the effect of humidity and then stored at room temperature until further use (Hameed et al., 2015c; Hamza et al., 2015). *N. sativa* seeds are washed with water, dried and ground into powder. *N. sativa* seeds powder was macerated using methanol for 1 × 24 h. Whatman No.1 filter paper was used to separate the extract of plant. The filtrates were used for further phytochemical analysis. It was again filtered through sodium sulphate in order to remove the traces of moisture (Hussein et al., 2015).

Gas chromatography-mass spectrum (GC-MS) analysis

The GC-MS analysis of the plant extract was made in a Agilent 7890 A instrument under computer control at 70 eV. About 1 µl of the methanol extract was injected into the GC-MS using a micro syringe and the scanning was done for 45 min. As the compounds were separated, they eluted from the column and entered a detector which was capable of creating an electronic signal whenever a compound was detected (Imad et al., 2014a; Hameed et al., 2015d). The greater the concentration in the sample, the bigger the signal obtained which was then processed by a computer. The time from when the injection was made (Initial time) to when elution occurred is referred to as the retention time (RT). While the instrument was run, the computer generated a graph from the signal called chromatogram. Each of the peaks in the chromatogram represented the signal created when a compound eluted from the gas chromatography column into the detector (Mohammed and Imad, 2013). The x-axis showed the RT and the y-axis measured the intensity of the signal to quantify the component in the sample injected. As individual compounds eluted from the gas chromatographic column, they entered the electron ionization (mass spectroscopy) detector, where they were bombarded with a stream of electrons causing them to break apart into fragments. The fragments obtained were actually charged ions with a certain mass .The mass/charge (M/Z) ratio obtained was calibrated from the graph obtained, which was called as the mass spectrum graph which is the fingerprint of a molecule (Imad et al., 2014b). Before analyzing the extract using GC-MS, the temperature of the oven, the flow rate of the gas used and the electron gun were programmed initially. The temperature of the oven was maintained at 100°C. Helium gas was used as a carrier as well as an eluent. The flow rate of helium was set at 1 ml/min. The electron gun of mass detector liberated electrons having energy of about 70eV.The column employed here for the separation of components was Elite 1(100% dimethyl poly siloxane). The identity of the components in the extracts was assigned by the comparison of their retention indices and mass spectra fragmentation patterns with those stored on the computer library and also with published literatures. Compounds were identified by comparing their spectra to those of the Wiley and NIST/EPA/NIH mass spectral libraries (Kareem et al., 2015; Imad et al., 2014c).

RESULTS AND DISCUSSION

Preparation of the extract was done by maceration method. Maceration was done using the appropriate solvent with several times shaking or stirring at room temperature (Rader et al., 2007). Maceration is a method that is suitable for compounds that do not withstand heating at high temperatures (Ramaa et al., 2006). The aim is to attract the chemical components based on the principle of mass transfer of substance into the solvent component, where the movement began to occur at the interface layer and then diffuses into the solvent (Sethi et al., 2008). Identification of the structure using a mass spectrometer conducted to determine the compounds contained in the samples analyzed can be seen from the relative abundance of mass fragments of molecules (m/e) of the molecular ion (M +). The more stable a molecular fragment that is formed is, then the fragment will be at a relative abundance of large and have a longer lifespan (Vuorela et al., 2004; Shama et al., 2009).

Gas chromatography and mass spectroscopy analysis of compounds was carried out in methanolic extract as shown in Table 1. The GC-MS chromatogram of the 28 peaks of the compounds detected are shown in Figure 1. Chromatogram GC-MS analysis of the methanol extract

Table 1. Major phytochemical compounds identified in methanolic extract of *Nigella sativa*.

S/N	Phytochemical compound	RT (min)	Formula	Molecular weight	Exact mass	Chemical structure	MS Fragment- ions	Pharmacological actions
1	ß-Pinene	3.173	$C_{10}H_{16}$	136	136.1252		53, 69, 93, 121	*Anti-inflammatory*
2	D-Glucose ,6-O-α-Dgalactopyranosyl	3.613	$C_{12}H_{22}O_{11}$	342	342.11621		60, 73, 85, 110, 126, 182, 212, 261	Anticoagulant, *anti*-infl 3matory, psychotomimetic and anticancer activities
3	O-Cymene	3.939	$C_{10}H_{14}$	134	134.10955		51, 58, 65, 77, 91, 103, 119, 134	*Anti-oxidant activity*
4	DL-Arabinose	4.815	$C_{5}H_{10}O_{5}$	150	150.052823		55, 60, 73, 85, 96, 119, 132, 149	*Antivirus* activity
5	Trans -4-methoxy thujane	4.952	$C_{11}H_{20}O$	168	168.151415		55, 59, 72, 81, 85, 93, 107, 125, 136, 153, 168	Antibacterial and *anti*-Candida *activities*

Table 1. Cont'd

#	Name							Activity
6	2-Propyl-tetrahydropyran-3-ol	5.742	$C_8H_{16}O_2$	144	144.115029		55, 73, 101, 116, 144	*Anti*-allergenic and *anti*-bacterial
7	Terpinen-4-ol	6.097	$C_{10}H_{18}O$	154	154.135765		55, 59, 71, 81, 86, 93, 111, 121, 136, 154	*Anti*-tumoral *activity*
8	α-D-Glucopyranoside,O-α-D-glucopyranosyl-(1.fwdarw.3)-ß-D-fruc	6.697	$C_{18}H_{32}O_{16}$	504	504.169035		60, 73, 85, 97, 113, 126, 145, 187	Anticarcinogenic antimutagenic, antineoplastic and *anti*-thrombotic
9	Thymoquinone	7.081	$C_{10}H_{12}O_2$	164	164.08373		53, 68, 77, 93, 96, 108, 121, 136, , 149, 164	*Anti*-cancer activity
10	2-Isopropylidene-5-methylhex-4-enal	7.378	$C_{10}H_{16}O$	152	152.120115		55, 67, 81, 95, 109, 137, 152	Good antioxidant and *anti*-inflammatory properties

Table 1. Cont'd

11	Limonen -6-ol ,pivalate	8.717	$C_{15}H_{24}O_2$	236	236.17763		57, 93, 107, 134, 185, 236	Antioxidant and *anti-* inflammatory
12	Longifolene	9.158	$C_{15}H_{24}$	204	204.1878		55, 67, 79, 94, 107, 119, 133, 147, 161, 175, 189, 204	Antifeedant, *anti* tumor, *anti* inflammatory, antioxidant and antibacterial
13	2-(4-Nitrobutyryl)cyclooctanone	9.839	$C_{12}H_{19}NO_4$	241	241.131408		55, 69, 97, 123, 153, 193, 213, 241	*Anti*-tumor activity
14	ß-Bisabolene	10.302	$C_{15}H_{24}$	204	204.1878		55, 69, 93, 109, 135, 161, 189, 204	*Anti*-ulcer activity

Table 1. Cont'd

	Name	RT	Formula	MW	Exact mass	Structure	m/z	Activity
15	1,1-Diphenyl-4-phenylthiobut-3-en-1-ol	10.440	$C_{22}H_{20}OS$	332	332.123486		55, 81, 105, 121, 135, 150, 179, 205, 233, 314	*Anti*-inflammatory properties
16	Phenol, 4-methoxy-2,3,6-trimethyl	11.069	$C_{10}H_{14}O_2$	166	166.09938		53, 67, 77, 83, 91, 107, 123, 135, 151, 166	Antioxidant, anticancer, *anti* inflammatory and sex hormone *activity*
17	Pyrrolidin -2-one-3ß-(propanoic acid , methyl ester),5-methylene-4α	12.625	$C_{16}H_{25}NO_5$	311	311.173273		57, 81, 110, 136, 149, 164, 196, 224, 255, 280, 311	Unknown
18	Cholestan-3-ol, 2-methylene-,(3ß,5α)	12.980	$C_{28}H_{48}O$	400	400.370516		69, 81, 95, 149, 175, 227, 260, 315, 400	*Anti*-inflammatory
19	l-(+)-Ascorbic acid 2,6-dihexadecanoate	15.246	$C_{38}H_{68}O_8$	652	652.49142		57, 73, 85, 98, 115, 129, 143, 157, 185, 199, 213, 227, 256, 297, 322, 353	Antioxidant, cardio protective, cancer preventive, flavour and *anti*-infertility

Table 1. Cont'd

					Structure	Fragment ions	Activity
20	9,12-Octadecadienoic acid (Z,Z)-, methyl ester	16.636	$C_{19}H_{34}O_2$	294	294.25588		55, 67, 81, 95, 109, 123, 150, 164, 178, 191, 220, 263, 294	Analgesic, *anti*-inflammatory and ulcerogenic
21	1-Heptatriacotanol	17.867	$C_{37}H_{76}O$	536	536.58962		55, 81, 95, 147, 161, 190, 257	Antioxidant, anticancer, *anti* inflammatory and to sex hormone *activity*
22	10,13-Eicosadienoic acid , methyl ester	18.387	$C_{21}H_{38}O_2$	322	322.28718		55, 67, 95, 109, 124, 150, 164, 192, 224, 248, 291, 322	*Anti*-bacterial and *anti*-candidal *activities*
23	E,E,Z-1,3,12-Nonadecatriene-5,14-diol	18.742	$C_{19}H_{34}O_2$	294	294.25588		55, 81, 95, 149, 262, 294	Antimicrobial *activity*
24	9-Octadecenamide ,(Z)	18.960	$C_{15}H_{35}NO$	281	281.271864		59, 72, 83, 114, 184, 212, 264, 281	*Anti*-inflammatory activity and antibacterial activity
25	2H-Benzo[f]oxireno[2,3-E]benzofuran-8(9H)-one,9-[[[2-(dimethylar	19.589	$C_{19}H_{32}N_2O_3$	336	336.241293		58, 81, 109, 149, 173, 204, 233, 278, 336	Unknown
26	Phthalic acid , decyl oct-3-yl ester	23.686	$C_{26}H_{42}O_4$	418	418.30831		57, 104, 149, 167, 193, 251, 307	*Anti*-inflammatory

Table 1. Cont'd

| 27 | 1,2-Benzenedicarboxylic acid , bis(8-methylnonyl) ester | 24.012 | $C_{28}H_{46}O_4$ | 446 | 446.33961 | 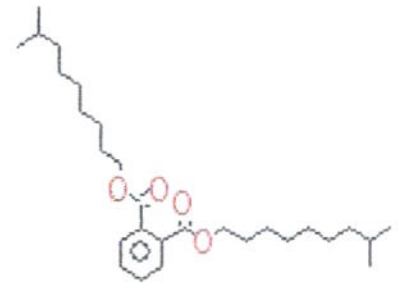 71, 99, 149, 167, 193, 228, 289, 307, 321, 361, 403, 446 | Antibacterial *activity* |
| 28 | Stiqmasterol | 29.007 | $C_{29}H_{48}O$ | 412 | 412.370516 | 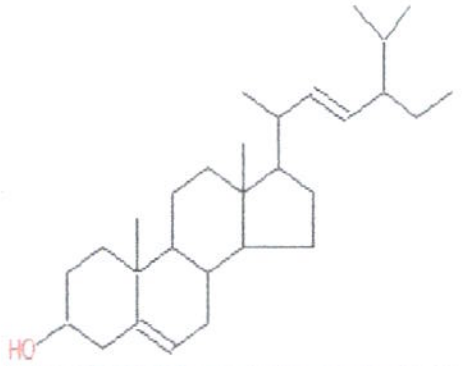 55, 69, 83, 133, 213, 255, 300, 351, 369, 412 | *Biological activities* such as *anti*-diabetic, *anti*-neoplastic, *anti*-hypertensive and *anti*-retroviral |

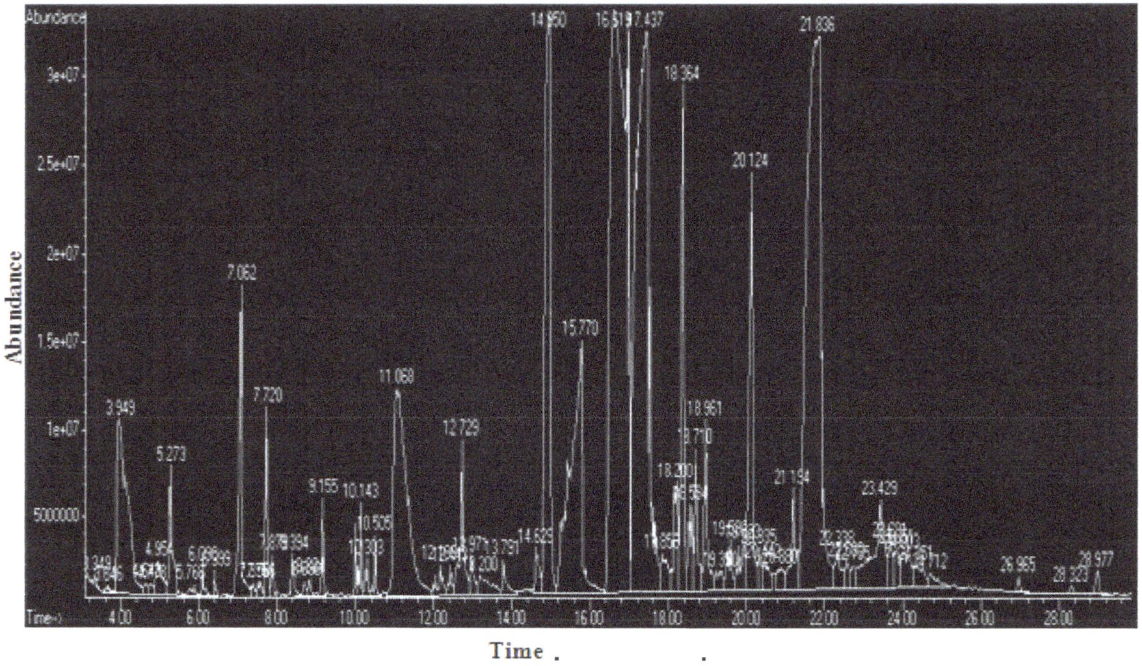

Figure 1. GC-MS chromatogram of methanolic seed extract of *Nigella sativa*.

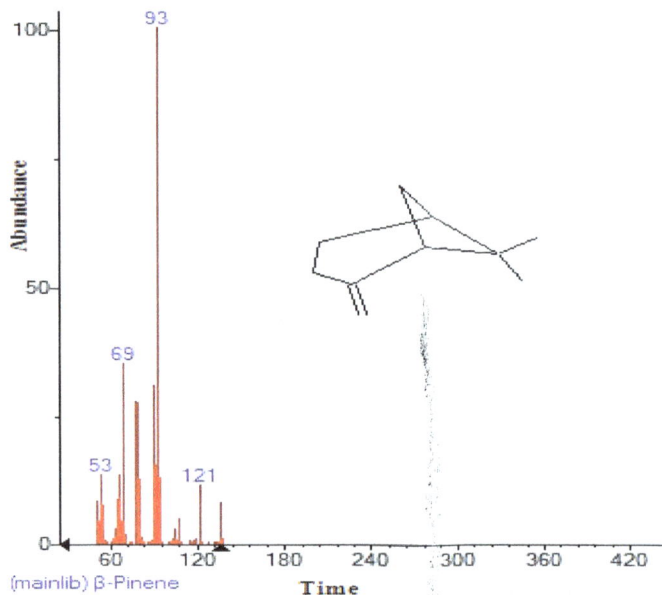

Figure 2. Structure of ß-Pinene present in the methanolic seeds extract of *Nigella sativa* by using GC-MS analysis.

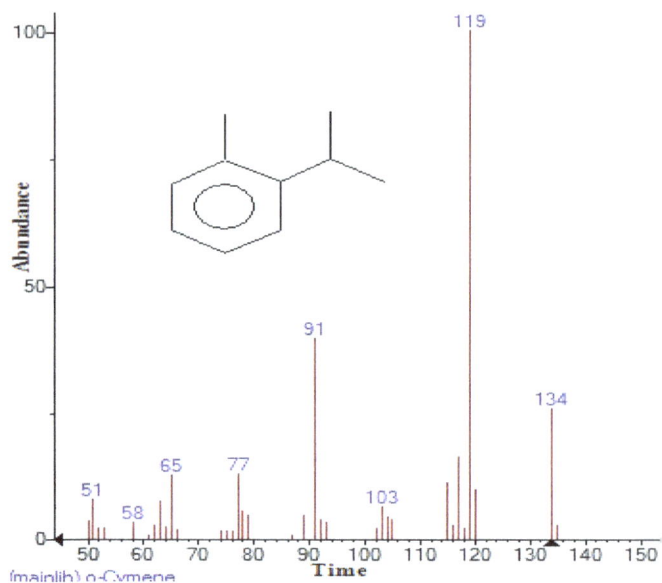

Figure 3. Structure of D-Glucose, 6-O-α-Dgalactopyranosyl present in the methanolic seeds extract of *Nigella sativa* by using GC-MS analysis.

of *N. sativa* showed the presence of 28 major peaks and the components corresponding to the peaks were determined as follows. The first setup peak were determined to be ß-Pinene (Figure 2). The second peak showed D-Glucose, 6-O-α-Dgalactopyranosyl (Figure 3). The next peaks was considered to be O-Cymene, DL-Arabinose, Trans -4-methoxy thujane, 2-Propyl-tetrahydropyran-3-ol, Terpinen-4-ol, α- D-Glucopyranoside, O-α-D-glucopyranosyl-(1.fwdarw.3)-ß-

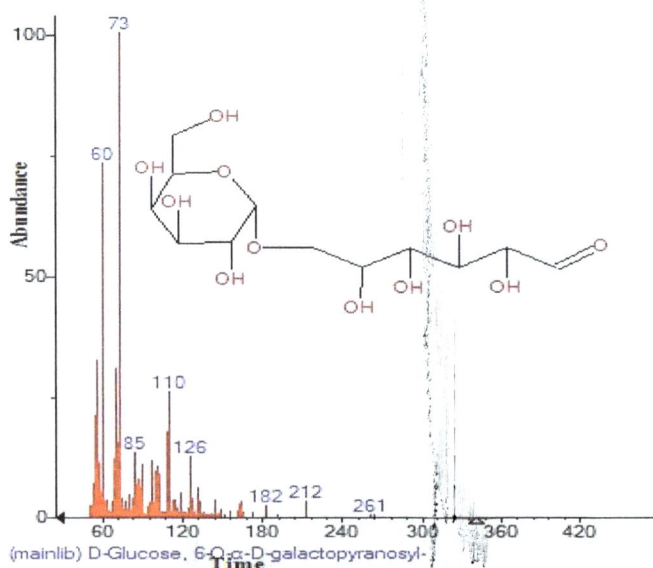

Figure 4. Structure of o-Cymene present in the methanolic seeds extract of *Nigella sativa* by using GC-MS analysis.

D-fruc, Thymoquinone, 2-Isopropylidene-5-methylhex-4 enal, Limonen-6-ol, pivalate, Longifolene, 2-(4- Nitrobutyryl cyclooctanone, ß-Bisabolene, 1,1-Diphenyl-4 phenylthiobut-3-en-1-ol, Phenol, 4-methoxy-2,3,6 trimethyl, Pyrrolidin -2-one-3ß-(propanoic acid, methy ester),5-methylene-4α, Cholestan-3-ol, 2-methylene ,(3ß,5α), l-(+)-Ascorbic acid 2,6-dihexadecanoate, 9,12 Octadecadienoic acid (Z,Z)-, methyl ester, 1 Heptatriacotanol, 10,13-Eicosadienoic acid, methyl ester E,E,Z-1,3,12-Nonadecatriene-5,14-diol, 9 Octadecenamide,(Z), 2H-Benzo[f]oxireno[2,3 E]benzofuran-8(9H)-one,9-[[[2-(dimethylar, Phthalic acid decyl oct-3-yl ester, 1,2-Benzenedicarboxylic acid, bis(8 methylnonyl) ester and Stiqmasterol (Figures 4 to 30) Plants are considered to be one of the natural bases fo the production of bioactive compounds, many of whicl are used to support health and fight against pathologica conditions and many of them are marketed as food o herbal medicines (Shama et al., 2009). The usage o herbal medicine has amplified dramatically for various diseases amongst general people over last few years no only because of their easy accessibility withou prescription, low cost and appointment to the health care specialists and more with the belief that natural remedies have less lethal effects as compared to syntheti medicines (Ashraf et al., 2011). A qualitative investigatior of *N. sativa* has revealed the presence of sterols triterpenes, tannins, flavanoids, cardiac glycosides alkaloids, saponins, volatile oils, volatile bases glucosinolates and anthraquinones (A1-Yahya, 1986) Qualitative evaluation of the black seed oil via capillary GC-MS technique has enabled the identification of 6 compounds, when classified into various functiona

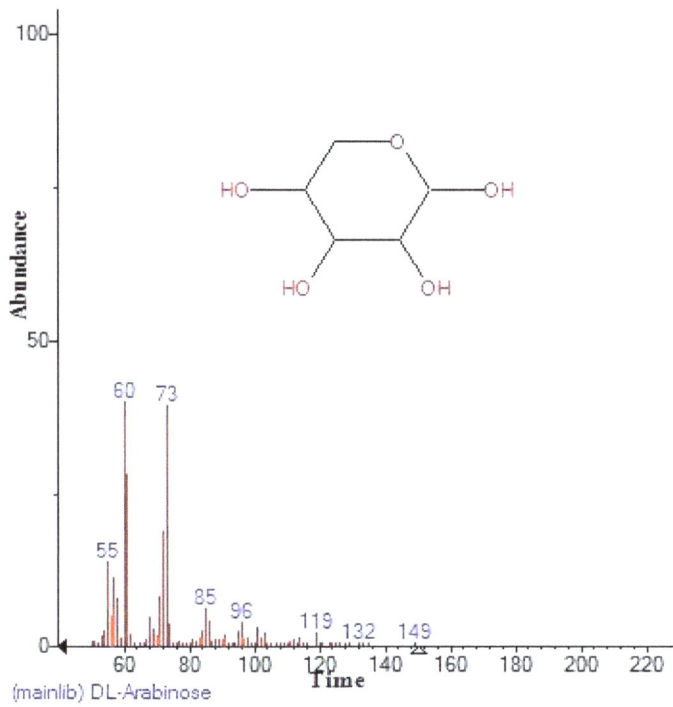

Figure 5. Structure of DL-Arabinose present in the methanolic seeds extract of *Nigella sativa* by using GC-MS analysis.

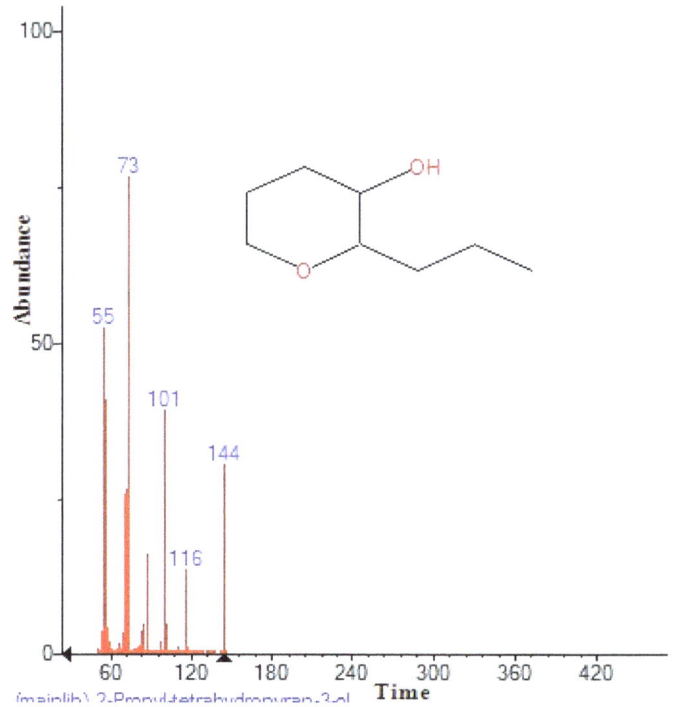

Figure 7. Structure of 2-Propyl-tetrahydropyran-3-ol present in the methanolic seeds extract of *Nigella sativa* by using GC-MS analysis.

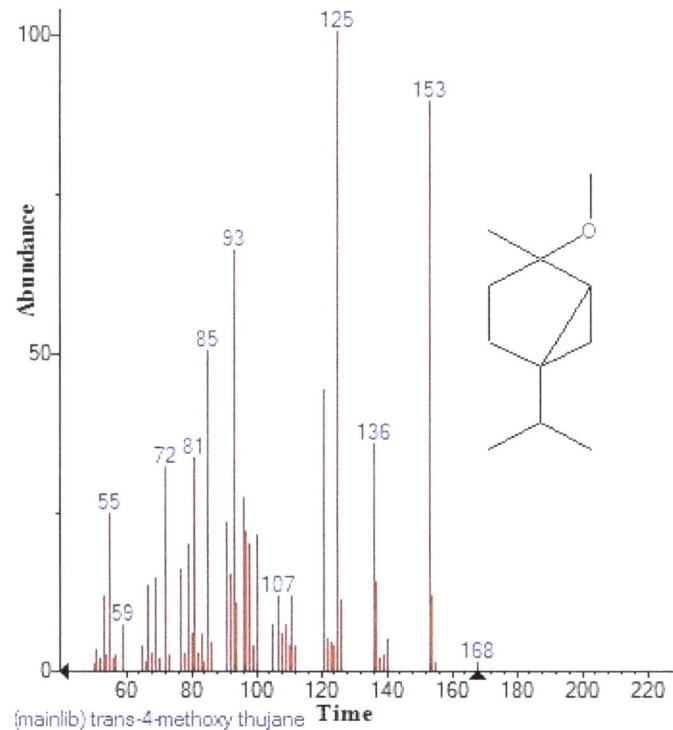

Figure 6. Structure of Trans -4-methoxy thujane present in the methanolic seeds extract of *Nigella sativa* by using GC-MS analysis.

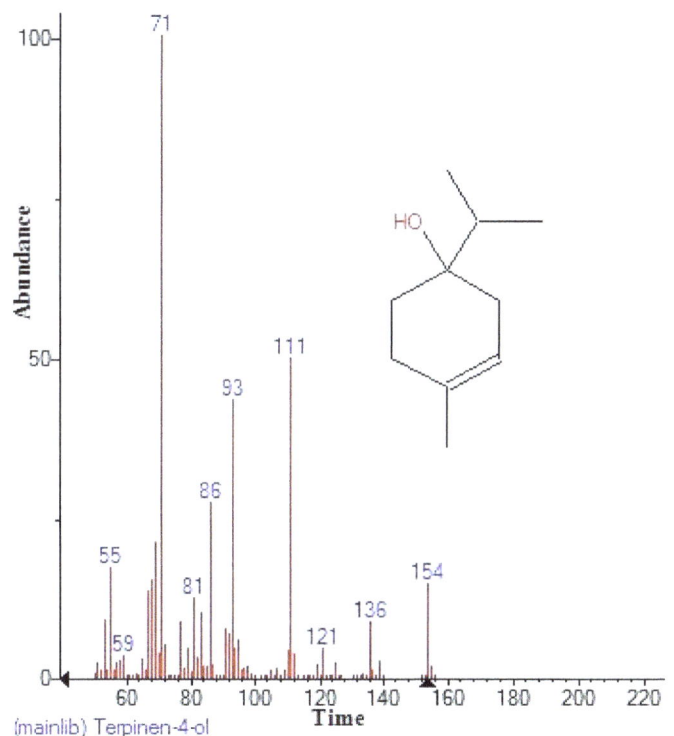

Figure 8. Structure of Terpinen-4-ol present in the methanolic seeds extract of *Nigella sativa* by using GC-MS analysis.

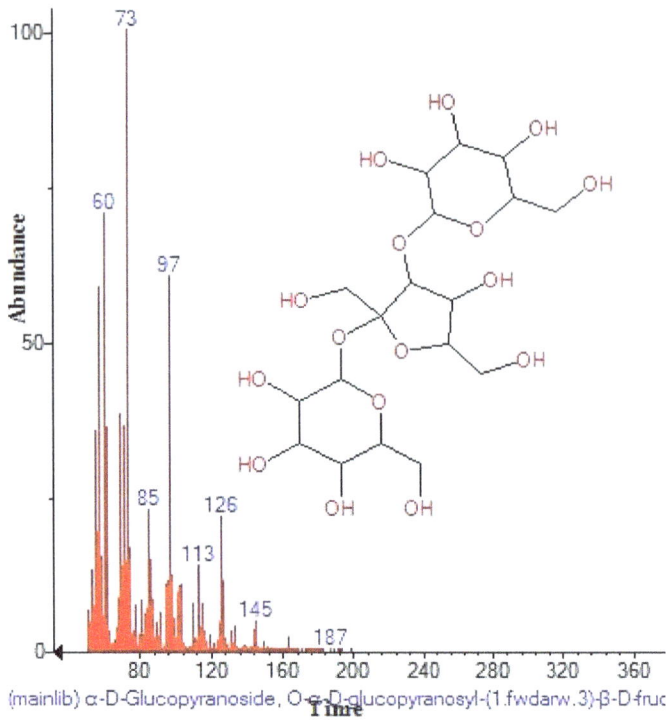

Figure 9. Structure of α- D-Glucopyranoside,O-α-D-glucopyranosyl-(1.fwdarw.3)-ß-D-fruc present in the methanolic seeds extract of *Nigella sativa* by using GC-MS analysis.

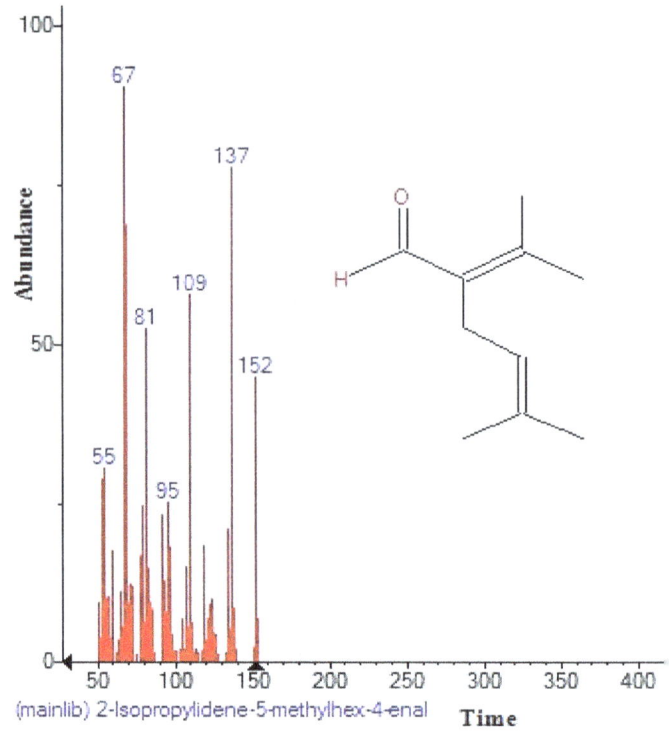

Figure 11. Structure of 2-Isopropylidene-5-methylhex-4-enal present in the methanolic seeds extract of *Nigella sativa* by using GC-MS analysis.

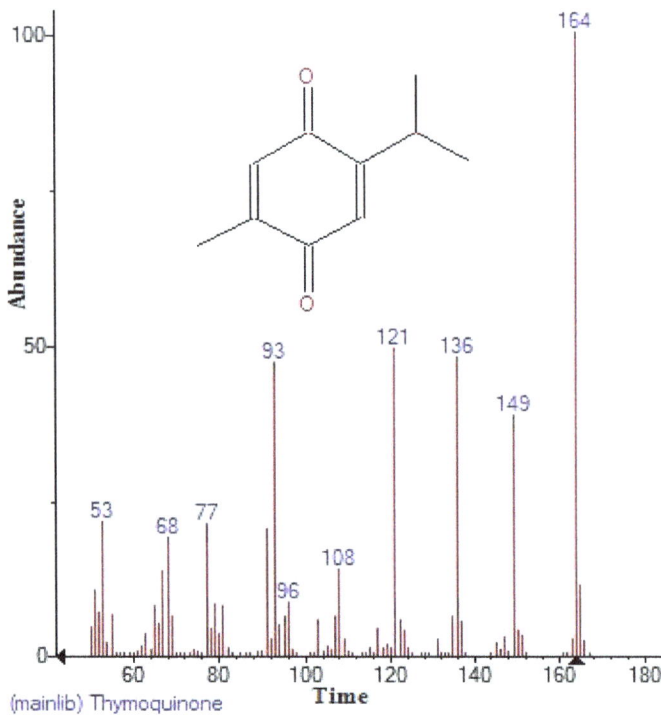

Figure 10. Structure of Thymoquinone present in the methanolic seeds extract of *Nigella sativa* by using GC-MS analysis.

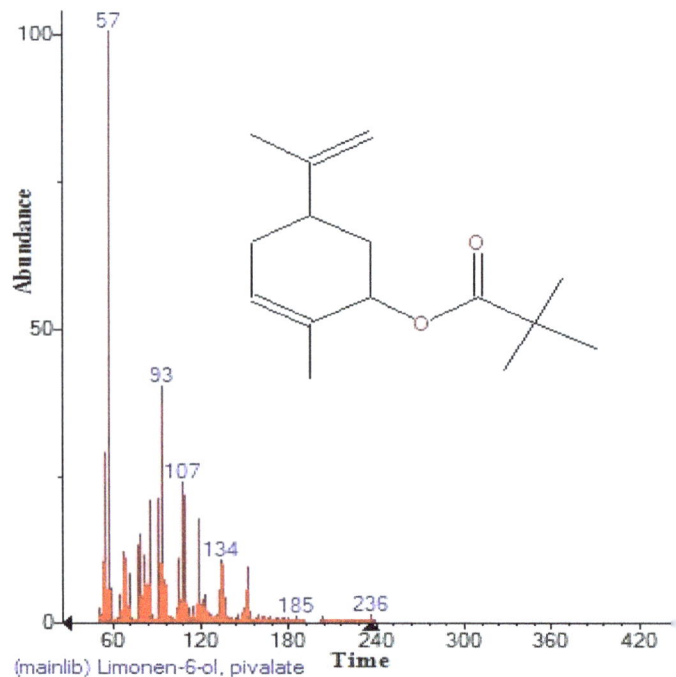

Figure 12. Structure of Limonen -6-ol ,pivalate present in the methanolic seeds extract of *Nigella sativa* by using GC-MS analysis.

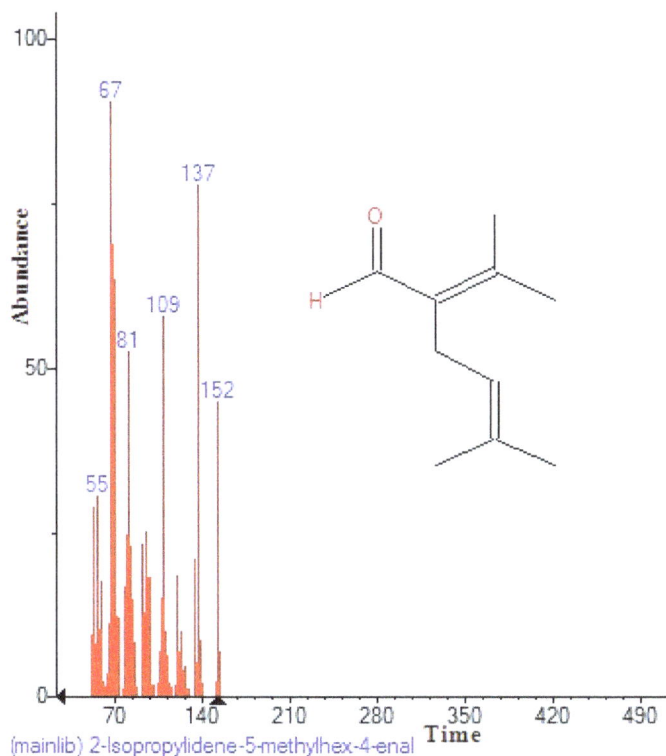

Figure 13. Structure of 2-Isopropylidene-5- methylhex-4-enal present in the methanolic seeds extract of *Nigella sativa* by using GC-MS analysis.

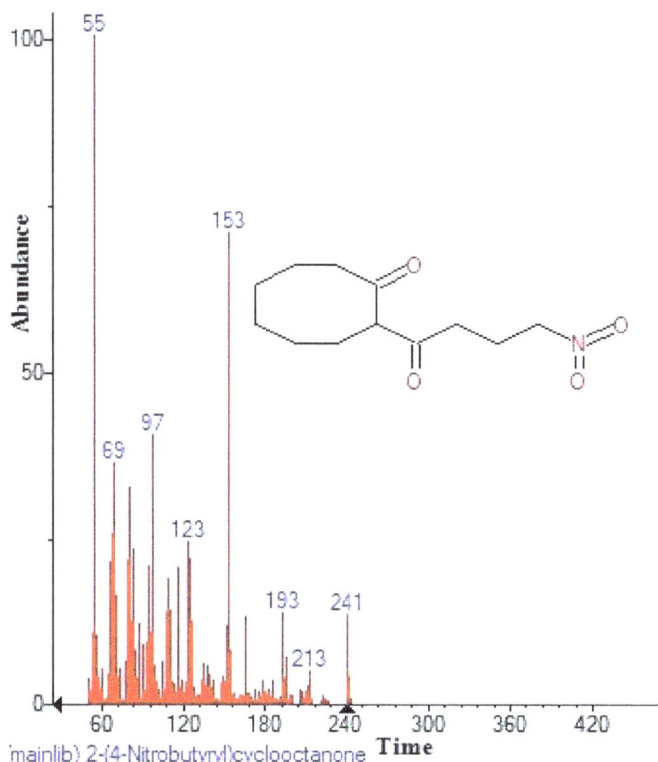

Figure 15. Structure of 2-(4-Nitrobutyryl) cyclooctanone present in the methanolic seeds extract of *Nigella sativa* by using GC-MS analysis.

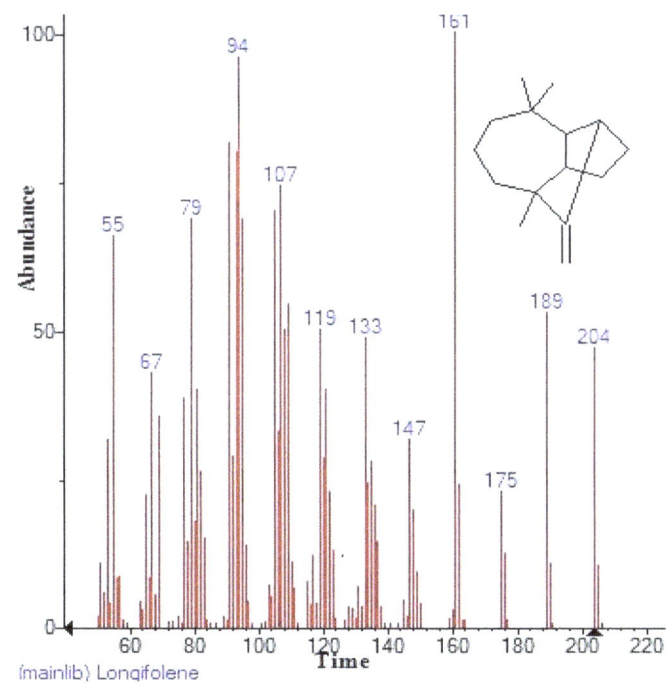

Figure 14. Structure of Longifolene present in the methanolic seeds extract of *Nigella sativa* by using GC-MS analysis.

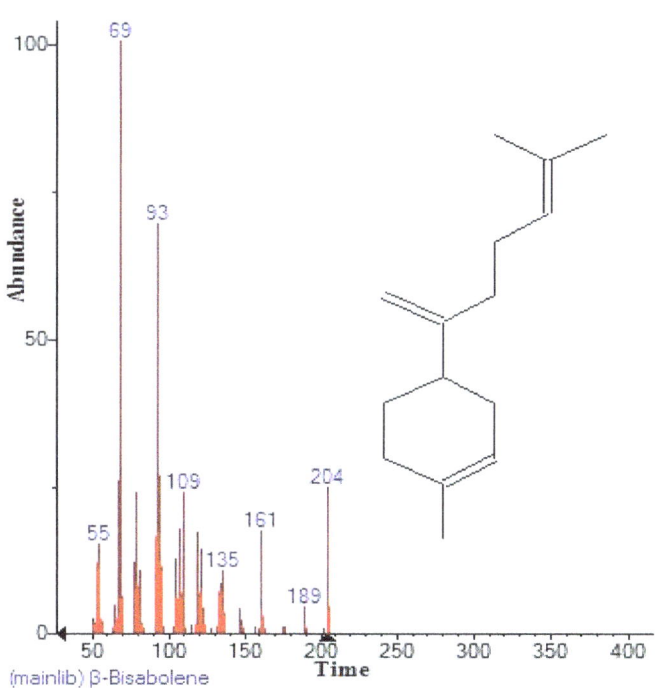

Figure 16. Structure of ß-Bisabolene present in the methanolic seeds extract of *Nigella sativa* by using GC-MS analysis.

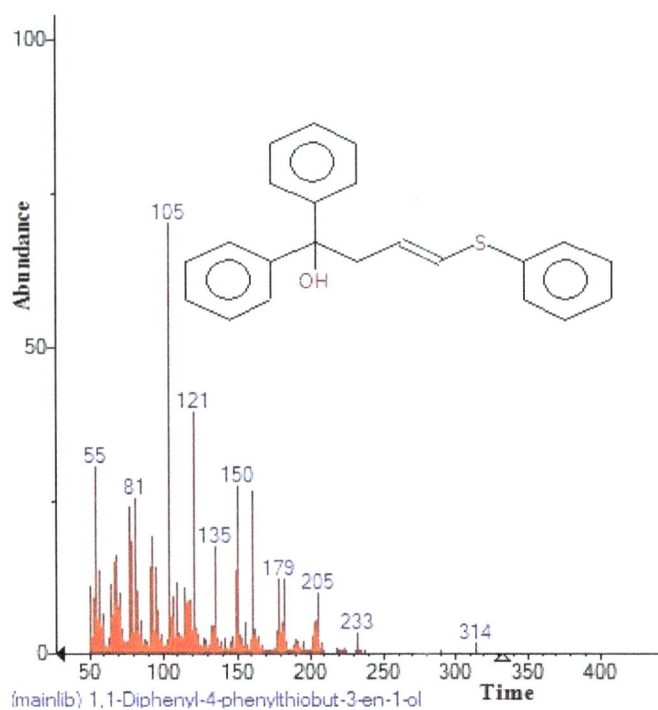

Figure 17. Structure of 1,1-Diphenyl-4-phenylthiobut-3-en-1-ol present in the methanolic seeds extract of *Nigella sativa* by using GC-MS analysis.

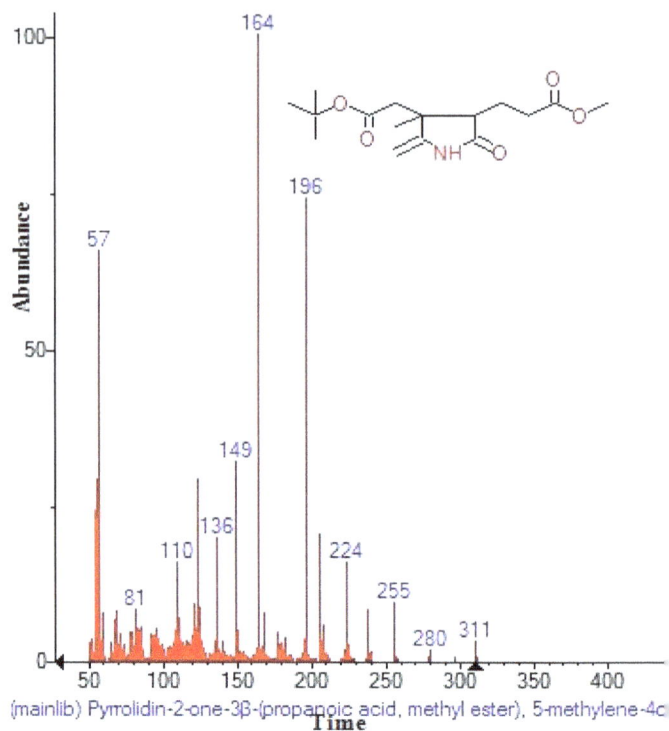

Figure 19. Structure of Pyrrolidin -2-one-3ß-(propanoic acid, methyl ester),5-methylene-4α present in the methanolic seeds extract of *Nigella sativa* by using GC-MS analysis.

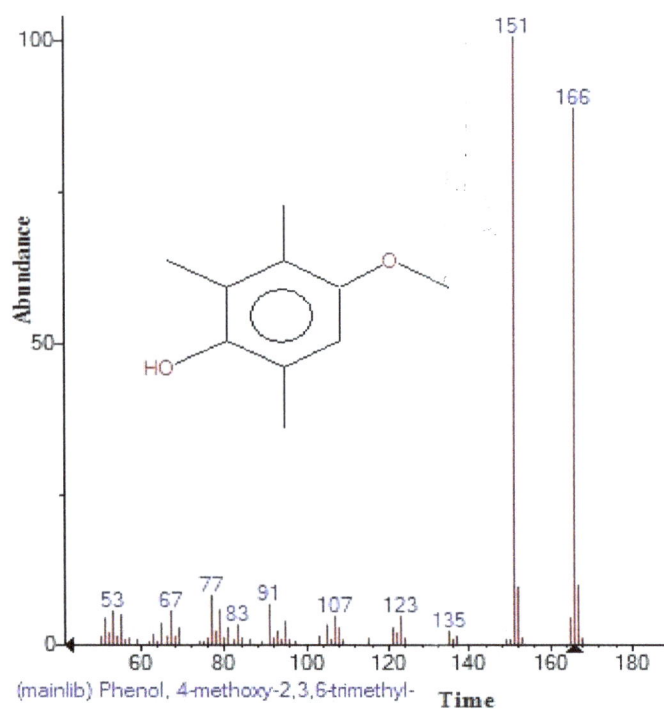

Figure 18. Structure of Phenol, 4-methoxy-2,3,6-trimethyl present in the methanolic seeds extract of *Nigella sativa* by using GC-MS analysis.

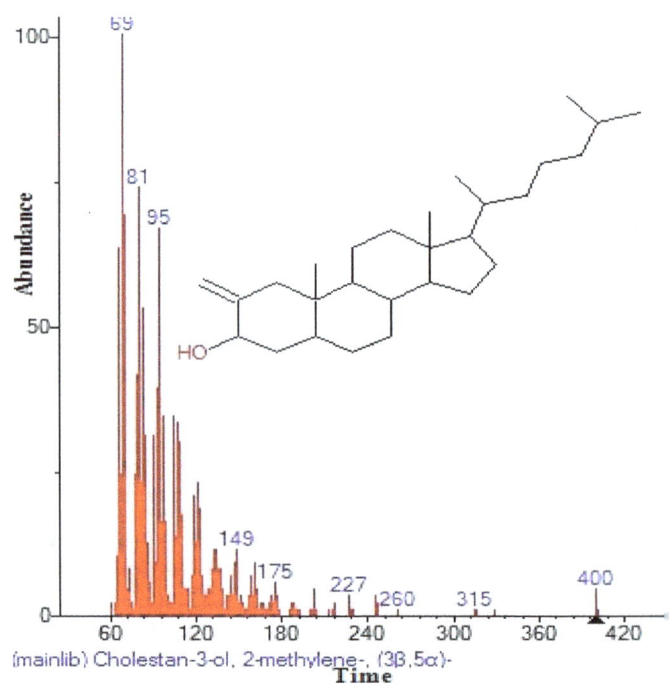

Figure 20. Structure of Cholestan-3-ol, 2-methylene-,(3ß,5α)- present in the methanolic seeds extract of *Nigella sativa* by using GC-MS analysis.

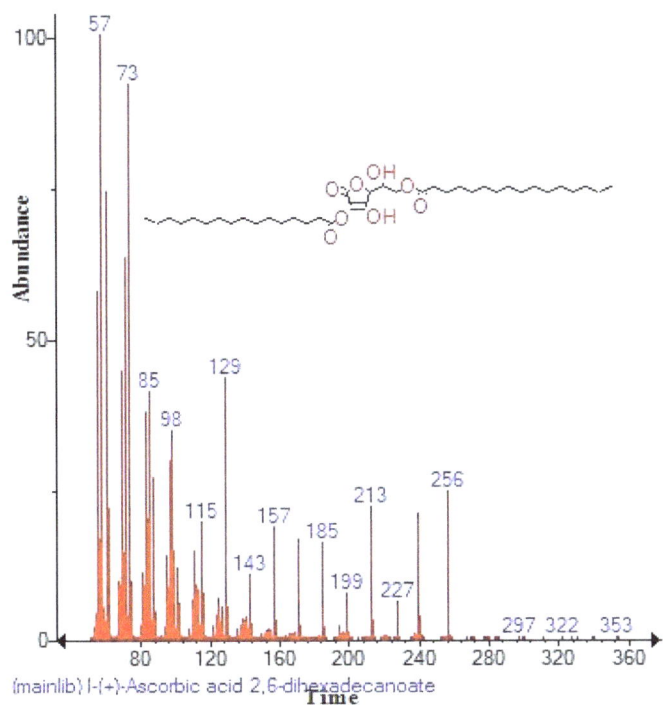

Figure 21. Structure of l-(+)-Ascorbic acid 2,6-dihexadecanoate present in the methanolic seeds extract of *Nigella sativa* by using GC-MS analysis.

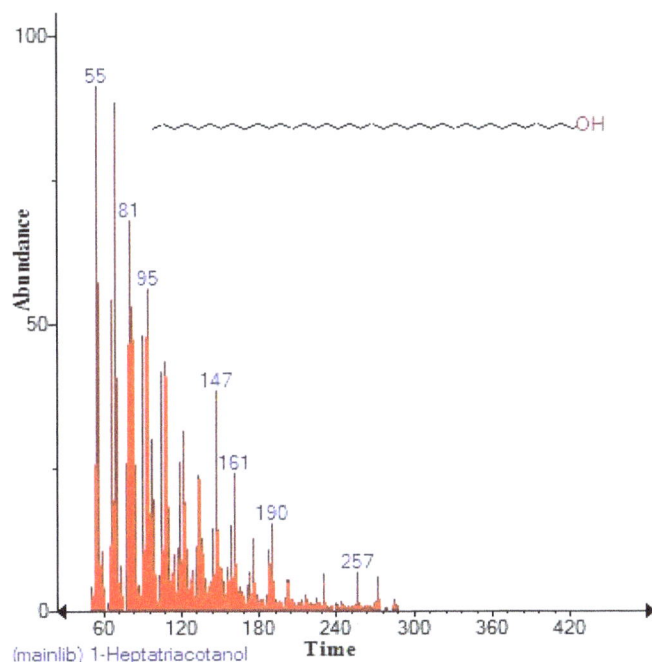

Figure 23. Structure of 1-Heptatriacotanol present in the methanolic seeds extract of *Nigella sativa* by using GC-MS analysis.

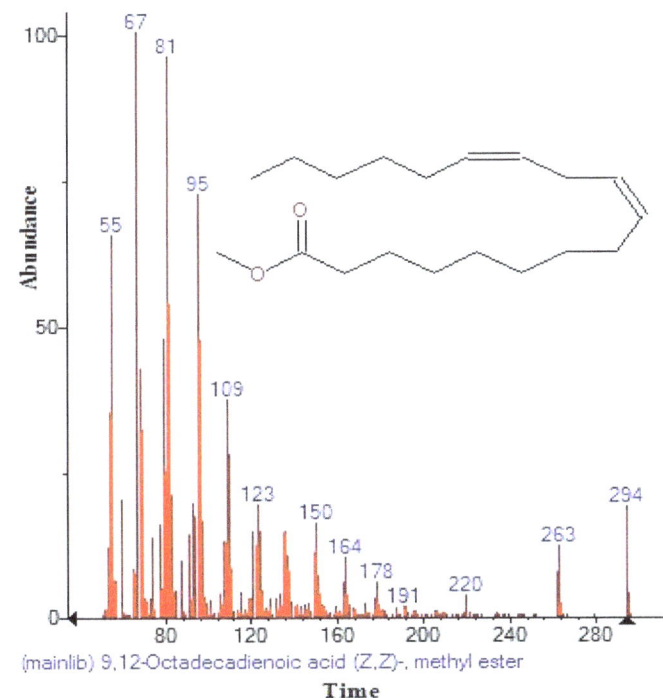

Figure 22. Structure of 9,12-Octadecadienoic acid (Z,Z)-, methyl ester present in the methanolic seeds extract of *Nigella sativa* by using GC-MS analysis.

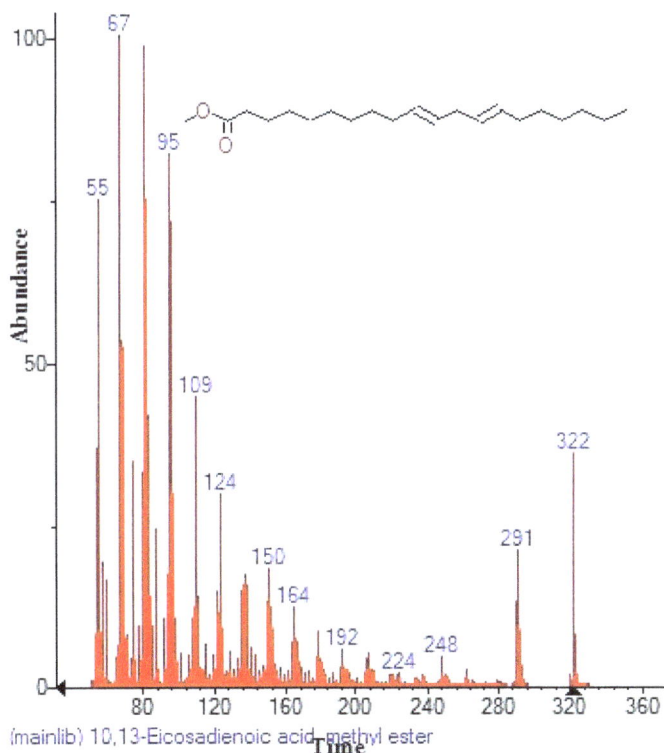

Figure 24. Structure of 10,13-Eicosadienoic acid, methyl ester present in the methanolic seeds extract of *Nigella sativa* by using GC-MS analysis.

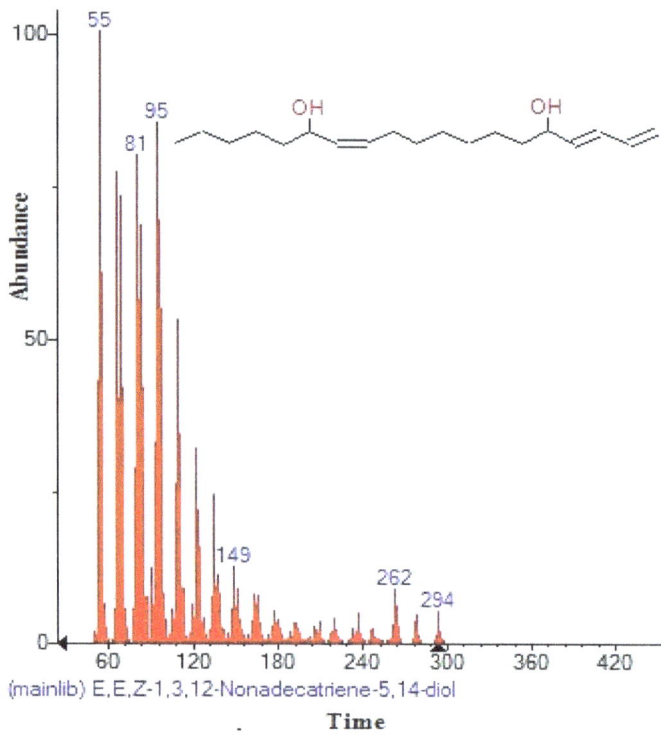

Figure 25. Structure of E,E,Z-1,3,12-Nonadecatriene-5,14-diol present in the methanolic seeds extract of *Nigella sativa* by using GC-MS analysis.

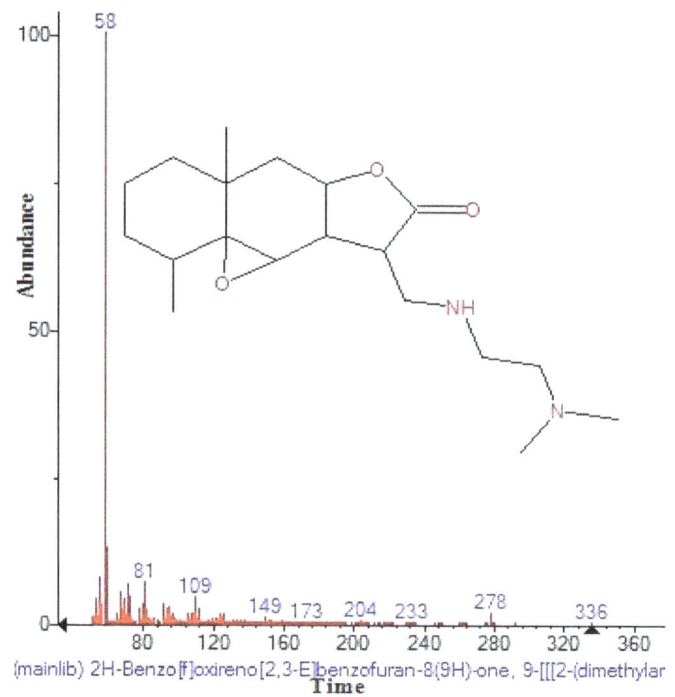

Figure 27. Structure of 2H-Benzo[f]oxireno[2,3-E]benzofuran-8(9H)-one,9-[[[2-(dimethylar present in the methanolic seeds extract of *Nigella sativa* by using GC-MS analysis.

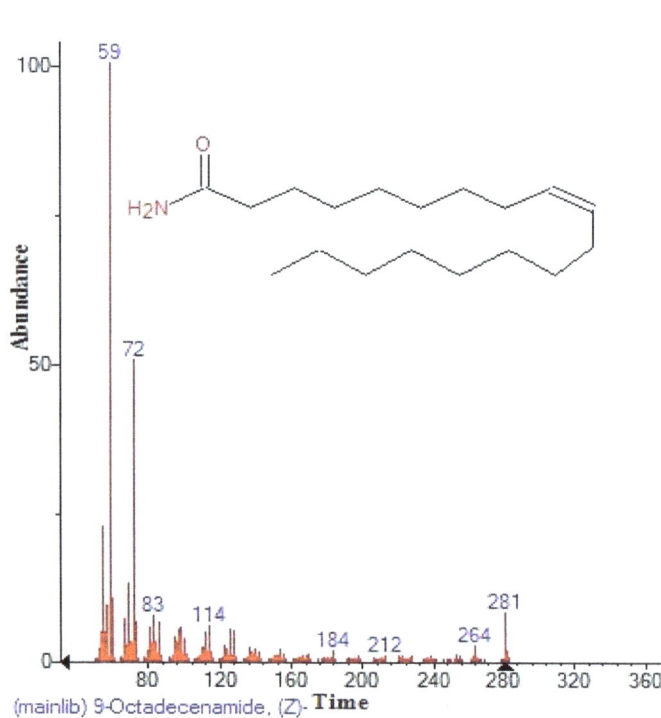

Figure 26. Structure of 9-Octadecenamide, (Z) present in the methanolic seeds extract of *Nigella sativa* by using GC-MS analysis.

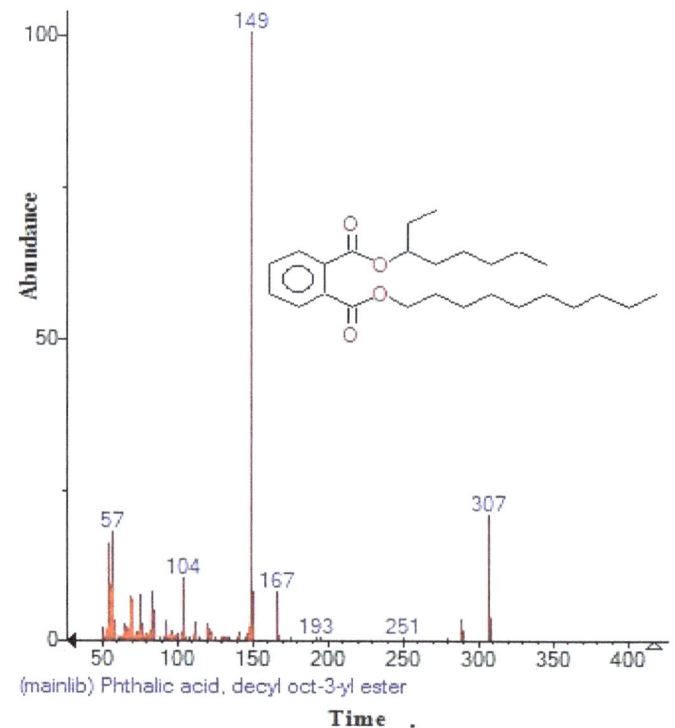

Figure 28. Structure of Phthalic acid, decyl oct-3-yl ester present in the methanolic seeds extract of *Nigella sativa* by using GC-MS analysis.

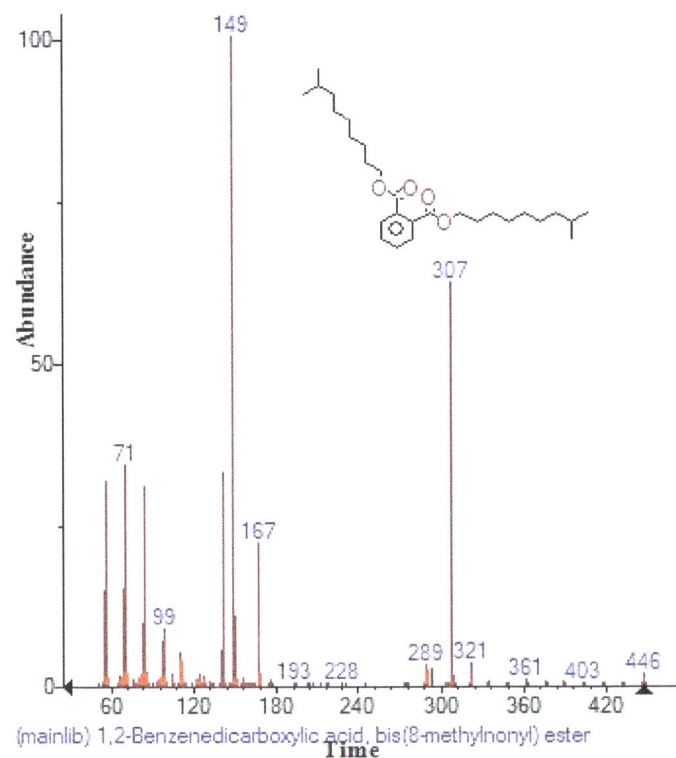

Figure 29. Structure of 1,2-Benzenedicarboxylic acid , bis(8-methylnonyl) ester present in the methanolic seeds extract of *Nigella sativa* by using GC-MS analysis.

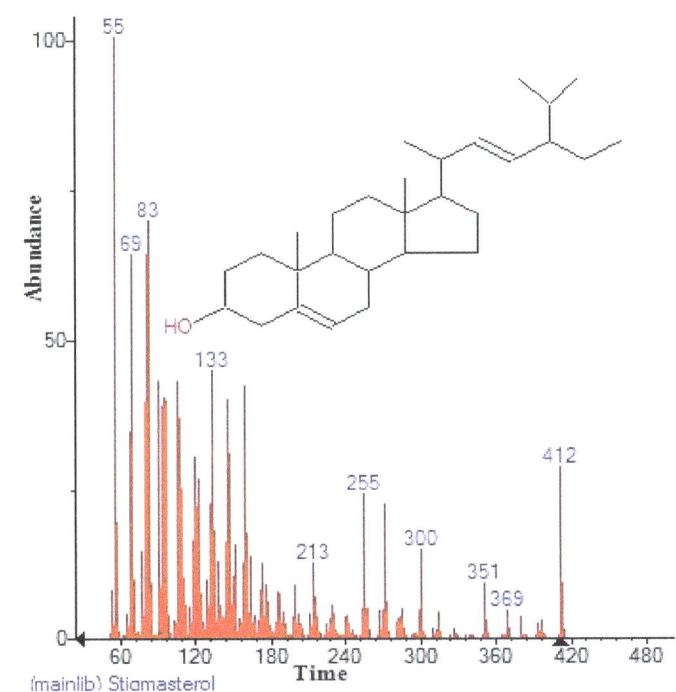

Figure 30. Structure of Stiqmasterol present in the methanolic seeds extract of *Nigella sativa* by using GC-MS analysis.

groups corresponding with the following data: monoterpenes (~46%); carbonyl compounds (~25%); phenols (~1.7%); alcohols (~0.9%) and esters (~16%) (Abu-Jadayil et al., 1999).

Conclusion

N. sativa seed is a promising source for active ingredients that would be with potential therapeutic modalities in different clinical settings. The efficacy of the active ingredients, however, should be measured by the nature of the disease. It contains chemical constitutions which may be useful for various herbal formulation as anti-inflammatory, analgesic, antipyretic, cardiac tonic and antiasthamatic.

ACKNOWLEDGEMENT

The authors thank Dr. Abdul-Kareem Al-Bermani, Lecturer, Department of Biology, for valuable suggestions and encouragement.

REFERENCES

Al-Yahya MA (1986). Phytochemical studies of the plants used in traditional medicine of Saudi Arabia. Fitoterapia 57(3):179-182.

Abdulelah HA, Abidin BA (2007). *In vivo* anti-malarial tests of *Nigella sativa* (black seed) Different extracts. Am. J. Pharm. Toxic. 2:46-50.

Aboul-Ela MA, El-Shaer NS, Ghanem NB (1996). Antimicrobial evaluation and chromatographic analysis of some essential and fixed oils. Pharmazie 51:993-4.

Abu-Jadayil S, Tukan SKH, Takruri HR (1999). Bioavailability of iron from four different local food plants in Jordan. Pl. Foods. Hum. Nutr. 54:285–294.

Ali A, Alkhawajah, Randhawa MA, Shaikh NA (2008). Oral and interaperitoneal LD50 of thymoquinone an active principal of *Nigella sativa* in mice and rats. J. Ayub Med. Coll. 20(2):25-27.

Ali BH, Blunden G (2003). Pharmacological and toxicological properties of *Nigella sativa*. Phytother Res. 17(4):299-305.

Al-Johar D, Shinwari N, Arif J, Al-Sanea N, Jabbar AA, El-Sayed R, Mashhour A, Billedo G, El-Doush I, Al-Saleh I (2008). Role of *Nigella sativa* and a number of its antioxidant constituents towards azoxymethane-inducedgenotoxic effects and colon cancer in rats. Phytother. Res. 22:1311-1323.

Al-Othman AM, Ahmad F, Al-Orf S, Al-Murshed SK, Arif Z (2006). Effect of dietary supplementation of *Ellataria cardamomum* and *Nigella sativa* on the toxicity of rancid corn oil in Rats. Int. J. Pharmacol. 2:60-65.

Altameme HJ, Hameed IH, Idan SA, Hadi MY (2015a). Biochemical analysis of *Origanum vulgare* seeds by Fourier-transform infrared (FT-IR) spectroscopy and gas chromatography-mass spectrometry (GC-MS). 7(9):221-237.

Altameme HJ, Hameed IH, Kareem MA (2015b). Analysis of alkaloid phytochemical compounds in the ethanolic extract of *Datura stramonium* and evaluation of antimicrobial activity Afr. J. Biotechnol. 14(19):1668-1674.

Ashraf M, Ali Q, Iqbal Z (2006). Effect of nitrogen application rate on the content and composition of oil, essential oil and minerals in black cumin (*Nigella sativa* L.) seeds. J. Sci. Food Agric. 86:871-876.

Ashraf R (2011). Plant (Garlic) Supplement with standard Antidiabetic agent provides better diabetic control in Type-II diabetes patients. Pak. J. Pharmaceut. Sci. 24(4):565-570.

Boskabady MH, Javan H, Sajady M, Rakhshandeh H (2007). The possible prophylactic effect of *Nigella sativa* seed extract in asthmatic patients. Fundam. Clin. Pharmacol. 21(5):559-566.

Burits M, Burcar F (2000). Antioxidant activity of *Nigella sativa* essential oil. Phytother. Res. 14(5): 323-8.

Chaudhry N, Tariq P (2008). *In vitro* antibacterial activities of Kalongi, Cumin and Poppy seed. Pak. J. Bot. 40(1):461-467.

Cheikh-Rouhou S, Besbes S, Hentati B, Blecker C, Deroanne C, Attia H (2007). *Nigella sativa* L.: Chemical composition and physicochemical characteristics of lipid fraction. Food Chem. 101:673–681.

Enomoto S, Asano R, Iwahori Y, Narui T, Okada Y, Singab AN, Okuyama T (2001). Hematological studies on black cumin oil from the seeds of *Nigella sativa* L. Biol. Pharm. Bull. 24:307–10.

Hameed IH, Hussein HJ, Kareem MA, Hamad NS (2015a). Identification of five newly described bioactive chemical compounds in methanolic extract of *Mentha viridis* by using gas chromatography-mass spectrometry (GC-MS). J. Pharmacogn. Phytother. 7 (7):107-125.

Hameed IH, Ibraheam IA, Kadhim HJ (2015b). Gas chromatography mass spectrum and Fourier-transform infrared spectroscopy analysis of methanolic extract of *Rosmarinus oficinalis* leaves. J. Pharmacog. Phytother. 7(6):90-106.

Hameed IH, Jasim H, Kareem MA, Hussein AO (2015c). Alkaloid constitution of *Nerium oleander* using gas chromatography-mass spectroscopy (GC-MS). J. Med. Plants Res. 9(9):326-334.

Hameed IH, Hamza LF, Kamal SA (2015d). Analysis of bioactive chemical compounds of *Aspergillus niger* by using gas chromatography-mass spectrometry and Fourier-transform infrared spectroscopy. J. Pharmacog. Phytother. 7(8):132-163.

Hamza LF, Kamal SA, Hameed IH (2015). Determination of metabolites products by *Penicillium expansum* and evaluating antimicobial activity. J. Pharmacogn. Phytother. 7(9):194-220.

Hussein AO, Hameed IH, Jasim H, Kareem MA (2015). Determination of alkaloid compounds of *Ricinus communis* by using gas chromatography-mass spectroscopy (GC-MS). J. Med. Plants Res. 9(10):349-359.

Imad H, Mohammed A, Aamera J (2014a). Genetic variation and DNA markers in forensic analysis. Afr. J. Biotechnol. 13(31):3122-3136.

Imad H, Mohammed A, Cheah Y, Aamera J (2014b). Genetic variation of twenty autosomal STR loci and evaluate the importance of these loci for forensic genetic purposes. Afr. J. Biotechnol. 13:1-9.

Imad H, Muhanned A, Aamera J, Cheah Y (2014c). Analysis of eleven Y-chromosomal STR markers in middle and south of Iraq. Afr. J. Biotechnol. 13(38):3860-3871.

Iqbal MS, Qureshi AS, Ghafoor A (2010). Evaluation of *Nigella sativa* L., for genetic variation and *Ex-situ* conservation. Pak. J. Bot. 42(4):2489-2495.

Jasim H, Hussein AO, Hameed IH, Kareem MA (2015). Characterization of alkaloid constitution and evaluation of antimicrobial activity of *Solanum nigrum* using gas chromatography mass spectrometry (GC-MS). J. Pharmacogn. Phytother. 7(4):56-72.

Kanter M (2008). Effects of *Nigella sativa* and its major constituent, thymoquinone onsciatic nerves in experimental diabetic neuropathy. Neurochem. Res. 33:87-96.

Kareem MA, Hussein AO, Hameed IH (2015). Y-chromosome short tandem repeat, typing technology, locus information and allele frequency in different population: A review. Afr. J. Biotechnol. 14(27):2175-2178.

Mansour MA, Nagi MN, El-Khatib AS, Al-Bekairi AM (2002). Effects of thymoquinone on antioxidant enzyme activities, lipid peroxidation and DT-diaphorase in different tissues of mice: a possible mechanism of action. Cell. Biochem. Funct. 20:143–51.

Mohammed A, Imad H (2013). Autosomal STR: From locus informatio to next generation sequencing technology. Res. J. Biotechno 8(10):92-105.

Rader JI, Delmonte P, Trucksess MW (2007). Recent studies o selected botanical dietary supplement ingredients. Anal. Bioana Chem. 389:27-35.

Ramaa CS, Shirode AR, Mundada AS, Kadam VJ (2006 Nutraceuticals an emerging era in the treatment and prevention o cardiovascular diseases. Curr. Pharm. Biotechnol. 7:15-23.

Saleh S (2006). Protection by *Nigella sativa* (Black seed) agains hyperhomo-cysteinemia in rats vascular disease. Preventia. 3:73-78.

Sethi G, Ahn K, Aggarwal B (2008). Targeting nuclear factor-kappa activation Pathway by thymoquinone: Role in suppression o antiapoptotic gene products and enhancement of apoptosis. Mo Cancer Res. 6:1059-1070.

Sharma NK, Ahirwar D, Jhade D, Gupta S (2009). Medicinal an pharmacological potential of *Nigella sativa*: A review. Ethnobot. Rev 13:946-55

Vuorelaa P, Leinonenb M, Saikkuc P, Tammelaa P, Rauhad JP Wennberge T, Vuorela H (2004). Natural products in the process o finding new drug candidates. Curr. Med. Chem. 11:1375–1389.

## 12

Evaluation of anti-bacterial activity and bioactive chemical analysis of *Ocimum basilicum* using Fourier transform infrared (FT-IR) and gas chromatography-mass spectrometry (GC-MS) techniques

Mohanad Jawad Kadhim[1], Azhar Abdulameer Sosa[2] and Imad Hadi Hameed[3]*

[1]Department of Genetic Engineering, Al-Qasim Green University, Iraq.
[2]College of Education for Women, Al-Qadisyia University, Iraq.
[3]College of Nursing, Babylon University, Iraq.

The objective of this research was to determine the chemical composition of aerial parts extract from methanol. The phytochemical compound screened by gas chromatography-mass spectrometry (GC-MS) method. Thirty one bioactive phytochemical compounds were identified in the methanolic extract of *Ocimum basilicum*. The identification of phytochemical compounds is based on the peak area, retention time molecular weight, molecular formula, MS fragment-ions and pharmacological actions. GC-MS and Fourier transform infrared (FT-IR) analyses of *O. basilicum* revealed the existence of Paromomycin, Stevioside, Campesterol and Ascaridole epoxide, aliphatic fluoro compounds, alcohols, ethers, carboxlic acids, esters, nitro compounds, alkanes, H-bonded H-X group, hydrogen bonded alcohols and phenols. Methanolic extract of bioactive compounds of *O. basilicum* was assayed for *in vitro* antibacterial activity against *Pseudomonas aerogenosa*, *Proteus mirabilis*, *Escherichia coli*, *Staphylococcus aureus* and *Klebsiella pneumonia* by using the diffusion method in agar. The zone of inhibition was compared with different standard antibiotics. The diameters of inhibition zones ranged from 5.70±0.10 to 0.55±0.29 mm for all treatments.

Key words: GC/MS, Bioactive compounds, Fourier transform infrared (FT-IR), *Ocimum basilicum*.

INTRODUCTION

Plants secondary metabolites have recently been referred to as phytochemicals. Phytochemicals are naturally occurring and biologically active plant compounds that have potential disease inhibiting capabilities (Rukayadi et al., 2006; Yoshikawa et al., 2007; Hameed et al., 2015a; Al-Marzoqi et al., 2016). It is believed that phytochemicals may be effective in combating or preventing disease due to their antioxidant

*Corresponding author. E-mail: imad_dna@yahoo.com.

effect (Halliwell and Gutteridge, 1992; Altameme et al., 2015a). Plant materials have played an important role in traditional methods of field crop and stored grain protection against insect pest infestation since time immemorial (Ogendo et al., 2003; Al-Marzoqi et al., 2015). *Ocimum* species contains a wide range of essential oils rich in phenolic compounds and a wide array of other natural products including polyphenols such as flavonoids and anthocyanins. The genus *Ocimum* comprises more than 150 species and is considered as one of the largest genera of the Lamiaceae family (Holm, 1996; Hameed et al., 2015b). *Ocimum basilicum* L. (sweet basil) is an annual herb which grows in several regions all over the world. The plant is widely used in food and oral care products. The essential oil of the plant is also used as perfumery (Bauer et al., 1997; Chiang, 2005). Kéita et al. (2000) reported *O. basilicum* and *O. gratissimum* to be potential insecticides. The leaves and seeds are rich in essential oils, which are repellent, toxic or growth inhibitory to many insects. A high degree of polymorphism in the genus *Ocimum* determines a large number of subspecies, different varieties and forms producing essential oils with varying chemical composition offering variable level of medicinal potential. Essential oils extracted from *Ocimum* plants have been reported to possess interesting biological properties. These volatile oils have been applied in perfumery, to inhibit growth of microorganisms, in food preservation and in aromatherapy. The potential uses of *O. basilicum, Ocimum canum Ocimum gratissimum* and *Ocimum sanctum* essential oils, particularly as antioxidant and antimicrobial agents have also been explored (Politeo et al., 2007; Koba et al., 2009; Zhang et al., 2009; Hameed et al., 2015c; Altameme et al., 2015b; Hussein et al., 2016a). *O. basilicum* has been traditionally used for the treatment of many ailments, such as headaches, coughs and diarrhea and it is generally recognized as safe and is a rich source of phenolic antioxidant compounds and flavonoids (Juliani and Simon, 2002). The aims of this study were to determine the phytochemical composition of aerial parts and evaluation of anti-bacterial activity.

MATERIALS AND METHODS

Collection and preparation of plant

The aerial parts were dried at room temperature for ten days and when properly dried then powdered using clean pestle and mortar, and the powdered plant was size reduced with a sieve (Altameme et al., 2015c; Hameed et al., 2015d; Hussein et al., 2016b). The fine powder was then packed in airtight container to avoid the effect of humidity and then stored at room temperature. About 9 g of the plant sample powdered were soaked in 100 ml methanol individually. It was left for 72 h so that alkaloids, flavonoids and other constituents if present will get dissolved (Jasim et al., 2015; Hadi et al., 2016; Hussein et al., 2016c). The methanol extract was filtered using Whatman No.1 filter paper and the residue was removed.

Gas chromatography–mass spectrum (GC-MS) analysis

The GC-MS analysis of the plant extract (*O. basilicum*) was made in a Agilent 7890 A instrument under computer control at 70 eV. About 1 µl of the methanol extract was injected into the GC-MS using a micro syringe and the scanning was done for 45 min. As the compounds were separated, they eluted from the column and entered a detector which was capable of creating an electronic signal whenever a compound was detected. The greater the concentration in the sample, bigger was the signal obtained which was then processed by a computer. The time from when the injection was made (Initial time) to when elution occurred is referred to as the retention time (RT). The M/Z (mass/charge) ratio obtained was calibrated from the graph obtained, which was called as the mass spectrum graph which is the fingerprint of a molecule. Before analyzing the extract using gas chromatography and mass spectroscopy, the temperature of the oven, the flow rate of the gas used and the electron gun were programmed initially. The temperature of the oven was maintained at 100°C. Helium gas was used as a carrier as well as an eluent. The flow rate of helium was set to 1 ml/min. The identity of the components in the extracts was assigned by the comparison of their retention indices and mass spectra fragmentation patterns with those stored on the computer library and also with published literatures. Compounds were identified by comparing their spectra to those of the Wiley and NIST/EPA/NIH mass spectral libraries (Yang et al., 2010).

Determination of antibacterial activity of crude bioactive compounds of *O. basilicum*

The test pathogens (*Pseudomonas aeruginosa, Klebsiella pneumoniae, Escherichia coli,* and *Staphylococcus aureus*) were swabbed in Muller Hinton agar plates. 60 µl of plant extract was loaded on the bored wells. The wells were bored in 0.5 cm in diameter. The plates were incubated at 37C° for 24 h and examined. After the incubation the diameter of inhibition zones around the discs was measured.

RESULTS AND DISCUSSION

Medicinal herbs are known as sources of active compounds that are widely sought after worldwide for their natural properties. They have been used since ancient times as sources of flavorings and for their pharmaceutical properties (Bais et al., 2002). Phytochemicals may be effective in combating or preventing disease due to their antioxidant effect (Halliwell and Gutteridge, 1992). A great number of organizations and scientists turn their attention to traditional therapies in order to find and conserve important resources and up to 80% of the population relies on traditional medicines or folk remedies for primary health care needs (Smith et al., 2010). Gas chromatography and mass spectroscopy analysis of compounds was carried out in methanolic aerial parts extract of *O. basilicum*, shown in Table 1. The GC-MS chromatogram of the 31 peaks of the compounds detected was shown in Figure 1. Chromatogram GC-MS analysis of the methanol extract of *O. basilicum* showed the presence of thirty one major peaks and the components corresponding to the peaks were determined

Table 1. Phytochemical compounds identified in methanolic extract of O. basilicum.

S/N	Phytochemical compound	RT (min)	Formula	Molecular weight	Exact mass	Chemical structure	MS Fragment- ions	Pharmacological actions
1	1,2,4-Triazole , 4-[N-(2-hydroxyethyl)-N-nitro]amino	3.196	$C_4H_7N_5O_3$	173	173.054889		55,70,83,113,127,173	*Biological* activities including *anti-* microbial activity
2	9-Acetoxynonanal	3.459	$C_{11}H_{20}O_3$	200	200.141245		55,81,97,112,157,200	Antimicrobial and *anti -* inflammatory
3	Paromomycin	3.567	$C_{23}H_{45}N_5O_{14}$	615	615.296303		57,67,80,94,109,124,162,191,21 0,227,244,262,287	*Anti*-bacterial
4	Stevioside	3.773	$C_{38}H_{60}O_{18}$	804	804.377964		60,73,85,98,113,121,144,163,18 5,214,260,285	Have *anti*-hyperglycemic, *anti*-hypertensive *anti*-inflammatory and *anti*-tumor
5	D-Limonene	3.985	$C_{10}H_{16}$	136	136.1252		53,68,79,93,136	*Anti*-stress effects

Table 1. Cont'd

No.	Name	RT	Formula		Exact mass	Fragment ions	Pharmacological and biological activities
6	Exo-2,7,7-Trimethylbicyclo[2.2.1]heptan-2-ol	4.300	$C_{10}H_{18}O$	154	154.135765	55,71,81,93,107,121,136,154	*Pharmacological and biological activities including anti-Candida, anti-inflammatory and anti-diabetic*
7	Dithiocarbamate , S-methyl-N-(2-methyl-3-oxobutyl)-	4.775	$C_7H_{13}NOS_2$	191	191.043856	57,72,85,91,117,143,191	*Anti-inflammatory effects*
8	1,6-Octadien-3-ol,3,7-dimethyl,	5.067	$C_{10}H_{18}O$	154	154.135765	55,71,80,93,107,121,136,154	Antioxidants
9	13,16-Octadecadiynoic acid , methyl ester	5.301	$C_{19}H_{30}O_2$	290	290.22458	55,74,164,199,242	Antifungal and Antialgal *effect*
10	Cyclohexanecarboxylic acid ,2-hydroxy-, ethyl ester	5.776	$C_9H_{16}O_3$	172	172.109944	57,73,81,101,127,144,154,172	Antipyretic and *anti-inflammatory*
11	Methyl 6-oxoheptanoate	6.011	$C_8H_{14}O_3$	158	158.094295	55,84,111,126,143	Unknown

Table 1. Cont'd

	Name	Retention time	Formula	Mass	Exact Mass	Structure	Identified in references	Activity
12	3,7-Octadiene-2,6-diol,2,6-dimethyl-	6.245	$C_{10}H_{18}O_2$	170	170.13068		55,59,67,71,82,91,109,125,137	*Anti*-tumour
13	Exo-2,7,7-trimethylbicyclo[2.2.1]heptan-2-ol	6.303	$C_{10}H_{18}O$	154	154.135765		55,81,93,121,136,154	*Anti-Candida, anti*-inflammatory and antidiabetic
14	Glycyl-D-asparagine	6.772	$C_6H_{11}N_3O_4$	189	189.074956		55,72,113,154	Acute *anti*-inflammatory effect
15	6-Acetyl-ß-d-mannose	6.932	$C_8H_{14}O_7$	222	222.073953		60,73,81,97,109,126,144,163,175,192	*Anti*-carcinogenic *effects*
16	2-Propenoic acid ,3-phenyl-,methyl ester , (E)-	7.744	$C_{10}H_{10}O_2$	162	162.06808		51,63,77,91,103,117,131,144,162	*Anti*-cancer agents

Table 1. Cont'd

#	Compound	RT	MW	Formula	Exact Mass	Structure	Fragment ions	Activity
17	Methyleugenol	8.980	178	$C_{11}H_{14}O_2$	178.09938		51,65,77,103,147,163	*Anti*-inflammatory
18	7-epi-cis-sesquisabinene hydrate	9.404	222	$C_{15}H_{26}O_2$	222.198365		55,69,82,93,105,119,133,147,161,175,204,222	Significant *anti*-microbial activities
19	Mannopyranose , 1-O-(triethylsilyl)-, 2,3:4,6-dibutaneboronate	13.163	384	$C_{17}H_{34}B_2O_6Si$	384.231075		55,75,103,139,157,213,228,257,313,341,369	New chemical compound
20	2,6-Bis[2-[2-S-thiosulfuroethylamino]eth oxy]pyrazine	16.133	478	$C_{12}H_{22}N_4O_8S_4$	478.032047		60,88,124,163,195,213,259,317,349	Unknown
21	9,12,15-Octadecatrienoic acid , (Z,Z,Z)-	17.031	278	$C_{18}H_{30}O_2$	278.22458		55,67,79,93,108,121,135,222,249,278	Antioxidant, *anti*-inflammatory, antimicrobial, pesticide and cancer preventive.

Table 1. Cont'd

No.	Name		Formula			Structure	m/z fragments	Activity
22	Lup-20(29)-en-28-oic acid , 3-hydroxy-, methyl ester , (3ß)-	17.317	$C_{31}H_{50}O_3$	470	470.375996		107,175,189,207,220,262,341,4 11,452,470	*Anti*-bacterial
23	Octadecanoic acid	17.186	$C_{18}H_{36}O_2$	284	284.27153		60,73,83,97,115,129,143,157,17 1,185,199,227,241,255,284	Antiviral and *anti*-inflammatory activities
24	2-[4-methyl-6-(2,6,6-trimethylcyclohex-1-enyl)hexa-1,3,5-trienyl]cyclol	17.369	$C_{23}H_{32}O$	324	324.245316		55,69,79,91,105,135,173,187,23 9,269,324	Unknown
25	9-Desoxo-9-x-acetoxy-3,8,12-tri-acetylingol	21.946	$C_{28}H_{40}O_{10}$	536	536.262146		55,69,122,207,236,297,357,417, 477	*Anti*-macrofouling
26	9,12-Cyclolanost-24-en-3-ol, acetate,(3ß)-	23.497	$C_{32}H_{52}O_2$	468	468.39673		55,69,81,95,175,203,231,286,40 8,468	*Anti*-inflammatory

Table 1. Cont'd

27	γ-Tocopherol	25.231	$C_{28}H_{48}O_2$	416	416.36543		57,107,135,151,191,205,232,26 0,288,316,344,372,416	Anti-inflammatory properties
28	Lup-20(29)-en-3-ol,acetate,(3ß)-	26.467	$C_{32}H_{52}O_2$	468	468.39673		55,69,81,95,189,218,249,298,35 7,408,453,468	Anti-inflammatory effects
29	Ethyl iso – allocholate	26.890	$C_{26}H_{44}O_5$	436	436.318874		55,69,81,95,253,400,418	Antimicrobial, anti-inflammatory, cancer preventive and antifouling agents
30	Campesterol	28.229	$C_{28}H_{48}O$	400	400.370516		55,81,145,161,213,255,289,315, 382,400	Anti-oxidative, anti-inflammatory, immunomodulatory and antiviral properties.
31	Ascaridole epoxide	7.167	$C_{10}H_{16}O_3$	184	184.109944		55,69,79,91,97,107,117,135,150 ,168	Anti-carcinogenic effects

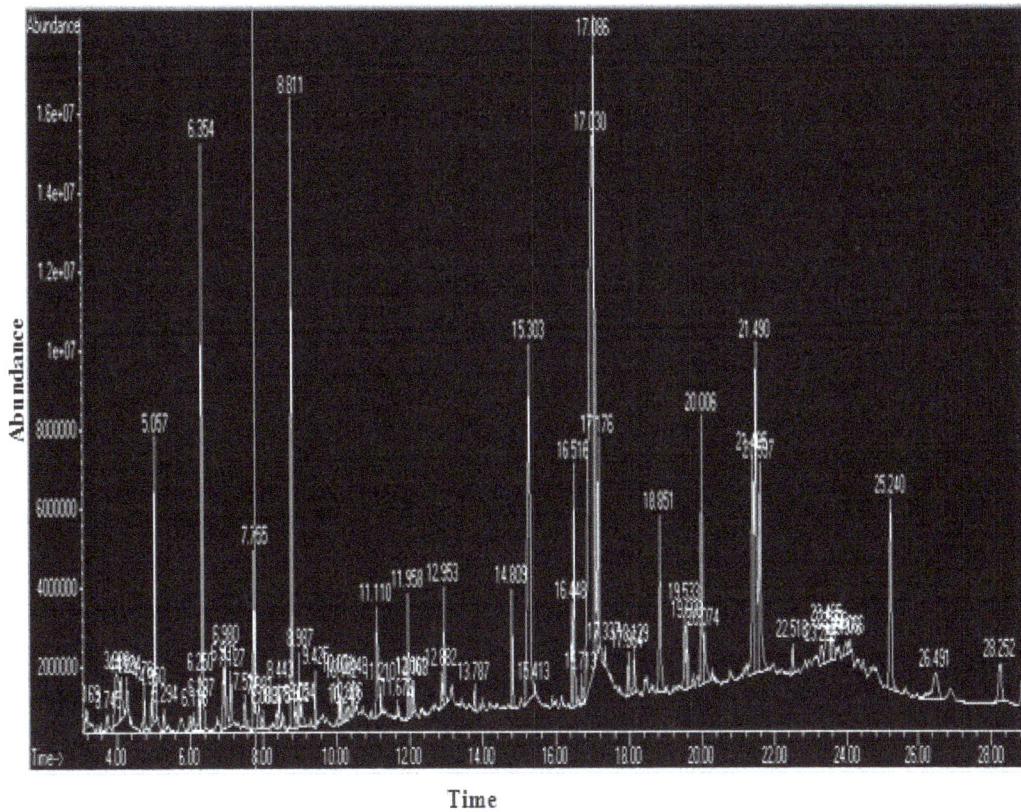

Figure 1. GC-MS chromatogram of methanolic extract of *Ocimum basilicum*.

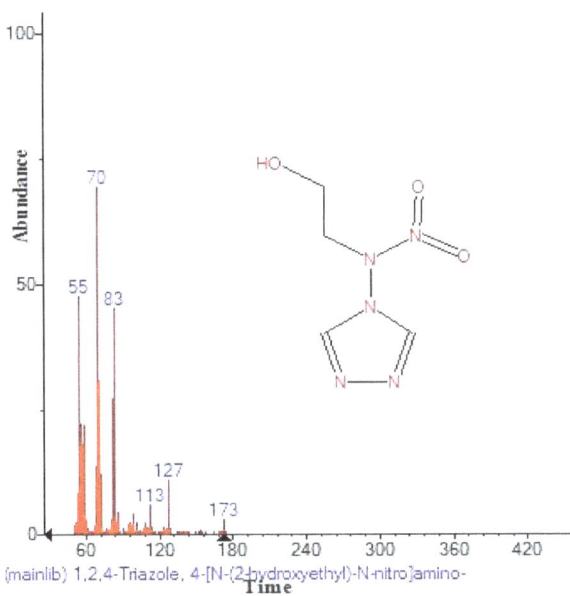

Figure 2. Structure of 1,2,4-Triazole, 4-[N-(2-hydroxyethyl)-N-nitro]amino with 3.196 (RT) present in *Ocimum basilicum*.

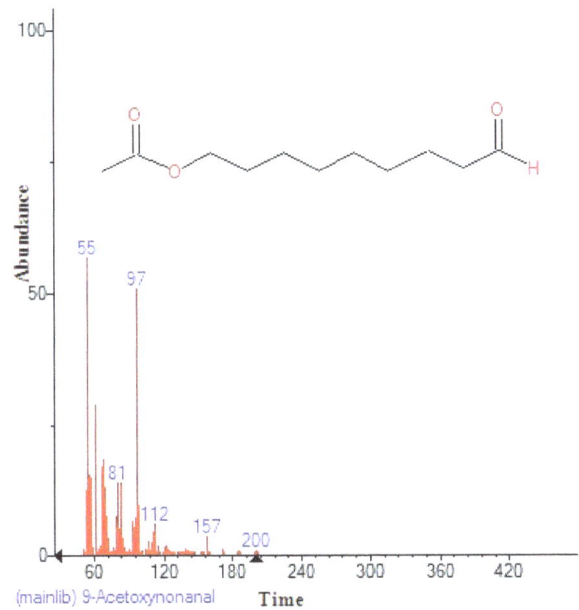

Figure 3. Structure of 9-Acetoxynonanal with 3.459 (RT) present in *Ocimum basilicum*.

as follows. The first set up peak were determined to be 1,2,4-Triazole (Figure 2). The second peak indicated to be 4-[N-(2-hydroxyethyl)-N-nitro]amino (Figure 3). The next peaks were considered to be, 9-Acetoxynonanal,

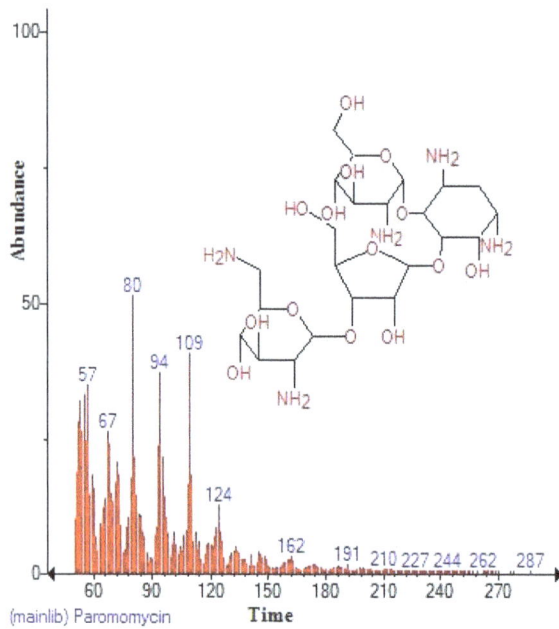

Figure 4. Structure of Paromomycin with 3.567 (RT) present in *Ocimum basilicum*.

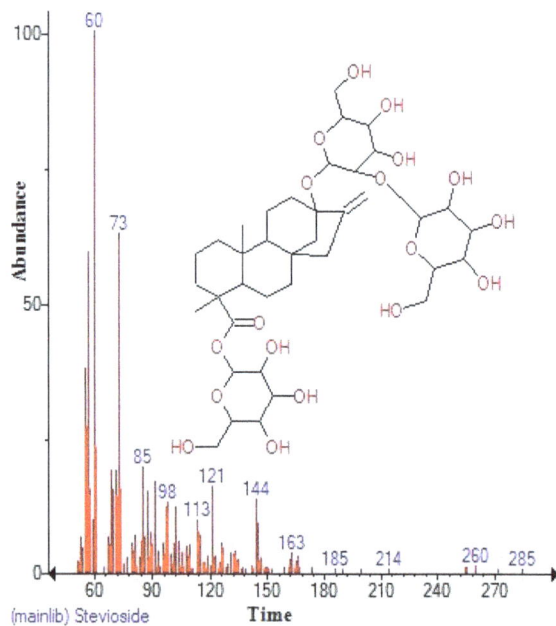

Figure 6. Structure of D-Limonene with 3.985 (RT) present in *Ocimum basilicum*.

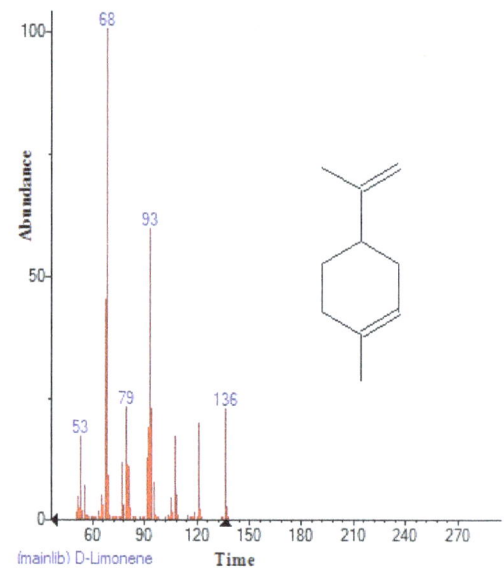

Figure 5. Structure of Stevioside with 3.773 (RT) present in *Ocimum basilicum*.

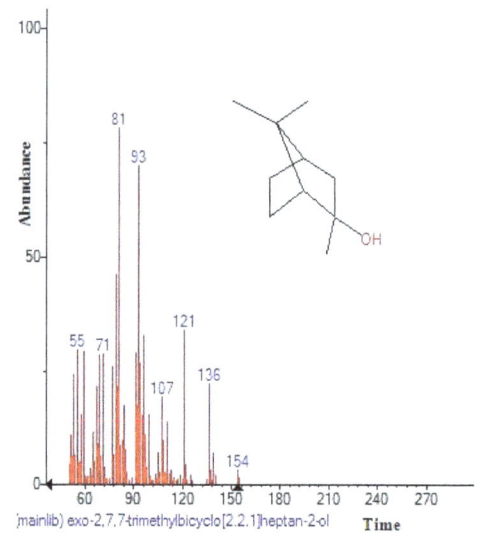

Figure 7. Structure of Exo-2,7,7-Trimethylbicyclo[2.2.1]heptan-2-ol with 4.300 (RT) present in *Ocimum basilicum*.

Paromomycin, Stevioside, D-Limonene, Exo-2,7,7-Trimethylbicyclo[2.2.1]heptan-2-ol, Dithiocarbamate, S-methyl-N-(2-methyl-3-oxobutyl)-, 1,6-Octadien-3-ol,3,7-dimethyl-, 13,16-Octadecadiynoic acid , methyl ester, Cyclohexanecarboxylic acid ,2-hydroxy-, ethyl ester, Methyl 6-oxoheptanoate, 3,7-Octadiene-2,6-diol,2,6-dimethyl-, Exo-2,7,7-trimethylbicyclo [2.2.1] heptan-2-ol,

Glycyl-D-asparagine, 6-Acetyl-ß-d-mannose, 2-Propenoic acid, 3-phenyl-,methyl ester, (E)-, Methyleugenol, 7-epi-cis-sesquisabinene hydrate, Mannopyranose, 1-O-(triethylsilyl)-, 2,3:4,6-dibutaneboronate, 2,6-Bis[2-[2-S-thiosulfuroethylamino] ethoxy]pyrazine, 9,12,15-Octadecatrienoic acid , (Z,Z,Z)-, Lup-20(29)-en-28-oic acid, 3-hydroxy-, methyl ester, (3ß)-, Octadecanoic acid, 2-[4-methyl-6-(2,6,6-trimethylcyclohex-1-enyl)hexa-1,3,5-trienyl]cyclol, 9-Desoxo-9-x-acetoxy-3,8,12-tri-acetylingol, 9,12-Cyclolanost-24-en-3-ol, acetate,(3ß)-, y-Tocopherol, Lup-20(29)-en-3-ol,acetate,(3ß)-, Ethyl iso – allocholate, Campesterol and Ascaridole epoxide (Figures 4 to 32).

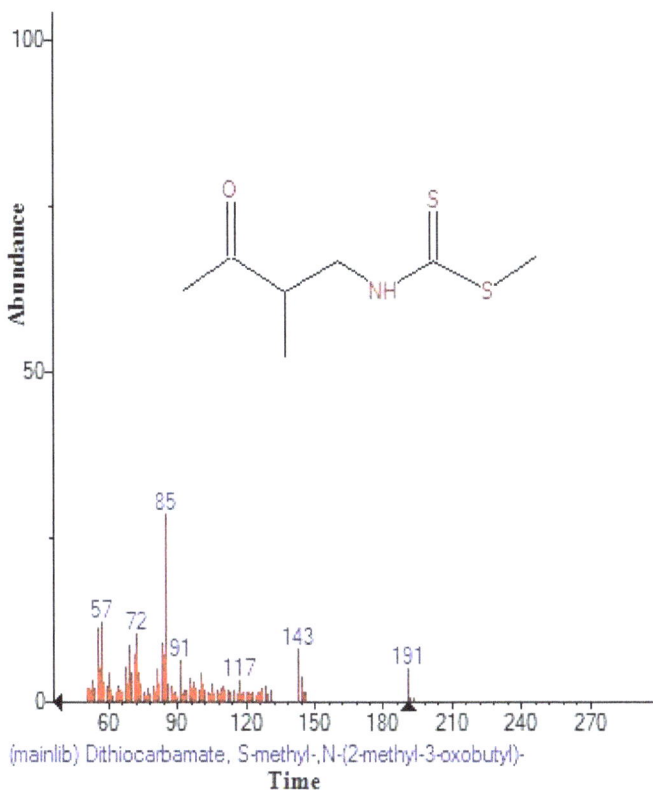

Figure 8. Structure of Dithiocarbamate , S-methyl-N-(2-methyl-3-oxobutyl) with 4.775 (RT) present in *Ocimum basilicum*.

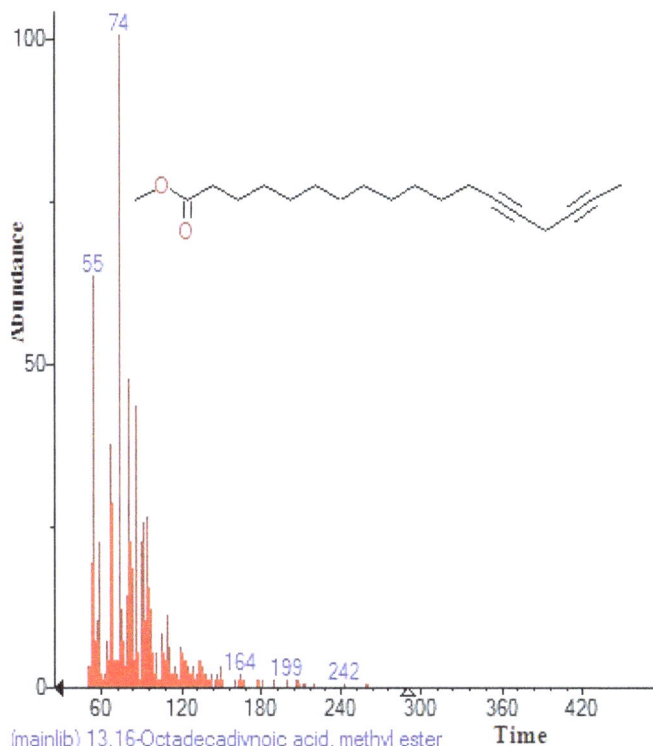

Figure 10. Structure of 13,16-Octadecadiynoic acid , methyl ester with 5.301 (RT) present in *Ocimum basilicum*.

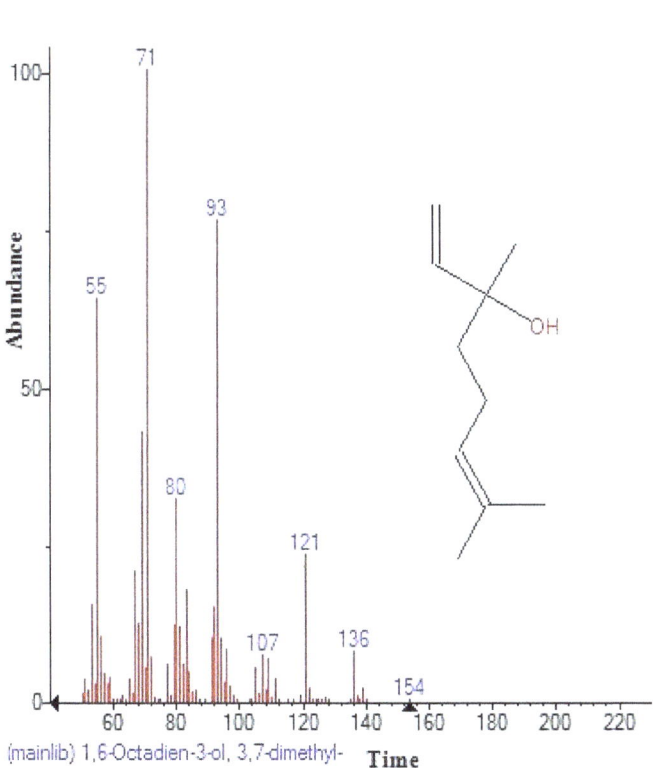

Figure 9. Structure of 1,6-Octadien-3-ol,3,7-dimethyl with 5.067 (RT) present in *Ocimum basilicum*.

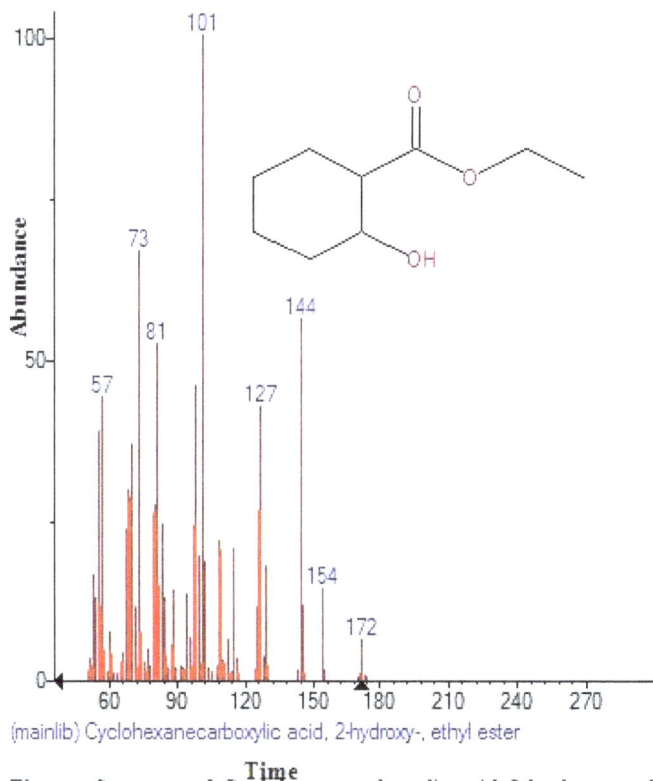

Figure 11. Structure of Cyclohexanecarboxylic acid ,2-hydroxy-, ethyl ester with 5.776 (RT) present in *Ocimum basilicum*.

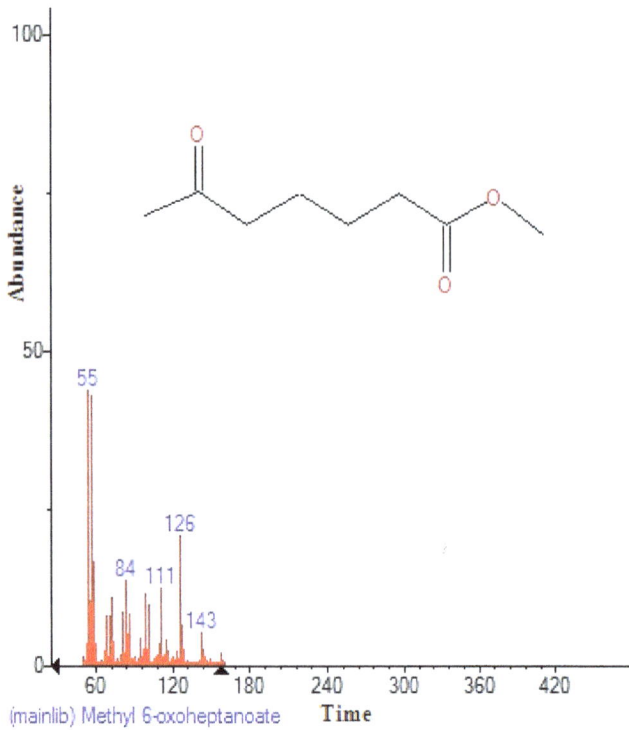

Figure 12. Structure of Methyl 6-oxoheptanoate with 6.011 (RT) present in *Ocimum basilicum*.

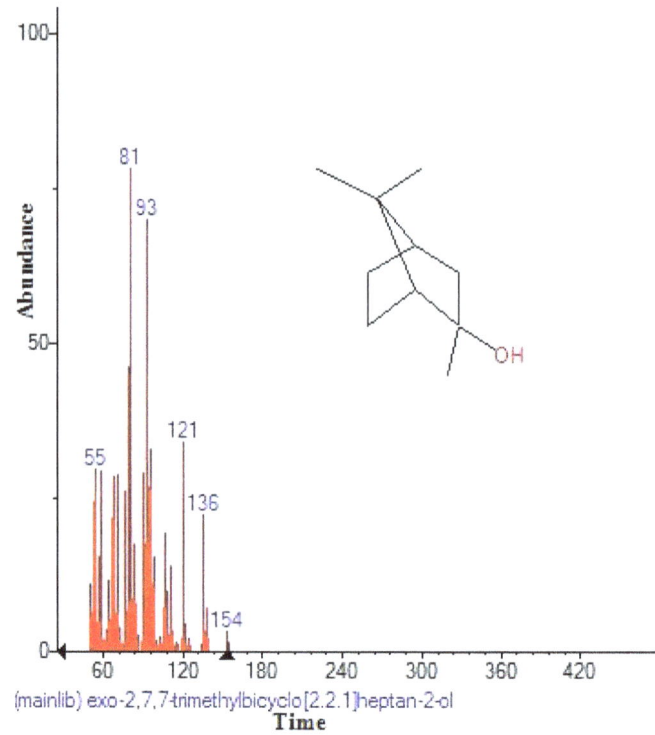

Figure 14. Structure of Exo-2,7,7-trimethylbicyclo[2.2.1]heptan-2-ol with 6.303 (RT) present in *Ocimum basilicum*.

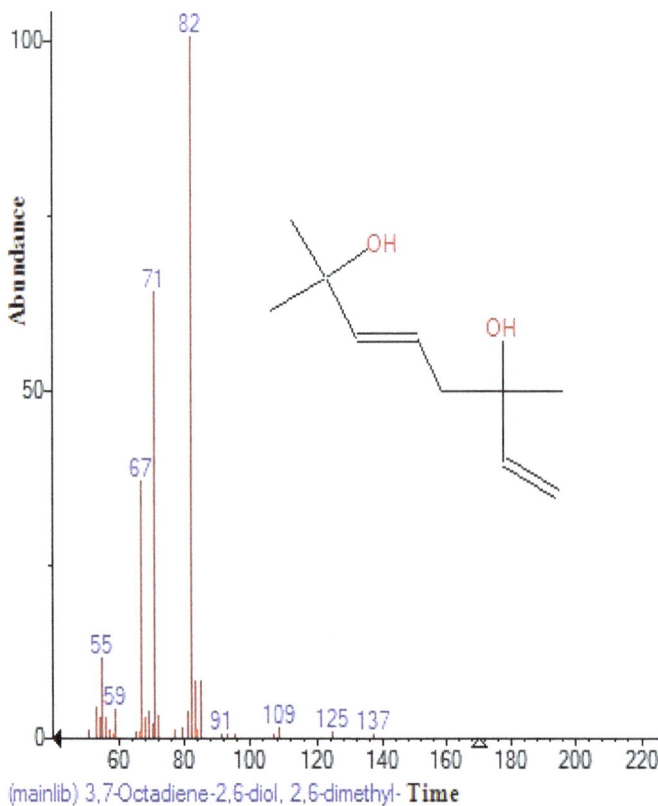

Figure 13. Structure of 3,7-Octadiene-2,6-diol,2,6-dimethyl with 6.245 (RT) present in *Ocimum basilicum*.

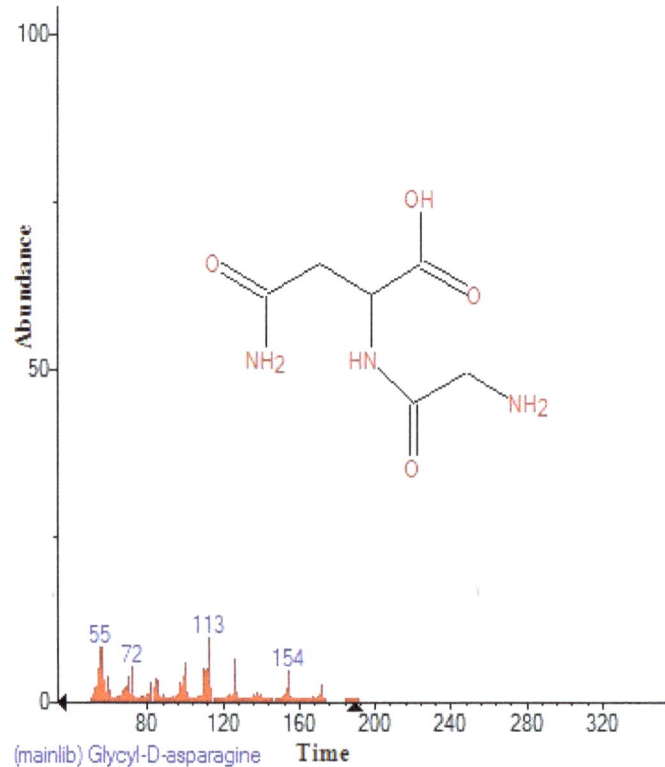

Figure 15. Structure of Glycyl-D-asparagine with 6.772 (RT) present in *Ocimum basilicum*.

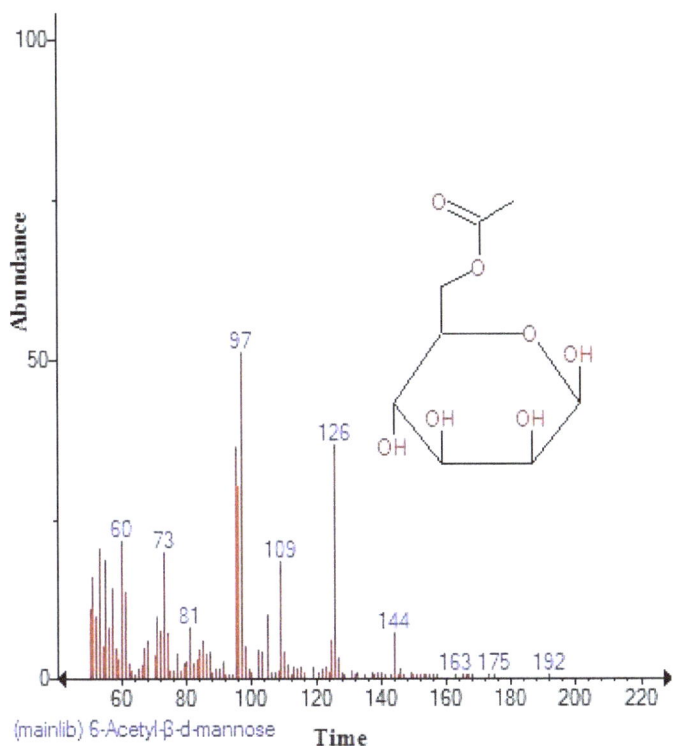

Figure 16. Structure of 6-Acetyl-ß-d-mannose with 6.932 (RT) present in *Ocimum basilicum*.

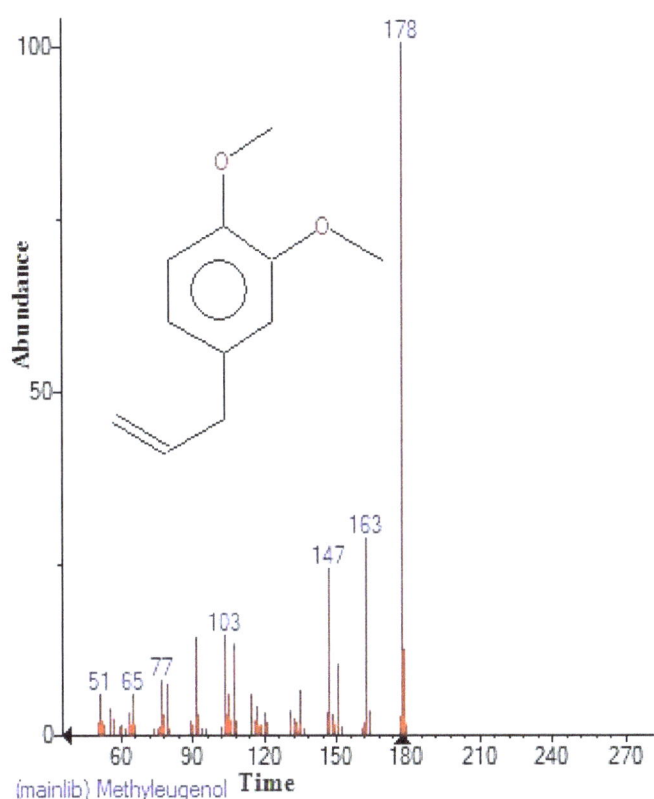

Figure 18. Structure of Methyleugenol with 8.980 (RT) present in *Ocimum basilicum*.

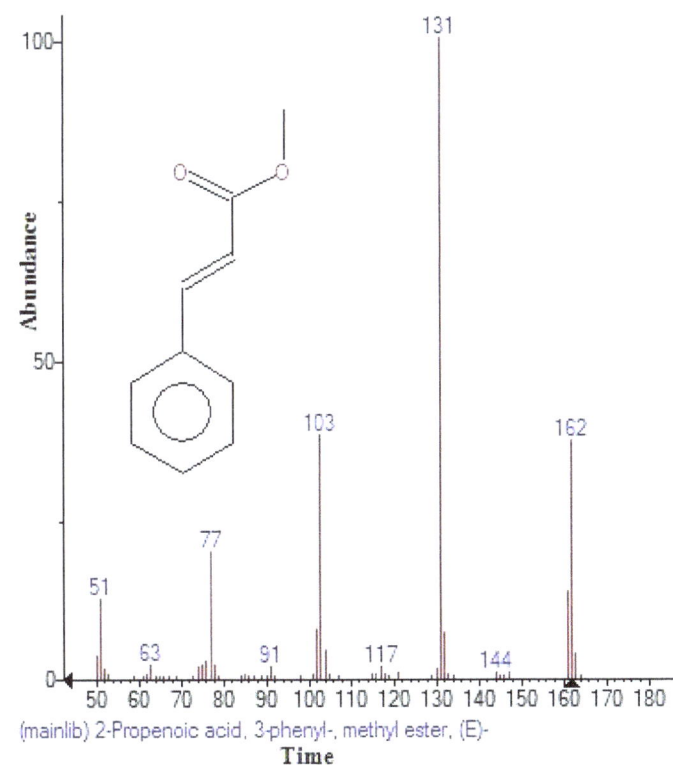

Figure 17. Structure of 2-Propenoic acid ,3-phenyl-,methyl ester , (E) with 7.744 (RT) present in *Ocimum basilicum*.

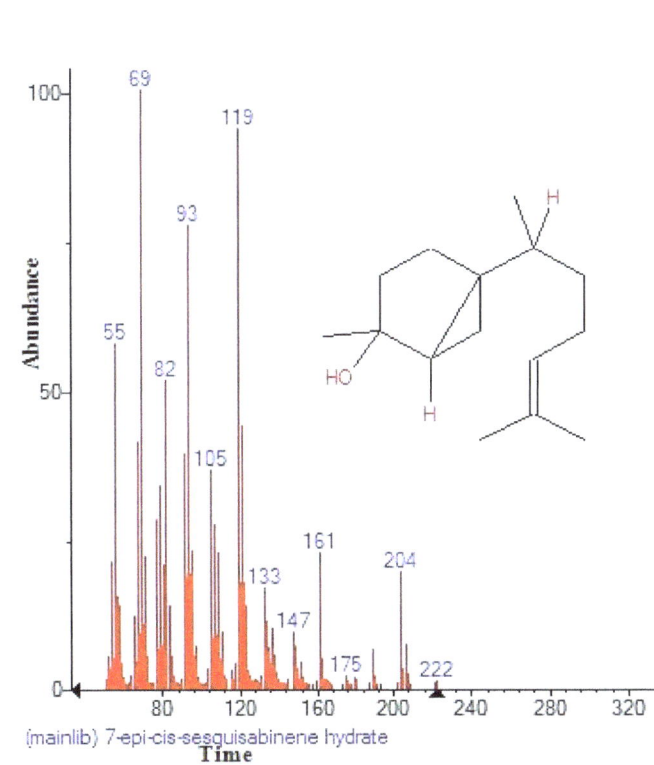

Figure 19. Structure of 7-epi-cis-sesquisabinene hydrate with 9.404 (RT) present in *Ocimum basilicum*.

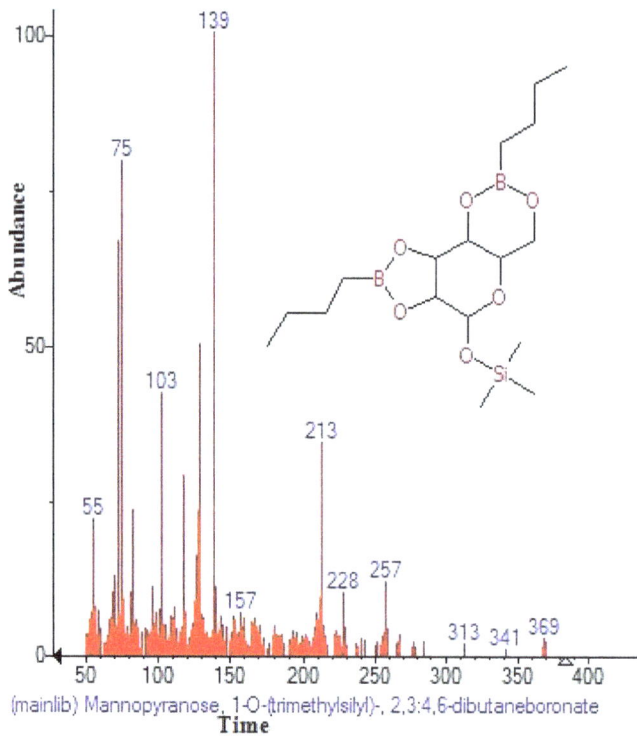

Figure 20. Structure of Mannopyranose , 1-O-(triethylsilyl)-, 2,3:4,6-dibutaneboronate with 13.163 (RT) present in *Ocimum basilicum*.

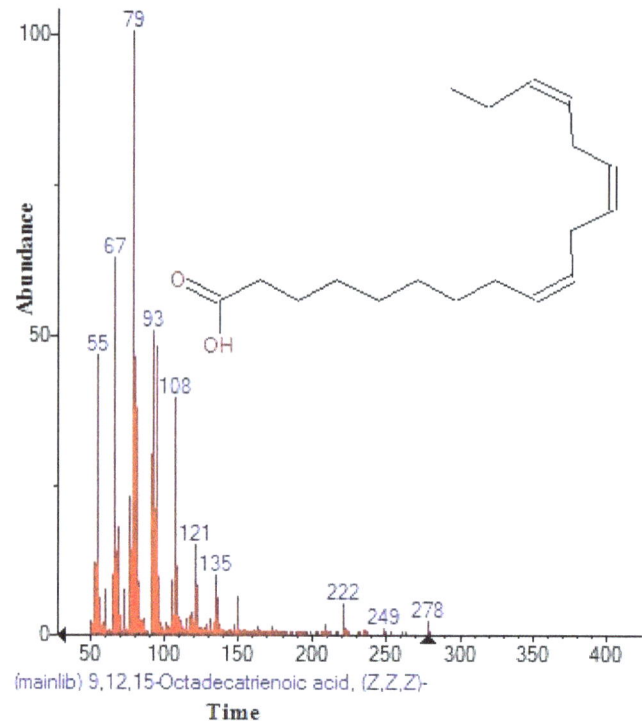

Figure 22. Structure of 9,12,15-Octadecatrienoic acid , (Z,Z,Z) with 17.031 (RT) present in *Ocimum basilicum*.

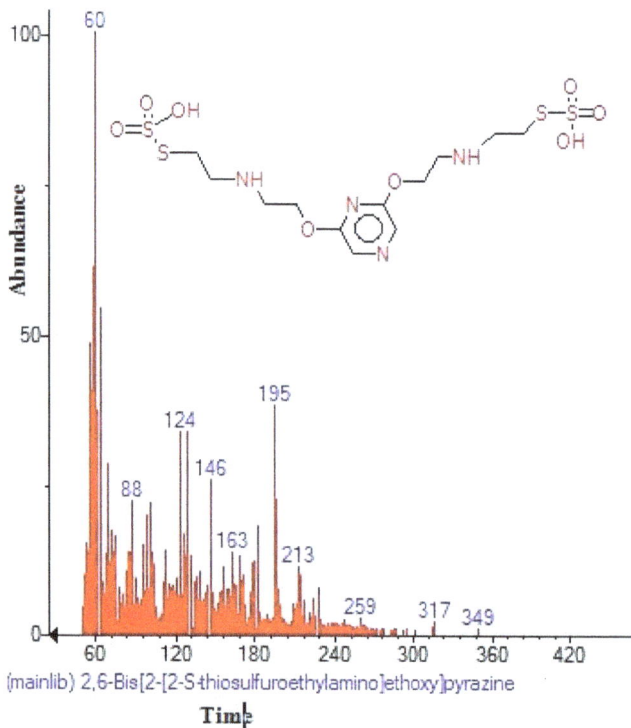

Figure 21. Structure of 2,6-Bis[2-[2-S-thiosulfuroethylamino]ethoxy]pyrazine with 16.133 (RT) present in *Ocimum basilicum*.

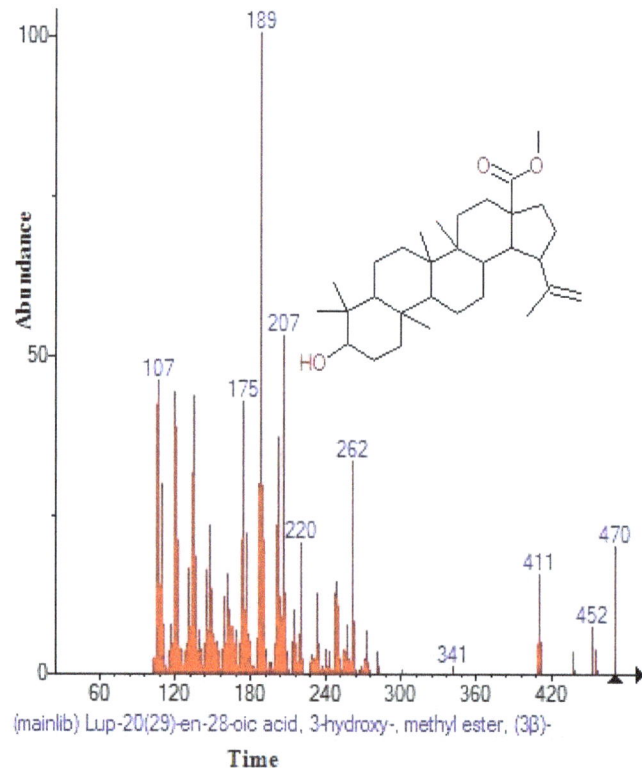

Figure 23. Structure of Lup-20(29)-en-28-oic acid , 3-hydroxy-, methyl ester , (3ß) with 17.317 (RT) present in *Ocimum basilicum*.

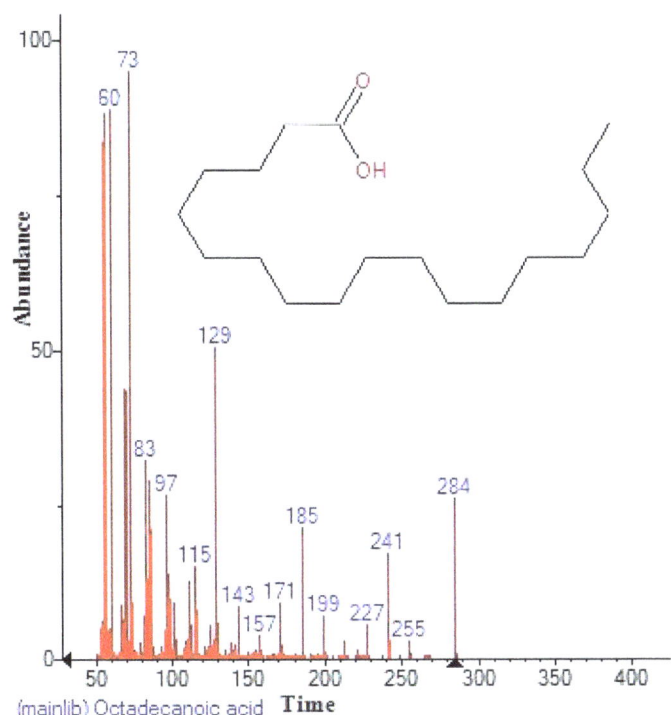

Figure 24. Structure of Octadecanoic acid with 17.186 (RT) present in *Ocimum basilicum*.

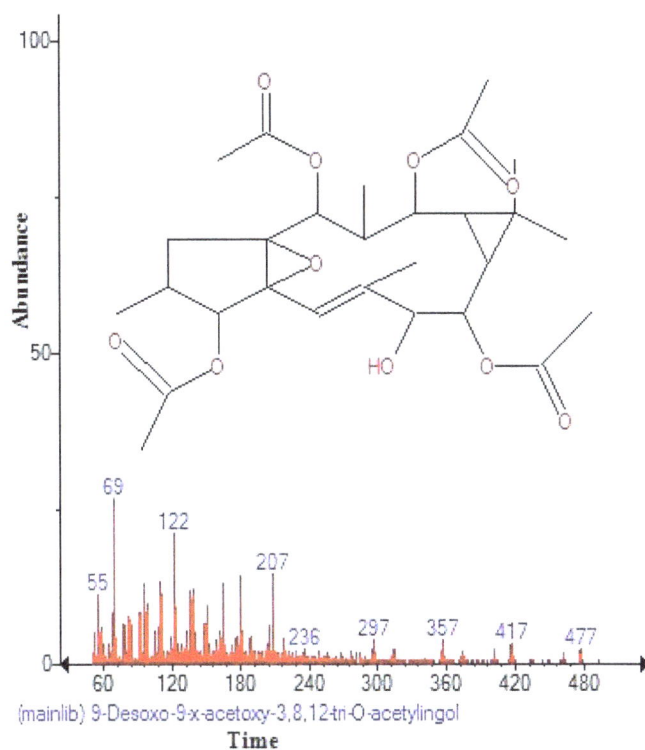

Figure 26. Structure of 9-Desoxo-9-x-acetoxy-3,8,12-tri-acetylingol with 21.946 (RT) present in *Ocimum basilicum*.

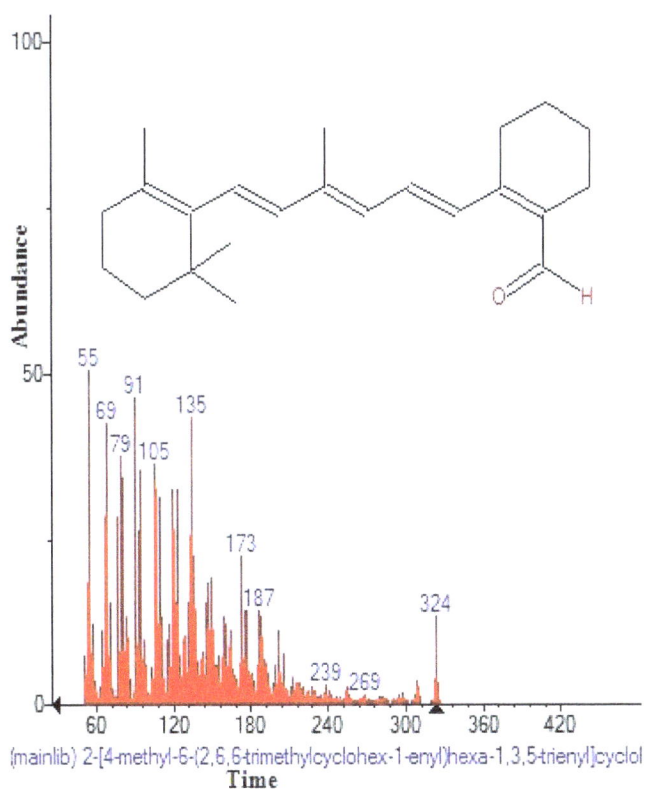

Figure 25. Structure of 2-[4-methyl-6-(2,6,6-trimethylcyclohex-1-enyl)hexa-1,3,5-trienyl]cyclol with 17.369 (RT) present in *Ocimum basilicum*.

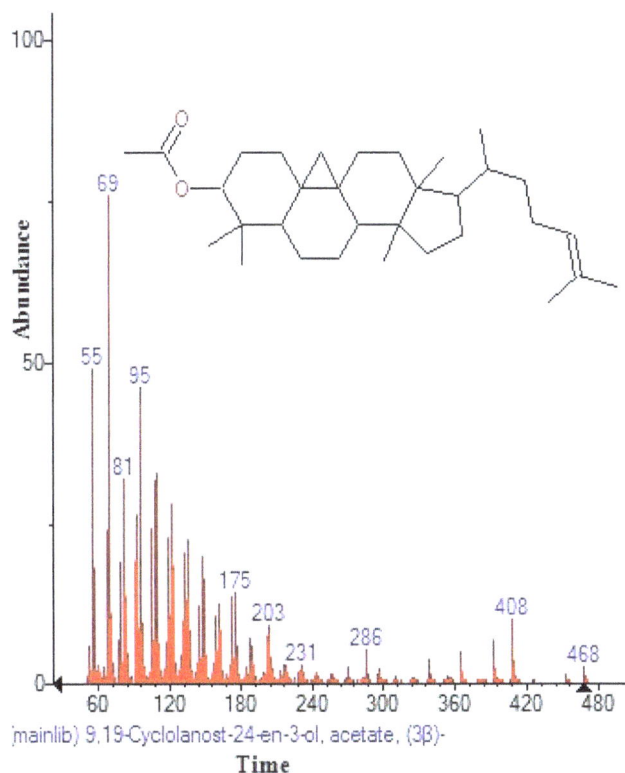

Figure 27. Structure of 9,12-Cyclolanost-24-en-3-ol, acetate,(3ß) with 23.497 (RT) present in *Ocimum basilicum*.

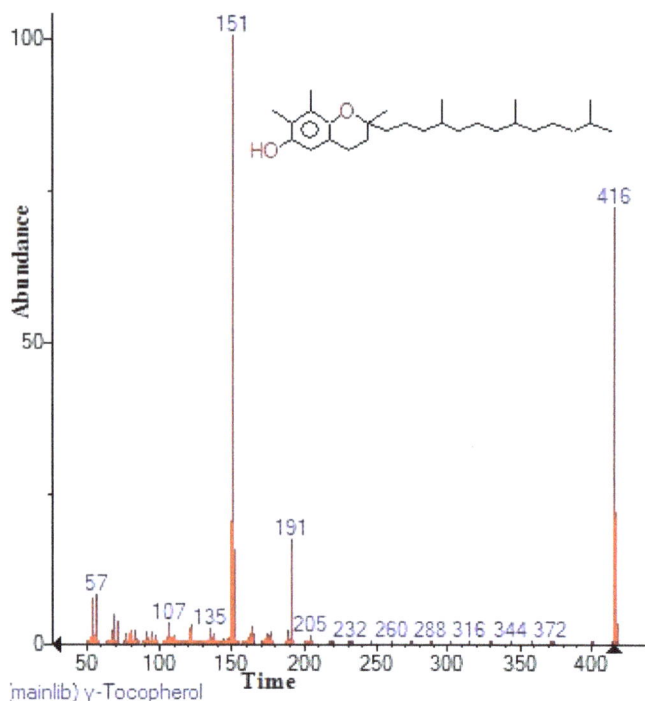

Figure 28. Structure of y-Tocopherol with 25.231 (RT) present in *Ocimum basilicum*.

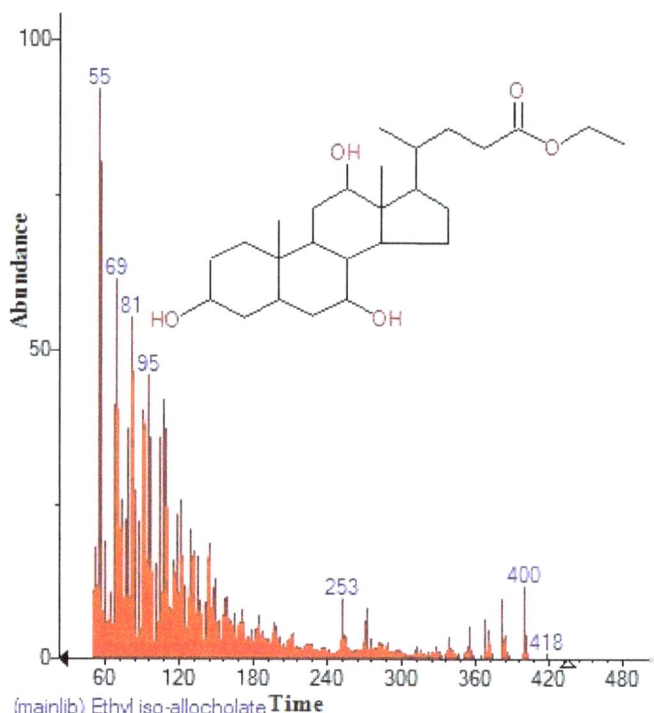

Figure 30. Structure of Ethyl iso – allocholate with 26.890 (RT present in *Ocimum basilicum*.

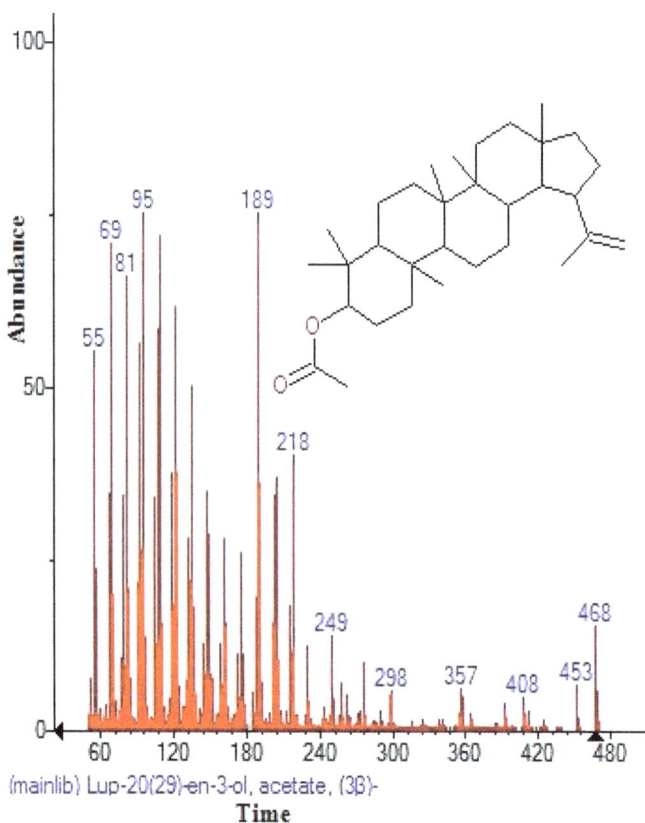

Figure 29. Structure of Lup-20(29)-en-3-ol,acetate,(3ß) with 26.467 (RT) present in *Ocimum basilicum*.

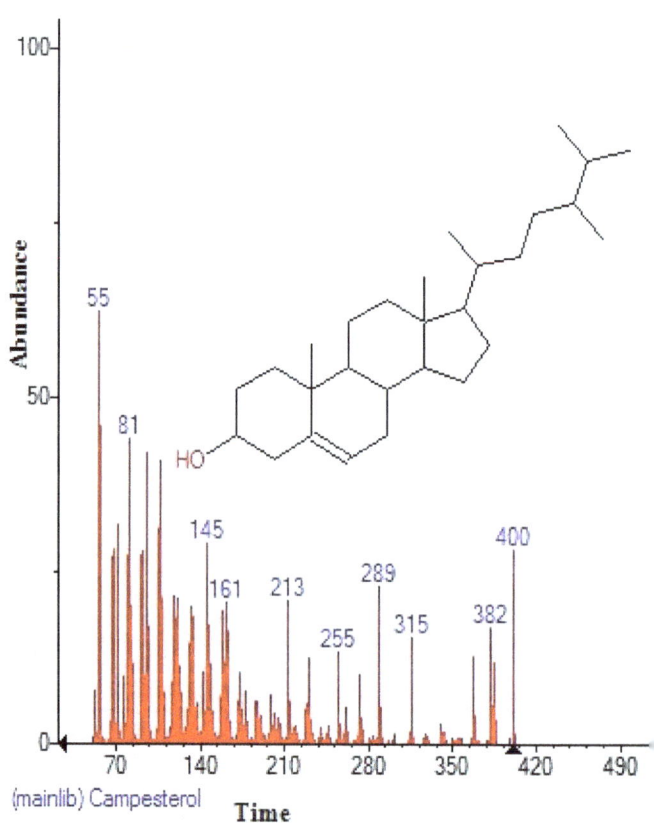

Figure 31. Structure of Campesterol with 28.229 (RT) present i *Ocimum basilicum*.

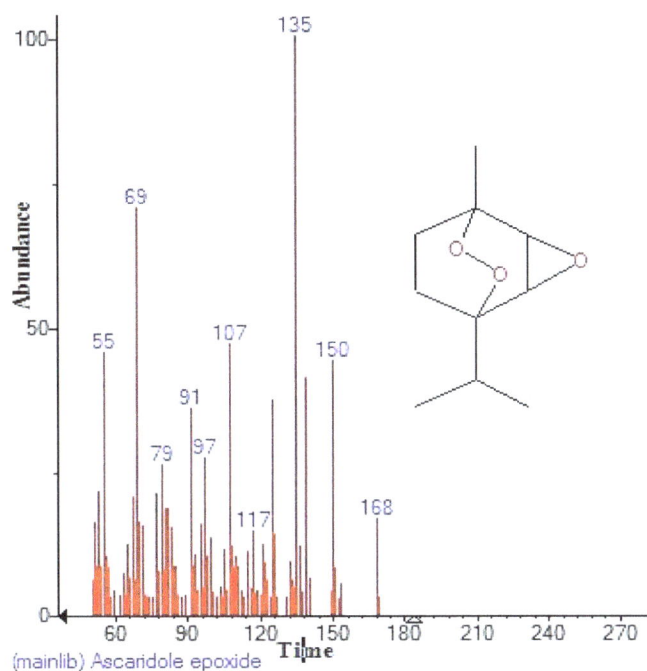

Figure 32. Structure of Ascaridole epoxide with 7.167 (RT) present in *Ocimum basilicum*.

Table 2. FT-IR peak values of *Ocimum basilicum* methanolic aerial parts extract.

No.	Peak (Wave number cm⁻ⁱ)	Intensity	Bond	Functional group assignment	Group frequency
1	665.44	61.240	-	Unknown	-
2	1028.06	60.648	C-F stretch	Aliphatic fluoro compounds	1000-1050
3	1095.57	64.096	C-O	Alcohols, ethers, carboxlic acids, esters	1050-1300
4	1139.93	67.976	C-O	Alcohols, ethers, carboxlic acids, esters	1050-1300
5	1155.36	67.976	C-O	Alcohols, ethers, carboxlic acids, esters	1050-1300
6	1238.30	72.739	C-O	Alcohols, ethers, carboxlic acids, esters	1050-1300
7	1317.38	76.675	NO₂	Nitro compounds	1300-1370
8	1361.74	75.877	NO₂	Nitro compounds	1300-1370
9	1396.46	75.235	C-H	Alkanes	1340-1470
10	1616.35	74.205	-	Unknown	-
11	1734.65	72.915	-	Unknown	-
12	2852.72	79.425	C-H	Alkanes	2850-2970
13	2924.09	73.457	C-H	Alkanes	2850-2970
14	3010.88	84.980	H-O	H-bonded H-X group	2500-3500
15	3196.05	83.617	H-O	H-bonded H-X group	2500-3500
16	3275.13	81.882	O-H	Hydrogen bonded alcohols, phenols	3200-3600

The FTIR analysis of *O. basilicum* aerial parts proved the presence of aliphatic fluoro compounds, alcohols, ethers, carboxlic acids, esters, nitro compounds, alkanes, H-bonded H-X group, hydrogen bonded alcohols and phenols which shows major peaks at 1028.06, 1095.57, 1238.30, 1317.38, 1396.46, 1396.46, 1616.35, 3010.88 and 3275.13 (Table 2 and Figure 33). Baritaux et al. (1992) isolated and analyzed essential oil from basil (*O.*

basilicum) by steam distillation, then it were recovered into a pentane/dichlorometane mixture containing known amounts of two internal standards, nonane and octadecane. Laakso et al. (1990) analyzed essential oil from holy basil by two extraction methods steam distillation and water distillation. The essential oil was identified into 20 different compounds by GC-MS and GCFTIR. They contained high amounts of eugenol

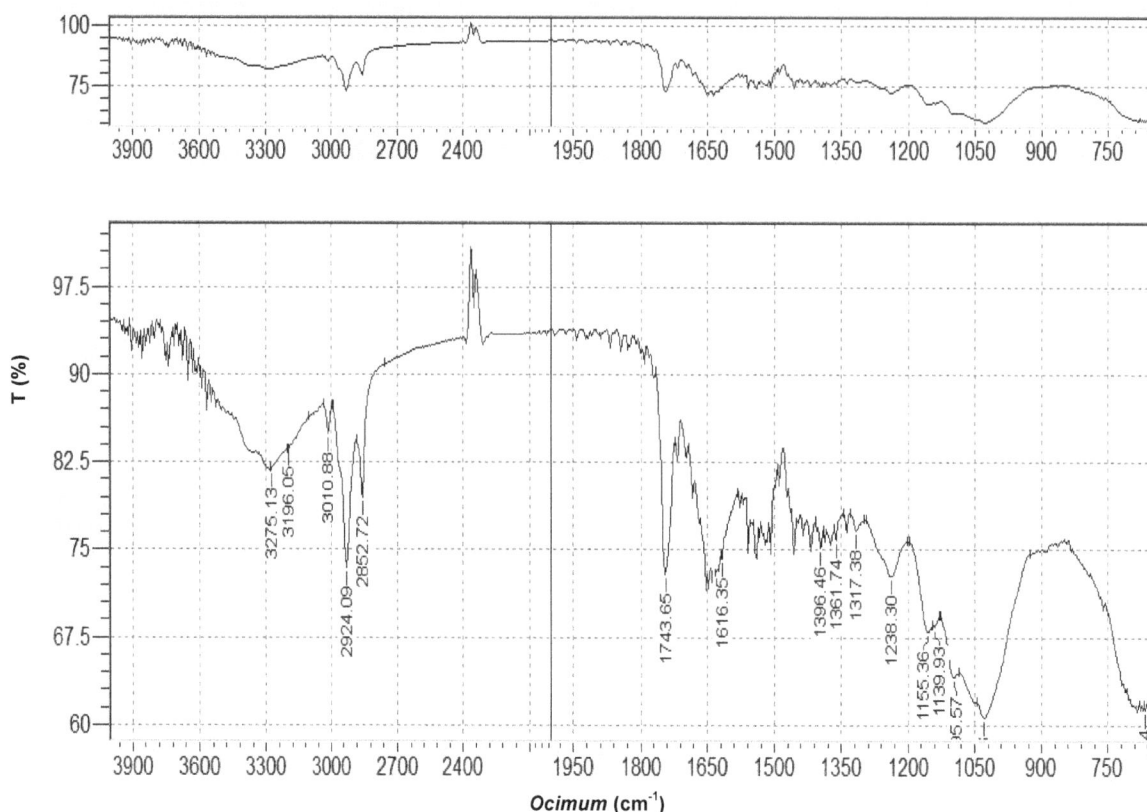

Figure 33. FT-IR peak values of *Ocimum basilicum*.

Table 3. Zone of inhibition (mm) of test bacterial strains to *Ocimum basilicum* bioactive compounds and standard antibiotics.

Ocimum basilicum antibiotics	Bacteria				
	Staphylococcus aureus	*Escherichia coli*	*Proteus mirabilis*	*Klebsiella pneumonia*	*Pseudomonas eurogenosa*
Ocimum basilicum	5.00±0.21	5.70±0.10	4.30±0.20	4.22±0.23	4.17±0.44
Rifambin	0.89±0.22	0.86±0.31	1.00±0.35	0.96±0.26	2.00±0.06
Streptomycin	1.09±0.33	1.44±0.29	0.99±0.28	1.00±0.47	1.64±0.30
Kanamycin	0.55±0.29	0.98±0.28	2.01±0.12	0.69±0.23	1.50±0.18
Cefotoxime	1.57±0.27	1.86±0.32	1.03±0.24	1.00±0.23	0.95±0.27

(24.2%), β-bisabolenes (15.4%), α-bisabolenes (10.6%) and methyl chavicol (11.16%), but methyleugenol could not be detected. Raju *et al.* (1999) analyzed bioactive chemical compounds isolated in the leaves of basil from India by GC and GC-MS. Twenty-five components were found from 98.7% total oil area. Eugenol (53.4%), β-caryophyllene (31.7%) and β-elemene were found as the major components. Essential oils are extracted from various aromatic plants generally located in temperate to warm countries, like Brazil, where they represent an important part of the traditional pharmacopoeia due to their important biological activities (Morales and Simon, 1996; Phippen and Simon, 1998). An important approach to discover new medicines is survey of natural products,

such as medicinal plants or their secondary metabolites that modulate painful conditions (Baratta et al., 1998 Chiang et al., 2005).

Previous studies (Bakkali et al., 2008; Quintans-Júnio et al., 2008; Oliveira et al., 2009; Li and Vederas, 2009 Venâncio et al., 2011) have demonstrated that severa *Ocimum* species are used to treat central nervous system (CNS) disorders in various regions of the world, mainly in developing countries, and their analgesic profile is frequently reported. In this study, five clinical pathogens were selected for antibacterial activity, namely, *S. aureus K. pneumoniae, P. aeruginosa, E. coli* and *Proteus mirabilis*. Maximum zone formation is against *E. col* (5.70±0.10) (Table 3). Essential oils derived from severa

Ocimum spp. have been reported to be active against several Gram-positive and Gram-negative bacteria as well as against yeasts and fungi due to their terpenic constituents. Recently, essential oils and extracts of certain plants have been shown to have antimicrobial effects as well as imparting flavour to foods (Zhang et al., 2009; Shareef et al., 2016; Kadhim et al., 2016). *Ocimum* spp. contain a wide range of essential oils rich in phenolic compounds and a wide array of other natural products including polyphenols such as flavonoids and anthocyanins. Antiviral and antimicrobial activities of this plant have also been reported (Li and Vederas, 2009; Venâncio et al., 2011).

Conclusion

The results of this study provide data on phytochemical characteristics of *O. basilicum*. *O. basilicum* is native plant of Iraq. It contains chemical constitutions which may be useful for various herbal formulation as anti-inflammatory, analgesic, antipyretic, cardiac tonic and antiasthamatic.

ACKNOWLEDGEMENT

The authors wish to express their deepest gratitude to Prof. Dr. Adul-Kareem for his valuable contributions and support throughout this study.

REFERENCES

Al-Marzoqi AH, Hadi MY, Hameed IH (2016). Determination of metabolites products by *Cassia angustifolia* and evaluate antimicobial activity. J. Pharmacogn. Phytother. 8(2):25-48.

Al-Marzoqi AH, Hameed IH, Idan SA (2015). Analysis of bioactive chemical components of two medicinal plants (*Coriandrum sativum* and *Melia azedarach*) leaves using gas chromatography-mass spectrometry (GC-MS). Afr. J. Biotechnol. 14(40):2812-2830.

Altameme HJ, Hadi MY, Hameed IH (2015a). Phytochemical analysis of *Urtica dioica* leaves by fourier-transform infrared spectroscopy and gas chromatography-mass spectrometry. J. Pharmacogn. Phytother. 7(10):238-252.

Altameme HJ, Hameed IH, Abu-Serag NA (2015b). analysis of bioactive phytochemical compounds of two medicinal plants, *Equisetum arvense* and *Alchemila valgaris* seed using gas chromatography-mass spectrometry and fourier-transform infrared spectroscopy. Malays. Appl. Biol. 44(4):47-58.

Altameme HJ, Hameed IH, Idan SA, Hadi MY (2015c). Biochemical analysis of *Origanum vulgare* seeds by fourier-transform infrared (FT-IR) spectroscopy and gas chromatography-mass spectrometry (GC-MS). J. Pharmacogn. Phytother. 7(9):221-237.

Bais HP, Walker TS, Schweizer HP, Vivanco JA (2002). 'Root specific elicitation and antimicrobial activity of rosmarinic acid in hairy root cultures of *Ocimum basilicum*'. Plant Physiol. Biochem. 40: 983-995.

Bakkali F, Averbeck S, Averbeck D, Idaomar M (2008). Biological effects of essential oils—A review. Food Chem. Toxicol. 46:446-475.

Baratta MT, Dorman HJD, Deans SG, Figueiredo AC, Barroso JG, Ruberto G (1998). Antimicrobial and antioxidant properties of some commercial essential oil. Flav Fragr J. 13:235-234.

Baritaux O, Richard H, Touche J, Derbesy H. (1992). Effects of drying and storage of herbs and spices on the essential oil. Part I. basil, *Ocimum bacilicum*. Flavour Fragr. J. 7:267-271.

Bauer K, Garbe D, Surburg H (1997). Common fragrance and flavor materials'. 3rd edition, Weinheim: Wiley- VCH. 171.

Chiang LC (2005). Antiviral activities of extracts and selected pure constituents of *Ocimum basilicum* . Clin. Exp. Pharmacol. Physiol. 32(10):811-816.

Chiang LC, Cheng PW, Chiang W, Lin CC (2005). Antiviral activity of extracts and selected pure constituents of *Ocimum basilicum*. Clin. Exp. Pharmacol. Physiol. 32:811-816.

Hadi MY, Mohammed GJ, Hameed IH (2016). Analysis of bioactive chemical compounds of *Nigella sativa* using gas chromatography-mass spectrometry. J. Pharmacogn. Phytother. 8(2):8-24.

Halliwell B, Gutteridge JM (1992). Free radicals, antioxidants and human diseases: where are we now? J. Lab. Clin. Med. 119:598-620.

Hameed IH, Abdulzahra AI, Jebor MA, Kqueen CY, Ommer AJ (2015a). Haplotypes and variable position detection in the mitochondrial DNA coding region encompassing nucleotide positions. Mitochondrial DNA 26(4):544-9.

Hameed IH, Hamza LF, Kamal SA (2015b). Analysis of bioactive chemical compounds of *Aspergillus niger* by using gas chromatography-mass spectrometry and fourier-transform infrared spectroscopy. J. Pharmacogn. Phytother. 7(8):132-163.

Hameed IH, Hussein HJ, Kareem MA, Hamad NS (2015c). Identification of five newly described bioactive chemical compounds in methanolic extract of *Mentha viridis* by using gas chromatography-mass spectrometry (GC-MS). J. Pharmacogn. Phytother. 7(7):107-125.

Hameed IH, Ibraheam IA, Kadhim HJ (2015d). Gas chromatography mass spectrum and fourier-transform infrared spectroscopy analysis of methanolic extract of *Rosmarinus oficinalis* leaves. J. Pharmacogn. Phytother. 7(6):90-106.

Holm Y (1999). Bioactivity of basil. In: Hiltunen, R. and Y. Holm (Eds.) Basil. The Genus Ocimum. Harwood Academic Publishers, Amsterdam. pp. 113-136.

Hussein AO, Mohammed GJ, Hadi MY, Hameed IH (2016a). Phytochemical screening of methanolic dried galls extract of *Quercus infectoria* using gas chromatography-mass spectrometry (GC-MS) and Fourier transform-infrared (FT-IR). J. Pharmacogn. Phytother. 8(3):49-59.

Hussein HJ, Hadi MY, Hameed IH (2016b). Study of chemical composition of *Foeniculum vulgare* using Fourier transform infrared spectrophotometer and gas chromatography - mass spectrometry. J. Pharmacogn. Phytother. 8(3):60-89.

Hussein HM, Hameed IH, Ibraheem OA (2016c). Antimicrobial activity and spectral chemical analysis of methanolic leaves extract of *Adiantum capillus-veneris* using GC-MS and FT-IR spectroscopy. Int. J. Pharmacogn. Phytochemical Res. 8(3).

Jasim H, Hussein AO, Hameed IH, Kareem MA (2015). Characterization of alkaloid constitution and evaluation of antimicrobial activity of *Solanum nigrum* using gas chromatography mass spectrometry (GC-MS). J. Pharmacogn. Phytother. 7(4):56-72.

Juliani HR, Simon JE (2002). Antioxidant activity of basil. In Trends in new crops and new uses, Janick, J. and A. Whipkey. Eds. ASHS Press. Alexandria. 575–579.

Kadhim MJ, Mohammed GJ, Hameed IH (2016). In vitro antibacterial, antifungal and phytochemical analysis of methanolic fruit extract of *Cassia fistula*. Oriental J. Chem. 32(2):10-30.

Koba K, Poutouli PW, Raynaud C, Chaumont JP, Sanda K (2009). Chemical composition and antimicrobial properites of different basil essential oils chemotyypes from Togo. Bangladesh J. Pharmacol. 4:1–8.

Laakso I, Seppanen T, Herrmann-Wolf B, Kuhnel N, Knobloch K (1990). Constituents of the essential oil from the holy basil or tulsi plant, *Ocimum sanctum*. Planta Med. 56:527.

Li JW, Vederas JC (2009). Drug discovery and natural products: End of an era or an endless frontier? Science 325:161–165.

Morales MR, Simon JE (1996). New basil selections with compact inflorescences for the ornamental market, In: Janick J (ed.), Progress in new crops. Arlington: ASHS Press;. p. 543-546.

Ogendo JO, Belma SR, Deng AL, Walker DJ (2003). Comparison of toxic and repellent effects of *Lantana camara* L. with *Tephrosia vogelii* Hook and a synthetic pesticide against *Sitophilus zeamais* Motschulsky (Coleoptera: Curculionidae) in stored maizegrain. Insect Science and its Application. 23:127-135.

Oliveira JS, Porto LA, Estevam, CS, Siqueira RS, Alves PB, Niculau ES, Blank AF, Almeida RN, Marchioro M, Quintans-Júnior LJ (2009). Phytochemical screening and anticonvulsant property of *Ocimum basilicum* leaf essential oil. *Bol. Latinoam. Caribe Plant. Med. Aromat.* 8:195–202.

Phippen WB, Simon JE (1998). Anthocyanins in basil (*Ocimum basilicum* L.). J. Agric. Food Chem. 46:1734–1738.

Politeo O, Jukic M, Milos M (2007). Chemical composition and antioxidant capacity of free volatile aglycones from basil (*Ocimum basilicum* L.) compared with its essential oil. Food Chem. 101:379–385.

Quintans-Júnior LJ, Souza T, Leite B, Lessa N, Bonjardim L, Santos M, Alves P, Blank A, Antoniolli A (2008). Phythochemical screening and anticonvulsant activity of *Cymbopogon winterianus* Jowitt (Poaceae) leaf essential oil in rodents. Phytomedicine 15:619–624.

Raju PM, Ali M, Velasco-Negueruela A, Perez-Alonso MJ (1999). Volatile constituents of the leaves of *Ocimum sanctum* L. J. Essent. Oil Res. 11:159-161.

Rukayadi Y, Yong D, Hwang JK (2006). In vitro anticandidal activity of xanthorrhizol isolated from *Curcuma xanthorrhiza* Roxb. J. Antimicrob. Chemother. 57:1231-1234.

Shareef HK, Muhammed HJ, Hussein HM, Hameed IH (2016). Antibacterial effect of ginger (*Zingiber officinale*) roscoe and bioactiv chemical analysis using gas chromatography mass spectrum Oriental J. Chem. 32(2):20-40.

Smith EE, Facelli E, Pope S, Smith FA (2010). Plant performance i stressful environments. Interpreting new and established knowledg of the roles of arbuscular mycorrhizas. Plant Soil 326: 3-20.

Venâncio AM, Marchioro M, Estavam CS, Melo MS, Santana MT Onofre AS, Guimarães AG, Oliveira MG, Alves PB, Pimentel HC (2011). *Ocimum basilicum* leaf essential oil and (−)-linalool reduc orofacial nociception in rodents: A behavioral an electrophysiological approach. Rev. Bras. Farmacogn. 21:1043-1051

Yang SA, Jeon SK, Lee EJ, Shim CH, Lee IS (2010). Comparativ study of the chemical composition and antioxidant activity of s essential oils and their components. Nat. Prod. Res. 24: 140-151.

Yoshikawa M, Morikawa T, Kobayashi H, Nakamura A, Matsuhira K Nakamura S, Matsuda H (2007). Bioactive saponins and glycoside Structures of new cucurbitane-type triterpene glycosides an antiallergic constituents from *Citrullus colocynthis*. Chem. Pharm Bull. l55:428-434.

Zhang JW, Li SK, Wu WJ (2009). The Main Chemical Composition an in vitro Antifungal Activity of Essential Oils of *Ocimum basilicum* Linr var. *pilosum* (Willd.) Benth. Molecules. 14(1):273-278.

## 13

In vivo anti-plasmodial activity and histopathological analysis of water and ethanol extracts of a polyherbal antimalarial recipe

Mojirayo Rebecca Ibukunoluwa

Department of Biology, Adeyemi College of Education, Ondo State, Nigeria.

Anthocleista djalonensis A. Chev. (stem bark), *Azadirachta indica* A. Juss (stem bark and leaf), *Cajanus cajan* (L.) Huth. (leaf), *Crescentia cujete* L. (stem bark), *Lawsonia inermis* L. (leaf), *Lophira alata* Banks ex C.F. Gaertn. (stem bark), *Myrianthus pruessii* Engl. (leaf), *Nauclea latifolia* Sm. (stem bark), *Olax subscorpioidea* Oliv. (root), and *Terminalia glaucescens* Planch ex Benth. (stem bark and root) are combined for use in the treatment of malaria in Akure, Southwestern Nigeria. The powdered plant samples were screened for phytochemical constituents, proximate composition and mineral elements according to standard protocols. *Plasmodium berghei* infected mice were screened for parasitemia and administered with water and ethanol extracts of the combined plant sample. Toxicity and histopathological studies were carried out on the liver and kidney sections of the mice. Data were statistically analyzed. The powdered herbal recipe contained appreciable phytochemicals and important minerals. The concentrations administered for LD_{50} did not elicit adverse reactions in the experimental animals, and no mortality was recorded. Histological studies revealed some pathology caused by the malaria parasite, as well as side effects of the extracts administered. This is discussed in relation to safety considerations.

Key words: Malaria, herbs, phytochemical, histopathology, Nigeria.

INTRODUCTION

Malaria, an infectious disease caused by *Plasmodium* species, has been a menace to the health conditions of both rural and urban populations in Nigeria (NGA, 2005). Although, it is a global epidemic the incidence and severity are higher in the tropics especially in the sub-Saharan Africa, where pregnant women and children are the most susceptible (Nmorsi et al., 2007; WHO, 2008; Nguta et al., 2010; Akanbi et al., 2012). It is prevalent in the tropical and subtropical regions because environmental factors such as rainfall, warm temperatures, and stagnant water provide the ideal habitats for the development of the mosquito that serve as the vector. Approximately 40% of the world's population is susceptible to malaria. Records have shown that 3.3 billion people all over the world live in areas at risk of malaria with episodes in 106 countries and

*Corresponding author. E-mail: mojibukun@yahoo.com.

territories (African Medical and Research Foundation - AMRF, 2012). In the year 2010, an estimated 655,000 people died of malaria - most of whom were young children in sub-Saharan Africa where one in every five childhood deaths is due to malaria (Ibrahim et al., 2004). Moreover, 91% of deaths in 2010 were in the African region, followed by the South-East Asian region (6%), and the Eastern Mediterranean region (3%), and about 86% of death in children globally (WHO, 2011). However, more than three million deaths and 300 to 500 million cases are still reported annually in the world (Sachs and Malaney, 2002).

In recent years, malaria has become more difficult to control and treat with conventional drugs of western medicine because malaria parasites have become resistant to drugs, and mosquitoes that transmit the disease have become resistant to insecticides. Plants, particularly herbs, are the basis for the development of modern drugs, and medicinal plants have been used for many years in daily life to treat diseases all over the world (Ates and Erdogrul, 2003). At present, traditional medicine is still the predominant means of health care in developing countries where about 80% of their total population depend on it for their wellbeing (WHO, 1978).

Ethnomedicinal investigation revealed that *Anthocleista djalonensis* A. Chev. (stem bark), *Azadirachta indica* A. Juss (stem bark and leaf), *Cajanus cajan* (L.) Huth. (leaf), *Crescentia cujete* L. (stem bark), *Lawsonia inermis* L. (leaf), *Lophira alata* Banks ex C.F. Gaertn. (stem bark), *Myrianthus pruessii* Engl. (leaf), *Nauclea latifolia* Sm. (stem bark), *Olax subscorpioidea* Oliv. (root), and *Terminalia glaucescens* Planch ex Benth. (stem bark and root) are combined for use as a polyherbal recipe in the treatment of malaria in Akure, Southwestern Nigeria.

Akure is a popular metropolis in Ondo State and supports a population of over 400,000 people. The mean annual rainfall is about 1350 mm with bimodal distribution spanning between March and November; the relative humidity averaged 80% with temperature range between 23 and 30°C which is suitable for agricultural production. Civil servants are the major inhabitants of the city which is the centre of administration of the Ondo State Government. However, farming and trading are other occupations of the residents who majored in food crops and livestock production.

This study aimed to screen the plant parts (root, stem bark, leaf) of some herbs used in the treatment of malaria and also to evaluate the toxicity and histopathological effects of the plant extracts on tissues of the kidney and liver using albino mice infected with *Plasmodium berghei* as a model.

MATERIALS AND METHODS

Procurement and identification of plant materials

Fresh samples of *A. djalonensis* (stem bark), *A. indica* (stem bark and leaf), *C. cajan* (leaf), *C. cujete* (stem bark), *L. inermis* (leaf), *L.*

alata (stem bark), *M. pruessii* (leaf), *N. latifolia* (stem bark), *O. subscorpioidea* (root), and *T. glaucescens* (stem bark and root) were bought from herb sellers in Akure and identified at the University of Ibadan herbarium by comparing them with representative specimens. Voucher specimens were deposited in the herbarium.

Preparation of plant samples

The fresh samples were air-dried for 2 to 3 weeks depending on the plant part. The dried plant samples were then pulverized to coarse powder using a laboratory mill (Model 4 Arthur Thomas, USA). The coarse powder was screened for phytochemical, proximate, and mineral compositions.

Phytochemical screening

The powdered plant samples were screened for alkaloids, anthraquinones, flavonoids, glycosides, polyphenols, saponins, and tannins according to the methods described by Harbone (1973), Evans (2002) and Sofowora (2008).

Mineral element analysis

The method of the Association of Analytical Chemists (AOAC, 1990) was used. Calcium (Ca), Sodium (Na), Potassium (K), Phosphorus (P), Copper (Cu), Iron (Fe), Zinc (Zn), Magnesium (Mg), Manganese (Mn), and Lead (Pb) were quantified. Sodium and potassium were estimated with Gallenkamp Flame Analyzer. Phosphorus was determined using phosphor-vanado-molybdate colorimetric techniques, whereas calcium, iron, magnesium, manganese, zinc, lead, and copper were determined using Spectrumlab 23A Spectrophotometer.

Preparation and concentration of extracts

combination (recipe) comprising 50 g each of the 10 powdered plant samples was dissolved in distilled water (500 g in 3 L of distilled water for 24 h) and ethanol (500 g in 3 L of 96% ethanol for 72 h) separately. The individual preparation was stirred every 2 h, decanted and filtered using Whatman No 1 filter paper. The solvent containing the extract was collected, filtered again and concentrated using a rotary evaporator at 40°C. The crude ethanolic extract was further concentrated in a vacuum oven set at 40°C with a pressure of 600 mmHg so as to further remove any traces of solvent. The crude extract of water solvent was further concentrated in a thermo-regulated water bath at 40°C. The concentrate was retrieved and weighed. The extract was refrigerated at 4°C prior to use.

Experimental animals (Swiss albino mice)

The Swiss albino mice weighing between eighteen and twenty-two grammes (18 to 22 g) were purchased from the Institute of Advanced Medical Research and Training (IAMRAT), College of Medicine, University of Ibadan. The animals were housed in iron cages in the animal house of IAMRAT. The animals were acclimatized for two weeks at room temperature with 12 h dark/light periodicity and fed with commercial chow (purchased from Cap Feeds Ibadan, Nigeria) and water *ad libitum*.

Experimental design

The experiment was in two phases (Phases 1 and 2). In Phase 1, the median lethal dose (LD$_{50}$) was determined and in Phase 2, the antiplasmodial activity of the recipe was examined.

Phase 1: Determination of median lethal dose

Twelve-four (24) mice were used. Four (4) mice received 1000 mg/kg body weight of water extract of the combined plant samples; another four (4) mice received 2000 mg/kg body weight; and still another four (4) mice received 3000 mg/kg body weight. The set-up was the same for the ethanol extract. All the animals were monitored for loss of appetite, pains, distress, change in respiration, behavioural manifestations, and most importantly death for a period of 24 h. Oral administration of extract was carried out using gastric feeding tube for 28 days, for long-term possible lethal outcomes (Lorke, 1983).

Phase 2: Antimalarial activity of plant extract

Forty (40) mice were used in all. Five (5) mice received 200 mg/kg body weight of water extract of the combined plant samples; another five (5) mice received 300 mg/kg body weight; and still another five (5) mice received 500 mg/kg body weight. The set-up was the same for the ethanol extract. The control groups were administered with distilled water (5 mice) and chloroquine (5 mice).

Malaria parasite specimen

P. berghei (NK65) was obtained from the Department of Parasitology, Institute of Advanced Medical Research and Training (IAMRAT), University College Hospital (UCH) Ibadan, Nigeria.

Ethical consideration

Ethical guidelines for the use of animal models in research were followed; clearance was sought and obtained from the University of Ibadan/University College Hospital Ethical Committee through the Institute of Advanced Medical Research and Training (IAMRAT), College of Medicine, University of Ibadan, Ibadan, Nigeria.

Inoculation of mice

A Swiss albino mouse (which served as the donor mouse) was intraperitoneally administered with a standard inoculum of *P. berghei* on day 0. On the 5th day (when the parasite had stabilized in the host mouse), blood was withdrawn from the heart of the donor mouse by cardiac puncture and diluted with isotonic saline. Normal saline and 0.1 ml of acid citrate dextrose (ACD) were drawn into the syringe to make inoculum for infecting experimental mice. Thereafter, the experimental mice were inoculated with 0.2 ml of parasite specimen (containing about 1×10^7 parasitized cells).

Determination of parasitemia

Blood was obtained from each of the experimental mice via a tail cut from which thin blood smears were prepared. Smears were fixed with methanol for 5 min and stained with 10% Geimsa. The slides were observed with compound microscope under x100 to determine the number of parasitized cell per magnification field. For each blood smear specific for a given mouse, four magnification fields were observed and the number of parasitized cells and the total number of cells in the magnification field were recorded. The data obtained was used to determine percentage parasitemia using

the method described by Hilou et al. (2006).

$$\% \text{ Parasitemia} = \frac{\text{Total number of parasitized red blood cells}}{\text{Total number of red blood cells}} \times 100\%$$

In vivo antimalarial study

By the 5th day from inoculation, parasites were fully established in the blood of infected mice. 200, 300 and 500 mg/kg body weight of water and ethanol extracts were administered to the experimental mice. Distilled water and 0.2 ml of Chloroquine were administered as negative and positive controls, respectively.

Evaluation of toxicity

On the 29th day, the experiment was discontinued. The mice were weighed, anaesthetized with chloroform and blood samples collected by cardiac puncture for serum biochemical and haematological analyses. Blood samples obtained by cardiac puncture were analyzed for white blood cells (WBC), red blood cells (RBC), platelet (Plt), haemoglobin (Hb), packed cell volume (PCV), mean corpuscular volume (MCV), mean corpuscular haemoglobin (MCH) and mean corpuscular haemoglobin concentration (MCHC). Serum biochemical parameters evaluated were total protein, albumin, globulin, aspartate amino transferase (AST), alanine amino transferase (ALT), alkaline phosphatase (ALP), bilirubin, creatinine, sodium, potassium, calcium, magnesium, and chloride ion (Dacie and Lewis, 1991; Bergmeyer et al., 1986; Roy, 1970).

Histopathological studies

The experimental mice were sacrificed and their liver and kidney were excised, weighed, trimmed and fixed in Bouin's solution. Fixed tissues were dehydrated, in ascending series of alcohol, cleared in xylene, and embedded in paraffin wax melted at 60°C. Serial sections (5 µm thick) were mounted in 3-aminopropyl triethsilane-coated slides and allowed to dry for 24 h at 37°C. The sections on the slides were de-paraffined, hydrated and stained with Mayer's haematoxylin and eosin dyes, dried and mounted, and thereafter examined under a light microscope (Drury et al., 1967).

Data analysis

Data were statistically analyzed and where necessary expressed as mean ± SD. Differences in means were assessed for significance with Duncan multiple range test (DMRT) at $p > 0.05$ using IBM SPSS Statistics version 20.

RESULTS

The medicinal plants profile

The plant profile of the ten (10) medicinal plants used in the treatment of malaria in Akure, Southwestern Nigeria is presented in Table 1.

Quantitative phytochemical composition

Table 2 shows the phytochemical constituents of the

Table 1. Plant profile of ten medicinal plants used in the management of malaria in Akure, Southwestern Nigeria.

S/N	Botanical name	Family	Local name (Yoruba)	Common name	Habit	Part used
1	*Anthocleista djalonensis* A. Chev	Loganiaceae	Sapo	Cabbage tree	Tree	Stem bark
2	*Azadirachta indica* A. Juss	Meliaceae	Dongoyaro	Neem	Tree	Stem bark, leaf
3	*Cajanus cajan* (L.) Huth.	Fabaceae	Otili	Pigeon pea	Shrub	Leaf
4	*Crecentia cujete* L.	Bignoniaceae	Igi-sogba	Calabash tree	Tree	Stem bark
5	*Lawsonia inermis* L.	Lythraceae	Laali	Henna	Shrub	Leaf
6	*Lophira alata* Banks ex C.F. Gaertn.	Ochnaceae	Ponhan	Red ironwood	Tree	Stem bark
7	*Myrianthus pruessii* Engl.	Urticaceae	Ogunsere	-	Tree	Leaf
8	*Nauclea latifolia* Sm.	Rubiaceae	Egbesi	African peach	Tree	Stem bark
9	*Olax subscorpioidea* Oliv.	Olacaceae	Ifon	-	Shrub	Root
10	*Terminalia glaucescens* Planch ex Benth.	Combretaceae	Idi	-	Tree	Stem bark, root

Table 2. Phytochemical constituents of combined medicinal plants used in the treatment of malaria in Akure, Southwestern Nigeria.

Parameter	Concentration (mg/100 g)
Alkaloids	0.78±0.01
Flavonoids	0.00±0.00
Saponins	0.31±0.01
Tannins	0.05±0.00
Polyphenols	0.18±0.00
Anthraquinones	0.00±0.00
Cardiac glycosides	0.35±0.00

Values are mean ± SD; n=3.

Table 3. Proximate composition of combined medicinal plants used in the treatment of malaria in Akure, Southwestern Nigeria.

Parameter	Composition (%)
Protein	16.52±0.30
Fat	12.28±0.20
Fibre	15.50±0.30
Ash	8.50±0.50
Carbohydrate	40.60±0.70
Moisture	6.60±0.50

Values are mean ± SD; n=3.

combined plant sample. The recipe contained appreciable quantity of alkaloids, saponins, tannins, polyphenols, and cardiac glycosides. Flavonoids and anthraquinones were altogether absent.

Proximate and mineral elements contents

The powdered recipe also contained important nutritive and mineral elements and are presented in Tables 3 and

4, respectively. Carbohydrate, protein, fat, and fibre were relatively high while ash and moisture were low. Phosphorus, calcium, magnesium, iron, and zinc were found to be high while sodium, potassium, and copper were found to be relatively low. Lead was absent.

Antiplasmodial activity of the combined plant sample

Figures 1 and 2 show the comparative antiplasmodia

Table 4. Quantitative mineral contents of combined medicinal plants used in the treatment of malaria in Akure, Southwestern Nigeria.

Parameter	Concentration (mg/kg)
Phosphorus	1800.50±15.00
Calcium	25280.00±30.50
Magnesium	4870.30±23.30
Sodium	0.90±0.03
Potassium	1.50±0.01
Manganese	95.60±2.80
Iron	770.37±16.77
Copper	21.64±0.60
Zinc	250.34±10.58
Lead	

Values are mean ± SD; n=3.

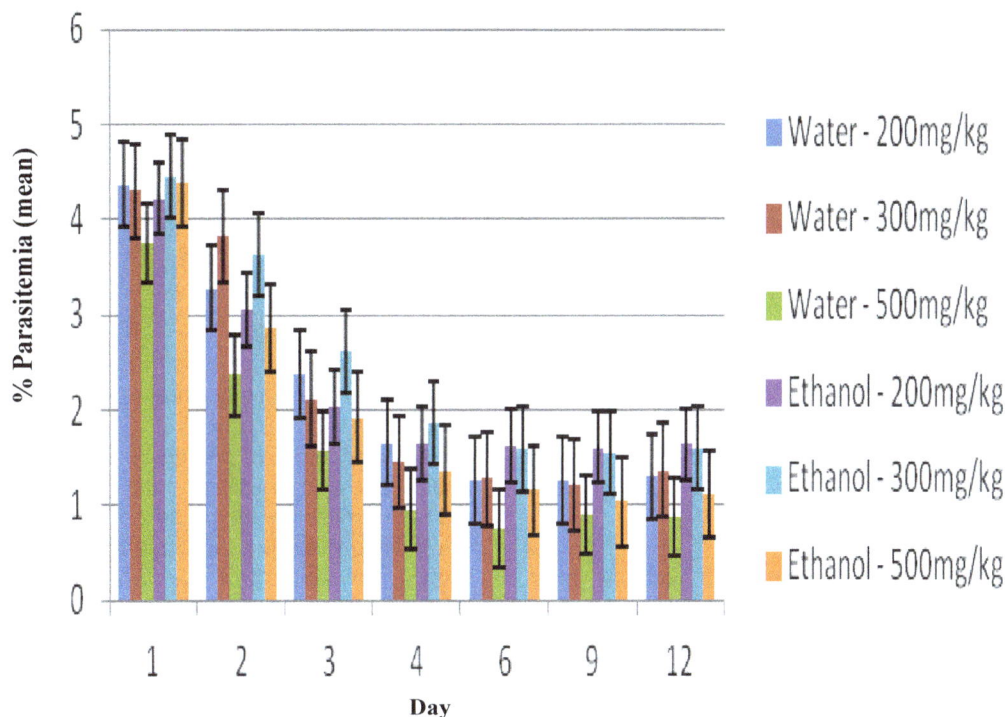

Figure 1. Comparative percentage parasitemia (mean) of *Plasmodium berghei* infected mice treated with water and ethanol extracts of the combined extract till 12th day post establishment.

activity of the recipe at graded concentrations of 200, 300, and 500 mg/kg body weight and the control group (negative and positive). Optimum activity was recorded on Day 4. Activity was highest with water extract of recipe at 500 mg/kg.

Serum biochemical, heamatological, and histopathological studies

Serum biochemical and haematological values are presented in Tables 5 and 6, respectively. Histological studies revealed some pathology caused by the malaria parasite and presentations of conditions after administration of extracts. These conditions (indicated on Plates 1 to 16) include interstitial nephritis, widespread severe flattening of the epithelium of renal tubules, congestion of interstitial renal blood vessels, hepatocellular necrosis, severe necrosis of epithelial renal tubules, nephrosis, congestion of hepatic sinusoids, and the presence of *Plasmodium* gametocytes (extra-erythrocytes). The damages were severe in the negative

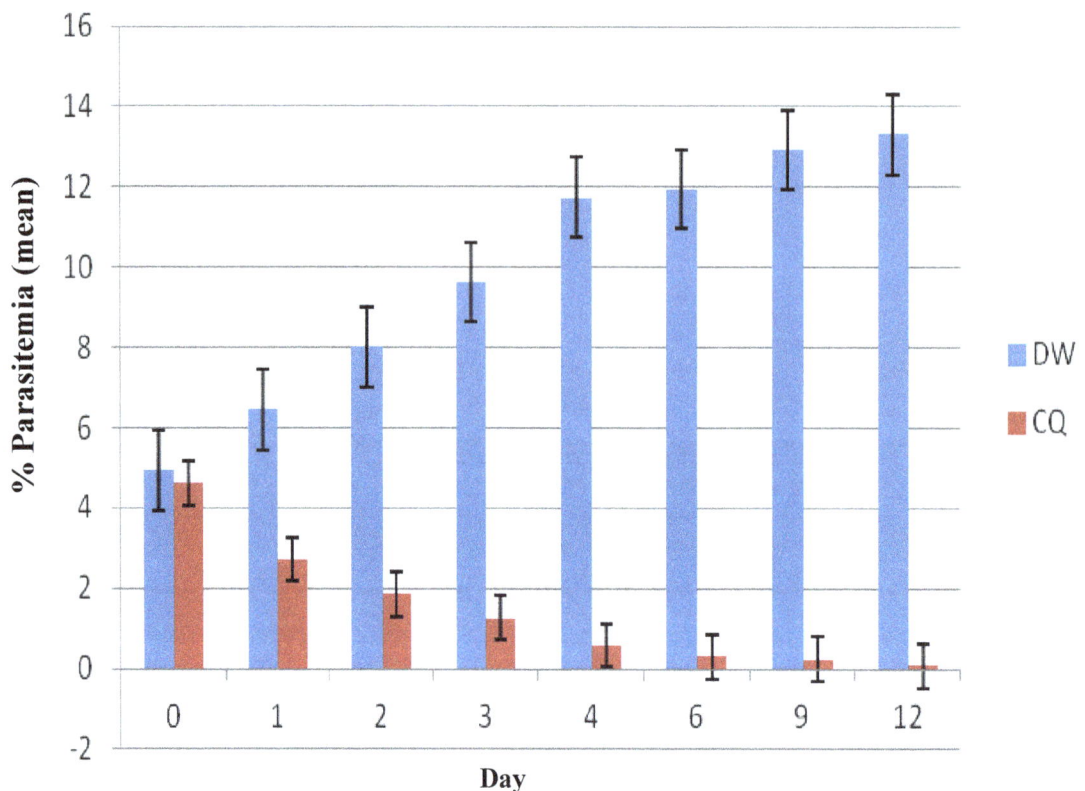

Figure 2. Comparative percentage parasitemia (mean) of *P. berghei* infected mice treated with distilled water and chloroquine till 12th day post establishment.

control (the group administered with distilled water after infection and establishment of malaria parasite).

DISCUSSION

This study reports the anti-plasmodial activity of a polyherbal recipe and serves as a ground breaking report of such combination. The traditional uses and the scientific justification of individual plants that formed the recipe used in this study have been reported. For example, the leaf and stem bark of *Nauclea latifolia* in the traditional treatment of yellow fever, toothache, dental caries, dysentery, septic, mouth, high blood pressure and diarrhoea have been reported by Benoit-Vicala et al. (1998) while Kayode (2006) reported anti-plasmodial activity of leaves, stem bark, root and seed of *Lophira alata*. Also, Priyanka et al. (2013) reported the antiplasmodial potentials demonstrated by *A. indica* in *P. berghei* infected mice model. Udobre et al. (2013) reported that the methanol leaf extract of *N. latifolia* reduced parasitemia in a dose dependent manner in albino mice infected with *P. berghei*. Akpanabiatu et al. (2005) also confirmed the vasodilatory property of the ethanol extract of *N. latifolia* and its action on aorta as well as the lipid profiles of rat upon administration with an increase in potassium concentration. All these reports are

in line with the activity obtained for the combination of the plants.

A polyherbal comprising *A. indica, C. papaya,* and *M. indica* showed antiplasmodial property (Ofori-Attah et al., 2012). Similar investigation on the prophylactic effect of a multi-herbal extract (*C. cajan* leaf, *E. laterifolia* leaf, *M. indica* leaf and stem, *Cymbopogon giganteas* leaf, and *Uvaria chamae* bark) by Nwabuisi (2002) gave noteworthy antimalarial activity with no apparent significant side effects. Binary combination of *Artocarpus altilis, Enantia chlorantha,* or *Murraya koenigii* with *N. latifolia* significantly increased the prophylactic and suppressive activities of the individual plants (Adebajo et al., 2014). In contrast, Arise et al. (2012) reported hepatotoxic and nephrotoxic potentials of the aqueous extract of *N. latifolia* stem. The toxic potentials of *N. latifolia* on the kidney and liver of the animals presents a great concern in the consumption of this plant since this study also reports the pathological changes observed upon administration of the plant extract.

Alkaloids, saponins, and flavonoids have been implicated to be responsible for antimalarial activity (Ettebong et al., 2015) as these secondary metabolites elicit bioactivity wholly or in combination with other plants (Shigemori et al., 2003). Malaria parasites in wreaking havoc synthesize protein and produce free radicals in the human body. These vices are corrected in the presence

Table 5. Serum biochemical of *Plasmodium berghei* infected mice after 12 days post infection treatment with water and ethanol extracts of antimalarial recipe.

Group	Total protein (g/dl)	Albumin (g/dl)	Globulin (g/dl)	Alb-Glob. ratio	AST (µl)	ALT (µl)	ALP (µl)	BUN (mg/dl)	Creatinine (mg/kg)	Sodium (mg/l)
Combination Water	7.35±0.47e	3.28±0.38g	4.07±0.32c	0.83±0.12abcd	88.67±5.45def	47.83±5.31a	88.83±12.70a	18.83±4.20abc	0.40±0.12a	133.33±11.45a
Combination Ethanol	8.32±0.61f	3.42±0.29g	4.90±0.35d	0.63±0.05a	89.17±10.26def	54.17±7.73a	142.00±24.75b	22.67±0.99d	0.98±0.22e	155.50±9.72d
Control DW	4.33±0.26a	1.88±0.07a	2.45±0.25a	0.80±0.06abc	52.83±13.41a	49.67±6.79a	89.83±13.81a	19.67±4.21abc	0.47±0.12abc	148.67±14.01cd
Contol CQ	7.40±0.76e	3.15±0.40g	4.25±0.06c	0.75±0.06abc	96.50±4.04f	57.00±4.62a	152.00±47.34b	21.00±1.16abcd	0.60±0.12d	168.00±17.32e

Values are mean ± SD; n = 15 except control where n = 5. Values with the same letter in the same column are not significantly different with Duncan's multiple range Test (DMRT), p>0.05.

Table 6. Haematological effects of water and ethanol extract of antimalarial recipe on *P. berghei* infected mice.

Group/Plant	PCV (%)	Hb (mg/dl)	WBC (10^3/mm³)	MCV (m³)	MCH (x 10^{-5})	MCHC (g %)	RBC (10^6/mm³)
Combination (water)	32.00	9.07	12.47	53.87	18.50	34.47	4.89
Combination (ethanol)	32.00	10.20	11.50	55.87	19.37	34.63	5.32
Control (Distilled water)	37.00	9.50	4.80	55.60	19.20	34.50	4.96
Control (CQ)	44.00	13.70	5.30	56.80	18.70	33.00	7.33

Values are mean of 6 determinations. PCV = Packed cell volume; Hb = Haemoglobin; WBC= White blood cell; MCV = Mean corpuscular volume; MCH = Mean corpuscular haemoglobin; MCHC = Mean corpuscular haemoglobin concentration; RBC = Red blood cell.

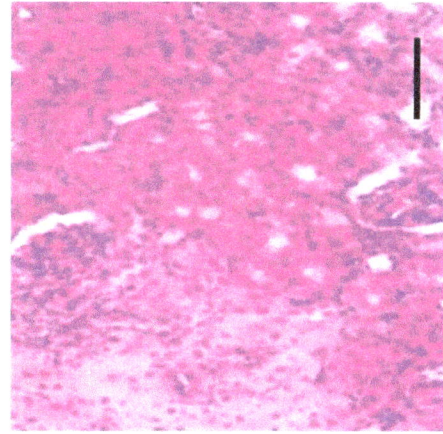

NVL except for a mild congestion of renal interstitial blood vessels

(H&E stain, X400). Scale bar: 20 µm

Plate 1. Effect of 200 mg/kg water extract of combination of plants on kidney.

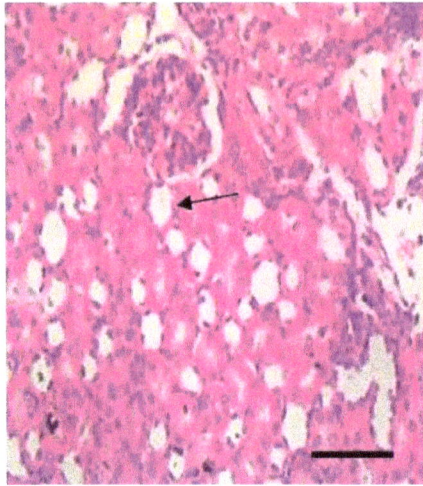

= Mild sloughing off of epithelium of tubules in the renal cortex.

(H&E stain, X400). Scale bar: 20 μm

Plate 3. Effect of 500 mg/kg water extract of combination of plants on kidney.

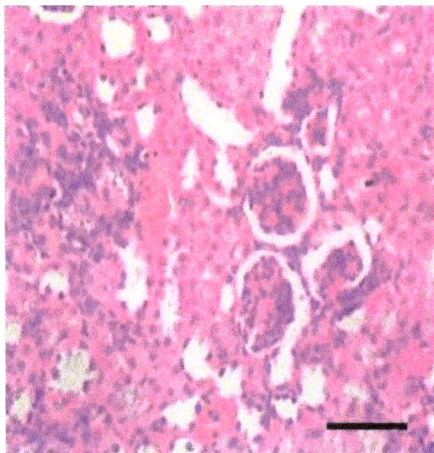

☆ = Moderate congestion of renal interstitial blood vessels

(H&E stain, X400). Scale bar: 20 μm

Plate 3. Effect of 500 mg/kg water extract of combination of plants on kidney.

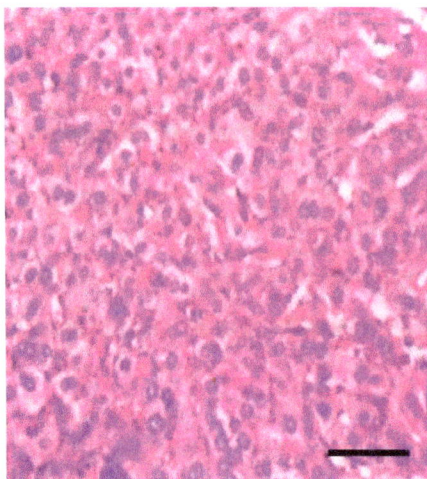

= Bile stasis within the canaliculi

= Widespread congestion of hepatic sinusoids

(H&E stain, X400). Scale bar: 20 μm

Plate 4. Effect of 200 mg/kg water extract of combination of plants on liver.

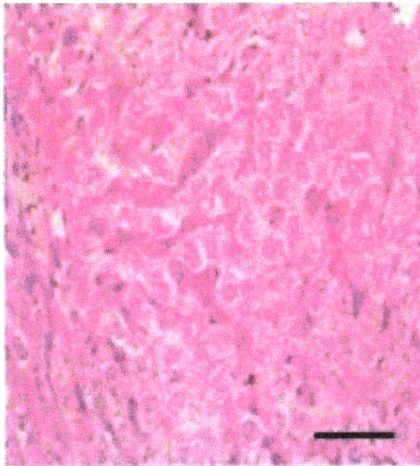

= Moderate KCH with some of the cells containing dark brown pigments.

(H&E stain, X400). Scale bar: 20 µm

Plate 5. Effect of 300 mg/kg water extract of combination of plants on liver.

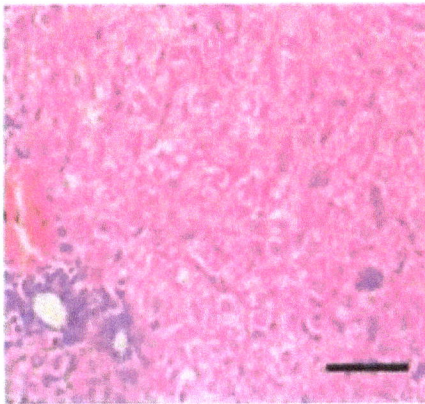

= Moderate KCH with some of the cells containing dark brown pigments and formation of multinucleated giant cells

= Widespread congestion of hepatic sinusoids and portal vessels.

(H&E stain, X400). Scale bar: 20 µm

Plate 6. Effect of 500 mg/kg water extract of combination of plants on liver.

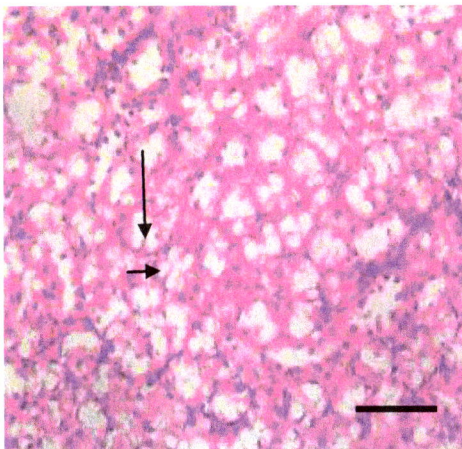

= Moderate vacuolar change of the epithelial cells of tubules in the renal medulla

(H&E stain, X400). Scale bar: 20µm

Plate 7. Effect of 200 mg/kg ethanol extract of combination of plants on kidney.

of alkaloids which block protein-synthesis of *Plasmodium* species, and flavonoid, saponin, and tannin which are involved in primary anti-oxidation of free radicals and other reactive oxygen species (David et al., 2004). In

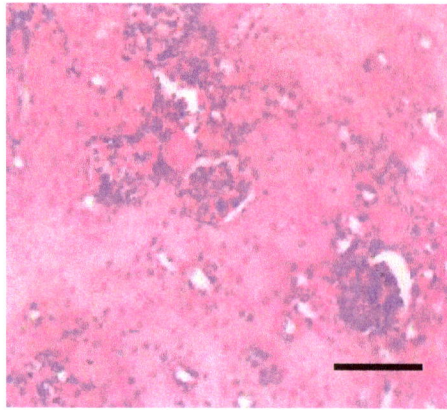

No visible lesion

(H&E stain, X400). Scale bar: 20 μm

Plate 8. Effect of 300 mg/kg ethanol extract of combination of plants on kidney.

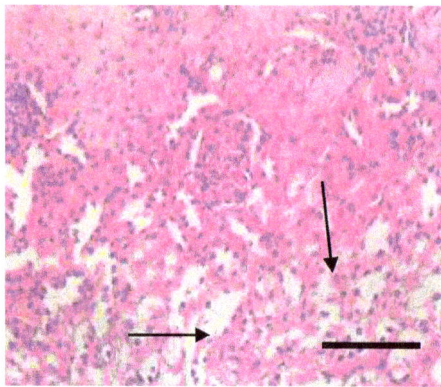

= A few foci of mild sloughing off of epithelial cells of tubules in renal cortex

(H&E stain, X400). Scale bar: 20 μm

Plate 9. Effect of 500 mg/kg ethanol extract of combination of plants on kidney.

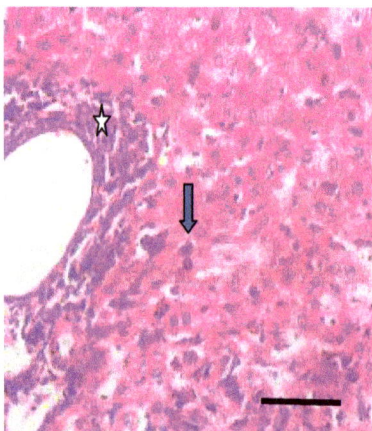

= Numerous round/oval dark structures likely to be *Plasmodium* gametocytes/extra-erythrocytic stages

☆ = Moderate aggregates of MNCs in portal tracts

(H&E stain, X400). Scale bar: 20μm

Plate 10. Effect of 200 mg/kg ethanol extract of combination of plants on liver.

many plants, antiplasmodial activity is associated with the presence of total polyphenols, flavonoids and alkaloids (Kaur et al., 2009). For instance, alkaloids occur in plants in association with characteristic acids (Evans, 2002) and are known to have anticancer, anti-aging and antiviral properties with marked physiological actions on man and animals. Tannins in the root of the plant could be an essential astringent. They act as astringent by

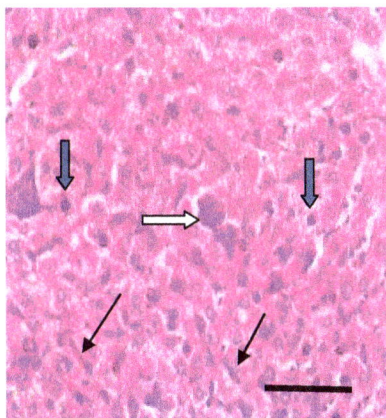

⬇ = Numerous round/oval dark structures likely to be *Plasmodium* gametocytes/extra-erythrocytic stages

⟹ = Moderate aggregates of MNCs in portal tracts

↙ = Moderate KCH with some of the cells containing dark brown pigments. **(H&E stain, X400). Scale bar: 20μm**

Plate 11. Effect of 300 mg/kg ethanol extract of combination of plants on liver.

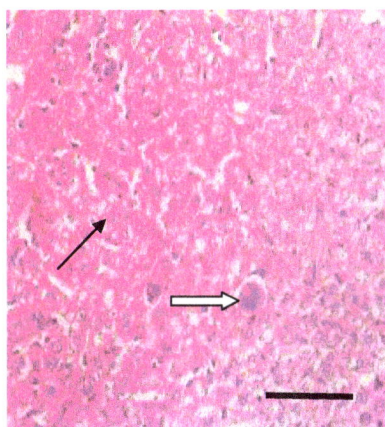

⟹ = Megakaryocyte suggestive of extra-medullary haematopoiesis

↗ = Mild widespread bile stasis in the bile canaliculi

(H&E stain, X400). Scale bar: 20μm

Plate 12. Effect of 500 mg/kg ethanol extract of combination of plants on liver.

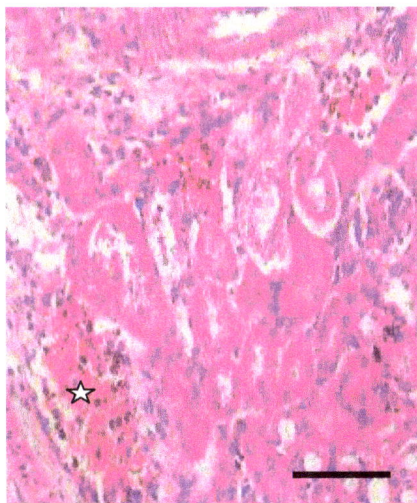

☆ = A few foci of haemorrhages in the renal medulla.

(H&E stain, X400). Scale bar: 20μm

Plate 13. Kidney section of control mouse administered with distilled water.

precipitating proteins in living tissues, on gastrointestinal tract and on skin abrasions (Sofowora, 2008). Polyphenols may aid in the prevention of age-associated diseases such as cardiovascular diseases, cancers, and

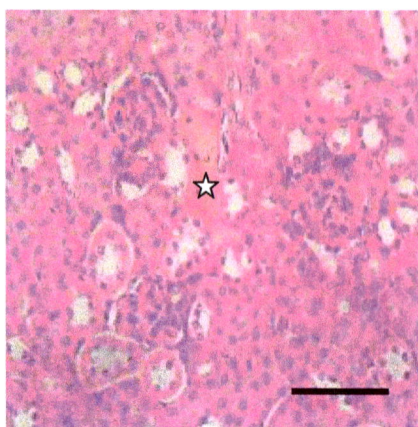

No visible lesion.

(H&E stain, X400). Scale bar: 20µm

Plate 14. Kidney section of control mouse administered with chloroquine

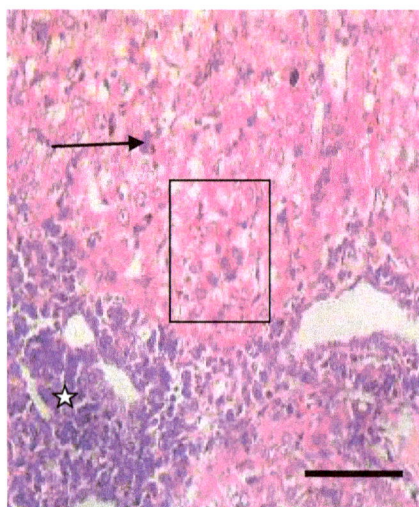

☐ = Multiple foci of moderate vacuolar change of hepatocytes

⟶ = Multinucleated giant cells

☆ = marked aggregates of MNCs in portal tracts.

(H&E stain, X400). Scale bar: 20µm

Plate 15. Liver section of control mouse administered with distilled water.

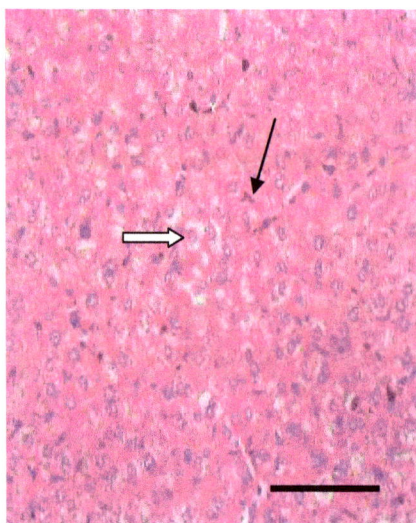

↙ = Moderate KCH with some of the cells containing dark brown pigments.

⟹ = A few foci of mild vacuolar change of hepatocytes

(H&E stain, X400). Scale bar: 20µm

Plate 16. Liver section of control mouse administered with chloroquine.

osteoporosis. The moisture content of the plant sample screened in this study was very low; this is an indication that the recipe could withstand long storage.

In food and drug industries, the evaluation of toxicity is important because it presents the likely physiological and pathological conditions associated with administration. The toxic effects noticed in animal models (mice, rats, rabbits etc.) could serve as baseline for comparison in mammalian anatomy and physiology. The concentrations administered for LD_{50} did not elicit adverse reactions in the animals, and no mortality was recorded. According to Hodge and Sterner (2005), these concentrations are practically safe. Ofori-Attah et al. (2012) evaluated the acute toxicity of aqueous leaf extract of *A. indica* by administering 12 mice with 1250, 2500 and 5000 mg/kg and found the concentrations to be safe. LD_{50} between 500 and 5000 mg/kg is considered as moderately toxic (Agaie et al., 2000), or may be classified as practically non-toxic, and fall within the safety margin considered acceptable (Hodge and Sterner Scale, 2005).

At the tested dosages, the recipe showed no significant lysis and could be said to boost the immune system of the mice. The haemoglobin concentration was fairly constant; this suggests that the oxygen-carrying capacity of the blood of the animals was not affected. The control (chloroquine) showed significantly high PCV and reduced WBC compared with the recipe. Histology of kidney and liver sections indicated that caution must be exercised in the use of the plants that make up the recipe especially in high doses. The combination of the plants (recipe) showed significant activity, although it compared less with the positive control (chloroquine).

ACKNOWLEDGEMENT

Special appreciation go to the research team at the Institute of Advanced Medical Research and Training (IAMRAT), College of Medicine, University of Ibadan, Nigeria. Thanks to Prof. O. G. Ademowo for granting laboratory space, facility, and the malaria parasite used for the study. The financial support from Tertiary Education Trust Fund (TETFund) through Adeyemi College of Education, Ondo, Ondo State is gratefully acknowledged.

REFERENCES

Adebajo CA, Odediran SA, Aliyu FA, Nwafor PA, Nwoko NT, Umana US (2014). *In vivo* antiplasmodial potentials of the combinations of four Nigerian antimalarial plants. Molecules 19:13136-13146.

African Medical and Research Foundation (AMRF) (2012). Malaria. New York, USA. Available at: http://www.usa.amref.org; accessed and retrieved: 17th June, 2012.

Agaie BM, Onyeyili PA, Muhammad BY, Ladan MJ (2007). Acute toxicity effects of the aqueous leaf extract of *Anogeissus leiocarpus* in rats. Afr. J. Biotechnol. 6(7):886-889.

Akanbi OM, Omonkhua AA, Cyril-Olutayo CA, Fasimoye RY (2012). The antiplasmodial activity of *Anogeissus leiocarpus* and its effect on oxidative stress and lipid profile in mice infected with *Plasmodium berghei*. Parasitol. Res. 110:219-226.

Akpanabiatu MI, Umoh IB, Udosen EO, Udoh AE, Edet EE (2005). Rat serum electrolytes lipid profile and cardiovascular activity of *Nauclea latifolia* leaf extract administration. Indian J. Clin. Biochem. 20(2):29-34.

Association of Analytical Chemists (AOAC) (1990). Official Methods of Analysis. Association of Analytical Chemists (15th Edition). Washington, DC, USA. pp.112-135.

Arise RO, Akintola AA, Olarinoye JB, Balogun EA (2012). Effects of aqueous extract of *Nauclea latifolia* stem on lipid profile and some enzymes of rat liver and kidney. Int. J. Pharmacol. 1-7.

Ates DA, Erdogrul OT (2003). Antimicrobial activities of various medicinal and commercial plant extracts. Turk. J. Biol. 27:157-162.

Benoit-Vicala F, Valentine A, Cournaca V, Pellisierb Y, Malliea M, Bastidea JM (1998). *In vitro* antiplasmodial activity of stem and root extracts of *Nauclea latifolia* Sm. (Rubiaceae). J. Ethnopharmacol. 61:173-178.

Bergmeyer HU, Horder M, Rej R (1986). International Federation of Clinical Chemistry (IFCC) Scientific Committee, analytical section: Approved recommendation (1985) on IFCC methods for the measurement of catalytic concentration of enzymes. Part 3 IFCC method for alanine aminotransferase (L- alanine: 2 oxoglutarate aminotransferase, EC 2.6.1.2). J. Clin. Chem. Biochem. 24:485-495.

Dacie JV, Lewis MS (1991). Practical Heamatology, 7th Edition. ELBS Churchill Livingstone, Edinburgh, England.

David AF, Philip JR, Simon LC, Reto B, Solomon N (2004). Antimalarial drug discovery: efficacy models for compound screening. Nature Rev. Drug Dis. 3:509-520.

Drury RAB, Wallington EA, Cameron B (1967). Carleton's Histological Techniques (4th Edition). Oxford University Press, New York, USA. pp. 279-280.

Ettebong EO, Edwin UPM, Edet EC, Samuel EU, Ezekiel AO, Dornu TV (2015). *In vivo* antiplasmodial activities of *Nauclea latifolia*. Asian J. Med. Sci. 6(3):6-11.

Evans WC (2002). Trease and Evans Pharmacognosy. 15th Edition. W.B. Saunders, London. pp. 214-393.

Harbone JB (1973). Phytochemical Methods. Chapman and Hall Ltd., London. pp. 49-188.

Hilou H, Nacoulma OG, Guiguemde TR (2006). *In vitro* antimalarial activity of extracts of *Amaranthus spinosus* L. and *Boerhavia erecta* L. in mice. J. Ethnopharmacol. 103:235-240.

Hodge A, Sterner B (2005). Toxicity classes in Canadian Centre for Occupational Health and Safety. Available at: http//www.ccohs.ca//ashanswers/chemicals/Ld50.htm; accessed: 3rd May, 2010.

Ibrahim HA, Imam IA, Bello AM, Umar U, Muhammad S, Abdullahi SA (2012). The potential of Nigerian medicinal plants as antimalarial agent: A review. Int. J. Sci. Tech. 2(6):600-605.

Kaur K, Meenakshi J, Terandeep K, Rahul J (2009). Antimalarials from nature. Bio-organic Med. Chem. 23(5):120-121.

Kayode J (2006). Conservation of indigenous medicinal botanicals in Ekiti State, Nigeria. J. Zhejiang Univ. Sci. 7:713-718.

Lorke D (1983). A new approach to practical acute toxicity testing. Arch. Toxicol. 54:275-287.

Nguta JM, Mbaria JM, Gakuya DW, Gathumbi PK, Kiama SG (2010). Antimalarial herbal remedies of Msambweni, Kenya. J. Ethnopharmacol. 128:424-432.

Nigeria Government in Action (NGA) 2005. Report from Presidential Research and Communication Unit, Office of Public Communication, Abuja.

Nmorsi OPG, Ukwandu NCD, Egwunyenga AO (2007). Antioxidant status of Nigerian children with *Plasmodium falciparum* malaria. Afr. J. Microb. Res. pp. 61-64.

Nwabuisi C (2002). Prophylactic effect of multi-herbal extract 'agbo-iba' on malaria induced in mice. East Afr. Med. J. 79(7):343-346.

Ofori-Attah K, Oseni LA, Quasie O, Antwi S. Tandoh M (2012). A comparative evaluation of *in vivo* antiplasmodial activity of aqueous leaf extracts of *Carica papaya, Azadirachta indica, Mangifera indica* and combination thereof using *Plasmodium* infected Balb/Mice. Int. J. Appl. Bio. Pharm. Tech. 3(3):373-378.

Priyanka J, Hingorani L, Nilima K (2013). Pharmacodynamic evaluation for antiplasmodial activity of *Holarrhena antidysentrica* (Kutaja) and *Azadirachta indica* (Neem) in *Plasmodium berghei* infected mice model. Asian Pacific J. Trop. Med. 520-524.

Roy AV (1970). Determination of alkaline phosphatase (ALP) in human serum. Clin. Chem. 16:431.

Sachs J, Malaney P (2002). The economic and social burden of malaria, Nature. 415(7):680-685.

Shigemori H, Kagata T, Ishiyama H (2003). New monoterpene alkaloids from *Nauclea latifolia*. Chem. Pharm. Bull. 51:58-61.

Sofowora A (2008). Medicinal plants and traditional medicine in Africa (3rd Edition). Spectrum Books Ltd., Ibadan, Nigeria. pp. 199-204.

Udobre AS, Udobang JA, Udoh AE, Anah VU, Akpan AE, Charles GE (2013). Effect of methanol leaf extracts on albino mice infected with *Plasmodium berghei berghei*. Afr. J. Pharmacol. Ther. 2(3):83-87.

World Health Organization (WHO) (1978). The promotion and development of traditional medicine. Technical Report Series 622. WHO, Geneva, Switzerland. 250p.

World Health Organization (WHO) (2008). World Malaria Report. WHO Press, Geneva, Switzerland. 250p.

World Health Organization (WHO) (2011). Malaria and HIV interactions and their implications for public health policy. WHO Press, Geneva, Switzerland. 180p.

## 14

Evaluation of antioxidant and anti-tyrosinase activities as well as stability of green and roasted coffee bean extracts from *Coffea arabica* and *Coffea canephora*

Kanokwan Kiattisin*, Thananya Nantarat and Pimporn Leelapornpisid

Department of Pharmaceutical Sciences, Faculty of Pharmacy, Chiang Mai University, Suthep Road, Chiang Mai, Thailand.

Coffea arabica (Arabica) and *Coffea canephora* (Robusta) are the economic plants in Thailand that are widely cultivated in Northern and Southern Thailand. This study aims to evaluate the antioxidant, anti-tyrosinase activities, toxicity, stability and identify chemical components of the coffee bean extracts. The best extract that showed good biological activities will be further used to develop cosmeceutical products. Green and roasted coffee beans from two species were extracted with hexane following ethanol by maceration. Their antioxidant activities were detected by 2,2-diphenyl-1-picryl hydrazyl (DPPH), 2,2'-Azino-bis(3-ethylbenzthiazoline-6-sulphonic acid) (ABTS) and lipid peroxidation inhibition assays. In addition, anti-tyrosinase activity was also evaluated. The results revealed that the ethanolic coffee bean extracts showed a higher level of antioxidant activity than in the hexane extracts. All extracts also possessed a considerable anti-tyrosinase activity, but less potent than kojic acid and arbutin. Chemical compounds of these extracts were determined using caffeine and chlorogenic acid as standards of reference by the thin layer chromatography and the high performance liquid chromatography. The green coffee bean extracts consisted of caffeine and chlorogenic acid while the roasted coffee bean extracts presented only caffeine due to a few chlorogenic acid content after the roasting process. The ethanolic coffee bean extracts that showed good activities were selected to be evaluated on toxicity and stability. The selected extracts were kept at various storage conditions to evaluate their stability using DPPH assay and anti-tyrosinase activity assay. The result showed that the extracts were not toxic to cells. Therefore, the extracts were safe to be components in skin care products. After the stability test, the extracts indicated a good stability and activities. These results led to the conclusions that the coffee bean extracts possess a good biological activities and are assumed to be promising natural active ingredients with a good stability profile for further development of cosmeceutical or anti-aging products.

Key words: *Coffea arabica, Coffea canephora,* green coffee bean, roasted coffee bean, antioxidant activity, anti-tyrosinase activity.

INTRODUCTION

Many factors such as environmental conditions, UV radiation, foods, stress as well as pollutants are all causes of free radicals formation in the body. Free radicals can induce many diseases such as different types of cancer, coronary artery disease, nervous system diseases, lung diseases and also rheumatoid arthritis (Devasagayam et al., 2004; Pham-Huy et al., 2008). Moreover, they play an important role in tissue aging, including skin aging (Farage et al., 2008; Poljsak et al., 2012). It is a never-ending endeavor for researchers in attempt to find the new active ingredients to counteract the aging process, especially the focus on antioxidant or anti-free radical capability and also anti-tyrosinase activity; which are involved in the prevention of skin aging and help to generate skin brightening. Numerous Thai plants have been used as health care and cosmetic products for many decades.

Coffee is one of the economic plants which is widely grown in Thailand. It is a native plant of Africa in Rubiaceae family and it is very popular around the world, especially Southeast Asia (Charrier and Berthaud, 2012). *Coffea arabica* (Arabica) is popularly cropped in the Northern part of Thailand while *Coffea canephora* (Robusta) is mostly cultivated in Southern Thailand. They are different in the seed shape, smell and taste (Chuakul et al., 1997). Robusta coffee is a major production in Thailand, with about 80,000-85,500 tons per year, whereas Arabica coffee production is only approximately 800-850 tons per year. Sixty percent of the Robusta coffee is exported and mostly used for instant coffee production. Most of Arabica coffee is used in roasted and ground coffee for the domestic market.

Previous studies showed that drinking coffee could reduce risk of Parkinson, Alzheimer, hypertension, diabetes type 2 and cancers, and also promote the liver function (Chu et al., 2011; Cano-Marquina et al., 2013; O'Keefe et al., 2013).

In addition, coffee beans serves as antioxidant, anti-inflammatory, for inhibition of albumin denature, UV radiation protection, and in anti-bacterial activities (Antonio et al., 2011; Wagemaker et al., 2011; Almeida et al., 2012; Chandra et al., 2012; Moreira et al., 2013; Liang et al., 2016). Therefore, coffee beans are an interesting option to select for the development of cosmeceutical products in the future. Previous phytochemical studies of coffee indicated that green coffee beans consisted of caffeine, caffeic acid, chlorogenic acid and trigonelline, whereas roasted coffee beans are composed of caffeine, trigonelline, chlorogenic acid, and melanoidin (Liu et al., 2011; Vignoli et al., 2011; Moreira et al., 2013). The chemical components that are mentioned above indicate that coffee beans are a great source for antioxidant.

The data from this research will be used to develop further cosmeceutical products. Therefore, the aims of to select the best extract from antioxidant, lipid peroxidation inhibition and anti-tyrosinase activities. This study are to

choose the good solvent extraction and research also shows toxicity of selected coffee bean extracts and stability at various storage conditions. Moreover, the research attempts to identify the chemical constituents of coffee bean extracts by thin layer chromatography and high performance liquid chromatography to confirm active compounds in the extracts.

MATERIALS AND METHODS

Plant materials, chemicals and enzymes

Green and roasted coffee beans (Arabica and Robusta) were obtained from a coffee farm in Chiang Mai province in the northern part of Thailand. The best geography and environment fo cultivating coffee include clay soil with high potassium, pH range between 4.5 and 6.5, and rainfall 1,500 and 2,300 ml per year. Arabica coffee is grown with the open-system without shade, the temperature of 15 and 26°C, 80% humidity at 1,000 to 1,700 m above sea level in Chiang Mai, Thailand. Arabica coffee cherries were harvested in October, they were prepared by the pulping process, the wet fermentation process, and the sun drying process. Green coffee beans were then transferred from a high efficiency hulling machine where the final layer of parchment was completely removed. Robusta coffee is grown with the open-system with shade, the temperature of 23 – 32°C, 90% humidity at 700 to 1,000 m above sea level in Chumphon province, Thailand. Robusta coffee cherries were harvested in November. Green coffee beans were prepared the same way as Arabica green coffee beans. Roasted coffee beans were prepared in a high quality, fully automated roaster and sealed in 4-layer-foil bags embedded with one way ai valves at 210 - 240°C for 10 to 20 min (medium roast). The green and roasted coffee beans were stored away from light at the room temperature.

Turmeric extract and mangosteen extract were obtained from a cosmetic laboratory at Chiang Mai University, Chiang Mai, Thailand. Caffeine, chlorogenic acid, mushroom tyrosinase and L-tyrosine were purchased from Sigma-Aldrich, USA. L-dopa was purchased from Isotec. Trolox, gallic acid, quercetin, 2,2-diphenyl-1-picry hydrazyl (DPPH), Folin-Ciocalteu reagent and linoleic acid were purchased from Sigma Chemical Co., (USA). 2,2'-Azino-bis(3 ethylbenzthiazoline-6-sulphonic acid) (ABTS) and 2, 2' azobis 2 amidinopropane dihydrochloride (AAPH) were purchased from Wako Pure Chemical Industries, Japan. RAW 264.7 cells were purchased from American Type Culture Collection (USA). MTT dye was purchased from Bio Basic (Markham, Canada). Dulbecco's Modified Eagle Medium (DMEM) was purchased from Gibco Acetonitrile and acetone were purchased from RCI Labscan Ltd. Thailand.

Extractions

Green and roasted coffee beans were grounded into powder before being extracted with hexane by maceration for three days. Then filtered with Whatman No. 1 filter paper and the filtrates were evaporated to concentrated extracts by rotary evaporator. The obtained extracts were named as hexane green Arabica bean extract (HGA), hexane roasted Arabica bean extract (HRA), hexane green Robusta bean extract (HGR) and hexane roasted Robusta

*Corresponding author. E-mail: ppp_pook@hotmail.com.

bean extract (HRR).

After that, each residue after hexane extraction was dried and extracted with 95% ethanol by maceration for three days, filtered and evaporated by rotary evaporator. The obtained extracts in this part were named as ethanolic green Arabica bean extract (EGA), ethanolic roasted Arabica bean extract (ERA), ethanolic green Robusta bean extract (EGR), and ethanolic roasted Robusta bean extract (ERR). All the extracts were kept in light resistant well-closed container in a freezer of a refrigerator for further investigations.

Determination of total phenolic content

The coffee bean extracts were determined for total phenolic content by Folin-Ciocalteu assay (Johnson et al., 2008; Garzón et al., 2009). Each sample was dissolved in ethanol (1 mg/ml) and then the 500 µl was transferred into a test tube, mixed with Folin-Ciocalteu reagent then Na_2CO_3 7.5% w/v was added. The mixtures were mixed with a vortex mixer and incubated for 30 min in the dark. The absorbance was measured at 765 nm using a spectrophotometer (Shimadzu UV-Vis 2450, Japan). The concentration of total phenolic content in all extracts was calculated as gallic acid equivalent (GAE), in milligram gallic acid/gram of a dry sample.

Determination of antioxidant activities

DPPH radical scavenging assay

The stable free radical DPPH (DPPH•) reacted with antioxidants and produced colorless 2,2-diphenyl-l-picryl hydrazine. The more colorless sample indicated the high antioxidant activity. Different concentrations of extracts were dissolved in ethanol and tested with freshly prepared 180 µl of DPPH• in ethanol. The mixtures were then mixed with a vortex mixer and incubated in the dark at room temperature for 30 min. The absorbance was measured spectrophotometrically at 520 nm with a microplate reader (DTX 880 multimode detector) (Brem et al., 2004). The percentage of inhibition was calculated by the equation:

Inhibition (%) = [($A_{control}$ − A_{sample}) / $A_{control}$] x 100

Where, $A_{control}$ is the absorbance of the control reaction and A_{sample} is the absorbance of the test sample. The half maximal inhibitory concentration (IC_{50}) was calculated from the curve between the percentage of inhibition and the concentration of extract. Gallic acid, trolox and quercetin were used as standard antioxidants.

ABTS cation radical scavenging assay

ABTS stock solution was prepared by mixing 7 mM ABTS with 140 mM $K_2S_2O_8$ and kept in the dark at room temperature for 16 h before use (Tang et al., 2004). The ABTS stock solution was diluted with deionized water to obtain the absorbance of 0.9±0.1 at 734 nm. The extracts were dissolved in ethanol and then 10 µl of each sample was mixed with 1 ml of ABTS solution. The mixture was kept for 6 min and was then measured for the absorbance at 734 nm using the spectrophotometer.

The absorbance was used to calculate percentage inhibition of antioxidant and IC_{50} value when compared with gallic acid, trolox and quercetin.

Lipid peroxidation inhibition (linoleic acid) assay

The extracts were diluted with ethanol before used. Each sample (200 µl) was mixed with 800 µl of phosphate buffer (pH 7.0), 200 µl of ethanol, 400 µl of deionized water, 400 µl of 2.5% linoleic acid and 80 µl of AAPH in a test tube. The mixture was incubated in the dark at 37°C for 24 h to generate the lipid peroxidation. After that, the mixture was tested by the ferric thiocyanate method. The mixture reacted with $FeCl_2$ and ammonium thiocyanate for 5 min. The absorbance was measured at 500 nm using a spectrophotometer.

The absorbance was used to calculate the percentage in the inhibition of lipid peroxidation activity and IC_{50} value when compared with gallic acid, trolox and quercetin.

Determination of mushroom tyrosinase inhibition activity

Each extract was dissolved in ethanol at the concentration of 2.5, 100 µl of each sample was added to the 96-well plate and then 40 µl of 2.5 mM L-dopa or 2.5 mM L-tyrosine solution were added to the well plate, then incubated at 37°C for 5 min before adding 60 µl of mushroom tyrosinase enzyme (Pomerantz et al., 1963). The mixture was incubated again at 37°C for 15 min before determining the absorbance at 450 nm with the microplate reader. Kojic acid, ellagic acid, α-arbutin and β-arbutin were used as reference tyrosinase inhibitors. The percentage inhibition of tyrosinase activity was calculated as followed:

inhibition (%) = [(A_a-A_b)/ A_a] × 100

Where A_a = absorbance without a test sample and A_b = absorbance with a test sample.

Cell culture and MTT assay

The cell culture was adapted from the previous study of Mueller et al. (2010). Briefly, RAW 264.7 cells were seeded at a density of 2 × 10^6 cells per well in 24 well plates, and incubated for 24 h at 37°C. On the following day, the extracts in ethanolic solution were added, and cells were incubated for a further 24 h at 37°C. Then, the media was removed and MTT was added to the cells, and the cells were incubated for 2 h at 37°C. The supernatant was then removed, and the cells were lysed with lysis buffer (10% SDS in 0.01 N HCl). The optical density at 570 nm, corrected by the reference wavelength 690 nm, was measured using a microplate reader.

Determination of TLC chromatogram

The extracts with good antioxidant and anti-tyrosinase activities were selected for TLC analysis. Caffeine and chlorogenic acid were used as standards. The extracts were performed for TLC fingerprints on Merck Silica gel 60 F254 plates. The solvent system was toluene : ethyl acetate : water : formic acid (15:90:5:5) (Adham, 2015). Then, the chromatogram was detected under short wavelength UV (246 nm) and R_f values were calculated when compared with caffeine and chlorogenic acid. The R_f values were calculated from the equation:

R_f = distance traveled by substances/distance traveled by solvent

Identification of chemical components of extracts using HPLC

Chlorogenic acid and caffeine were determined using HPLC model 1100 (Agilent®, USA). All samples were filtered with 0.45 µm filter paper. Ten microliters of samples was injected into a C18 column (Mightysil®, Japan). The mobile phase consisted of acetonitrile and

Table 1. Percentage yield of coffee bean extracts.

Extracts		Yield (%)	Physical appearances	pH
Hexane	Green Arabica (HGA)	4.82	Yellow color extract	5
	Roasted Arabica (HRA)	11.37	Brown color extract	5
	Green Robusta (HGR)	1.93	Yellow color extract	5
	Roasted Robusta (HRR)	12.07	Brown color extract	5
Ethanol	Green Arabica (EGA)	1.93	Yellow color extract	5
	Roasted Arabica (ERA)	6.51	Dark brown color extract	5
	Green Robusta (EGR)	2.17	Green color extract	5
	Roasted Robusta (ERR)	5.43	Dark brown color extract	5

1% acetic acid (pH 3) with ratio of 15:85 at a flow rate of 1.0 ml/min (Ayelign et al., 2013). Chromatograms were recorded at 280 nm. Identification of chlorogenic acid and caffeine in extracts was performed by comparing the retention time and chromatogram with their reference standard compounds.

The stability of coffee bean extracts

The extracts with good biological activities were selected for a stability study in which the extracts were kept at various storage conditions: room temperature (RT), room temperature in the dark (DRT), 4 and 45°C for 3 months. In addition, they were kept in accelerated conditions: heating-cooling cycling: 45°C for 48 h and then moved to 4°C for 48 h (1 cycle) for 6 cycles. After each condition, the extracts were analyzed on their antioxidant activity by DPPH assay and anti-tyrosinase activity.

Statistical analysis

All the experiments were done in triplicate and data were showed as mean ± standard deviation (sd). One-way analysis of variance (ANOVA) was carried out to determine the significant difference of the data between the green and roasted coffee bean extracts and standards at the level of p-value < 0.05 using software SPSS (Version 19.0, IBM).

RESULTS AND DISCUSSION

The yield of extracts

The coffee bean extracts obtained from hexane and ethanol maceration were calculated with percentage yield which ranged between 1.93 and 12.07% as shown in Table 1. The results showed that HGA, HGR and EGA were semisolid with a yellow color and unique odor. HRA, HRR, ERA and ERR were semisolid with brown or dark brown color and coffee odor whereas the EGR was green semisolid with a unique odor. All the extracts had pH of 5 which is suitable for skin care application. HRR possessed the highest percentage yield (12.07%) while HGR and EGA showed the lowest (1.93%). The hexane extracts from both green and roasted coffee beans showed higher percentage yield than ethanolic extracts.

This might be due to the non-polar property of hexane that could extract most of the lipid contents from the coffee bean. Additionally, the roasted coffee bean showed higher lipid contents than the green coffee bean in both species corresponding to their percentage yield (Farah, 2012).

Determination of total phenolic content

Total phenolic contents of all the extracts were determined by Folin-Ciocalteu assay. The total phenolic contents of both ethanolic green and roasted coffee extracts were statistically different. From the results, ERR presented the highest phenolic content (287.54 mg gallic acid/g extract) followed by EGA, EGR and ERA, respectively (255.99, 238.94 and 90.95 mg gallic acid/g extract) as shown in Table 2. In contrast, for hexane extracts, their total phenolic contents were not detectable. The results showed that total phenolic content of the green coffee bean extract was significantly higher than roasted coffee beans, except ERR. This might be due to auto-oxidation or degradation during the roasting process, leading to the decreased of polyphenol level in roasted coffee beans (Cheong et al., 2013). Generally, many research papers presented that the phenolic compounds were the good free radical scavenger. In addition, previous studies showed that coffee bean contained many polyphenolic compounds such as chlorogenic acid, mangiferin and hydroxycinnamic acid esters (Vignoli et al., 2011; Campa et al., 2012; Moreira et al., 2013). The major phenolic acid in all coffee samples was chlorogenic acid (Cheong et al., 2013). Therefore, the extracts that revealed a high total phenolic content tends to present a high level of antioxidant activity.

The determination of antioxidant activities

The coffee bean extracts' antioxidant activity was evaluated by DPPH, ABTS and lipid peroxidation inhibition (linoleic acid) assays when compared with

Table 2. Total phenolic contents and antioxidant activities of coffee bean extracts evaluated by DPPH, ABTS and lipid peroxidation inhibition assays.

Samples		Total phenolic (mg gallic acid/g extract)	IC$_{50}$ (mg/ml)		
			DPPH assay	ABTS assay	Lipid peroxidation inhibition assay
Hexane extract	Green Arabica (HGA)	ND	6.970±0.16[a]	0.790±2.29[a]	8.240±0.01[a]
	Roasted Arabica (HRA)	ND	4.880±0.12[b]	1.920±0.80[b]	10.030±0.01[b]
	Green Robusta (HGR)	ND	10.340±0.51[c]	5.010±1.29[c]	9.786±0.01[c]
	Roasted Robusta (HRR)	ND	5.750±0.32[d]	1.940±0.08[d]	8.230±0.02[d]
Ethanolic extract	Green Arabica (EGA)	255.99±2.05[a]	0.050±0.01[e]	0.016±0.01[e]	1.246±0.85[e]
	Roasted Arabica (ERA)	90.95±1.93[b]	0.180±0.01[f]	0.024±0.01[e,f]	0.405±0.02[f]
	Green Robusta (EGR)	238.94±0.44[c]	0.070±0.01[g]	0.014±0.01[e]	2.632±1.71[g]
	Roasted Robusta (ERR)	287.54±4.30[d]	0.090±0.01[h]	0.023±0.01[e,g]	5.144±0.01[h]
Natural extracts	Turmeric extract	-	0.040±0.01[e]	0.03±0.04[f,g]	2.414±0.52[i]
	Mangosteen extract	-	0.36±0.00[i]	0.06±0.50[h]	2.018±1.00[j]
Standard	Trolox (µg/ml)	-	0.005±0.19[j]	0.864±0.01[i]	0.047±0.01[k]
	Gallic acid (µg/ml)	-	0.002±0.31[j]	0.599±0.01[i]	0.124±0.01[k]
	Quercetin (µg/ml)	-	0.006±0.18[j]	0.538±0.03[i]	0.083±0.02[k]

ND = Not detectable, mean values with different letters in the same column are significantly different in Tukey's test (p ≤ 0.05).

natural extracts (turmeric extract and mangosteen extract) and standards: trolox, gallic acid and quercetin. DPPH assay is widely used for testing the ability of compounds that act as free radical scavengers or hydrogen donors. Turmeric extract and mangosteen extract are widely used as active ingredients in anti-aging products due to their antioxidant activity. Therefore, researchers selected these extracts to compare biological activities with coffee bean extracts. The results are shown in Table 2. A lower IC$_{50}$ value revealed a good antioxidant activity. Ethanolic extracts showed the higher antioxidant activity was significantly different from hexane extracts due to the presence of phenolic compounds that could be extracted by a more polar solvent (Prieto and Vázquez, 2014). Therefore, the research focus on the results of ethanolic extracts. Ethanolic green coffee bean extracts showed higher activity than ethanolic roasted coffee bean extracts in the same species that may be related to the higher polyphenol contents, especially chlorogenic acid (Yashin et al. 2013). Chlorogenic acid is a major component in green coffee beans and is reduced by the roasting process. There are many antioxidant

experiments which prove that the phenolic compounds were the good free radical scavenger as mentioned above (Sendra, 2009). These results also strongly indicated that phenolic compounds in coffee bean are major contributors to their antioxidant capacity. The results also showed no significant differences in the antioxidant capacity of EGA and turmeric extract. Additionally, the ethanolic extracts of both species revealed a better antioxidant activity than in the mangosteen extract. The results from ABTS assay exhibited the same trend as DPPH assay. The hexane extracts revealed IC$_{50}$ value much significantly higher than the ethanolic extracts. Additionally, the EGA and EGR presented better activity than turmeric extract while all ethanolic extracts presented a significantly higher level of activity than in the mangosteen extract. The results from lipid peroxidation inhibition assay also showed that ethanolic extracts significantly inhibited lipid peroxidation better than hexane extracts. The ethanolic roasted arabica bean extract showed a better activity than green arabica bean extract. This result might be due to the roasted coffee bean containing higher caffeine (lipophilic

Table 3. Percentage inhibition of coffee bean extracts evaluated by mushroom tyrosinase inhibition activity.

Samples		Inhibition (%) (concentration 2.5 mg/ml)	
		L-tyrosine	L-dopa
Hexane extract	Green Arabica (HGA)	13.50 ± 0.01^a	2.53 ± 0.02
	Roasted Arabica (HRA)	17.15 ± 0.02^b	12.07 ± 0.02
	Green Robusta (HGR)	12.12 ± 0.05^c	2.61 ± 0.05
	Roasted Robusta (HRR)	ND	14.43 ± 0.02
Ethanolic extract	Green Arabica (EGA)	44.27 ± 0.01^d	ND
	Roasted Arabica (ERA)	20.93 ± 0.01^e	ND
	Green Robusta (EGR)	23.20 ± 0.05^f	ND
	Roasted Robusta (ERR)	11.17 ± 0.02^g	ND
Natural extract	Turmeric extract	3.97 ± 0.02^h	ND
	Mangosteen extract	ND	ND
Standard	Kojic acid (0.25 mg/ml)	92.79 ± 0.23^i	86.07 ± 0.58
	α-arbutin (0.25 mg/ml)	58.91 ± 0.11^j	ND
	β-arbutin (0.25 mg/ml)	49.06 ± 1.16^k	ND
	Ellagic acid (0.25 mg/ml)	ND	70.61 ± 0.83

ND = not detectable, Mean values with different letters in the same column are significantly different in Tukey's test ($p \leq 0.05$).

agent) than the green coffee bean that could better react with linoleic acid and inhibit lipid peroxidation. On the other hand, the ethanolic green Robusta bean extract exhibited high activity than the roasted Robusta bean extract due to synergism effect of phenolic compounds. Moreover, EGA and ERA showed a good anti-lipid peroxidation activity as compared to turmeric and mangosteen extracts. However, all the extracts showed a lower antioxidant activity than the standards. The ethanolic coffee bean extracts revealed good antioxidant activity with different assays as mentioned earlier. They could also inhibit lipid peroxidation which is a major cause of skin aging. Therefore, the ethanolic extracts were selected for further study.

Determination of mushroom tyrosinase inhibition activity

Tyrosinase enzyme plays an important role in melanin synthesis. It can change tyrosine to L-dopa, then convert to dopaquinone and with several polymerization reactions, eumelanin and pheomelanin are formed (Chang, 2009). Compounds that can inhibit tyrosinase enzyme are used as skin brightening agent. The results are shown in Table 3. When tyrosine was used as substrate, EGA revealed the highest activity (%inhibition = 44.27%). HRR, mangosteen extract and ellagic acid showed no activity. The coffee bean extracts presented a higher activity than turmeric extract. However, all the extracts presented a lower activity than kojic acid and arbutin. These indicated that antioxidant compounds might promote the tyrosinase inhibition activity due to their antioxidative synergistic (Chang, 2009). Therefore, the extracts which consist of high amounts of total phenolic compounds possessed a good inhibition to

tyrosinase enzyme. In the part of L-dopa substrate, HRR showed the highest percentage of inhibition, whereas the ethanolic extracts showed no activity. Interestingly, the hexane extracts could inhibit tyrosinase enzyme in the step of converting L-dopa to dopachrome while α-arbutin and β-arbutin could not. It may be due to the components of triglycerides in the hexane extracts that are binding with some sites of the tyrosinase enzyme (Chang, 2009). It could be concluded that the ethanolic coffee bean extracts were the alternative ingredients in whitening products or mixing with other brightening natural ingredients.

The effect of coffee bean extracts on cell viability

The cytotoxicity of coffee bean extracts was measured in RAW 264.7 cells using MTT assay. Percentage of cell viability between samples and the control at the same concentration (100 mg/ml) is shown in Figure 1. Caffeine and chlorogenic acid were used as controls. The results revealed that all extracts showed no toxicity on cells including caffeine, whereas chlorogenic acid presented only 61.37% of cell viability due to its acidity. Additionally, the extracts showed a higher percentage of cell viability than 100 which is in accordance with the effect of caffeine on cell viability. This result improves the assertion that the selected extracts are safe and can be developed as skin care products.

Determination of TLC chromatogram and the identification of chemical components of extracts using HPLC

The ethanolic extracts showed good biological activities

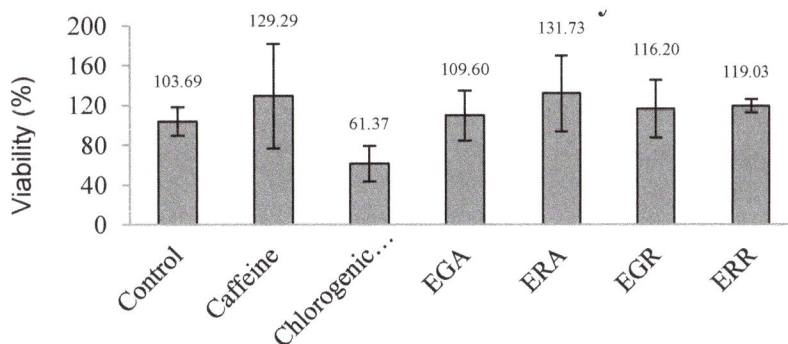

Figure 1. Percentage viability of RAW 264.7 cells treated with extracts and detected by MTT assay.

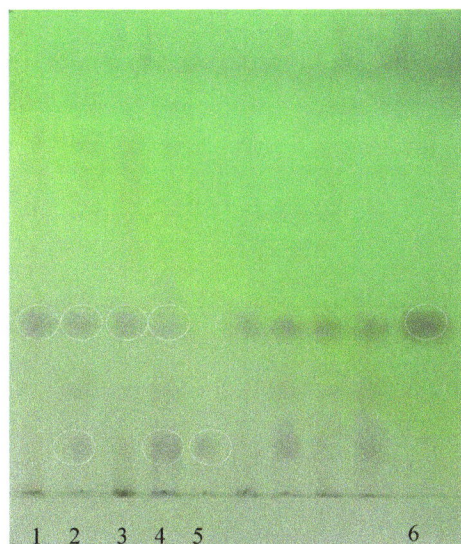

Figure 2. TLC chromatogram detected with UV 254 nm (1 = roasted Robusta (ERR), 2 = green Robusta (EGR), 3 = roasted Arabica (ERA), 4 = green Arabica (EGA), 5 = chlorogenic acid (R_f = 0.1), caffeine (R_f = 0.35).

therefore they were selected to further analyze major constituent by TLC. Coffee bean extracts, caffeine and chlorogenic acid were spotted on Merck Silica gel 60 F254 plate and developed with the mobile system of toluene: ethyl acetate : water : formic acid (15:90:5:5). Then, the chromatograms were detected under a short UV wavelength (246 nm). The TLC plates emitted green light where the compounds absorbed the light, and indicated as the dark areas. All the coffee bean extracts showed a deep dark spot with the same retardation factors with caffeine (R_f = 0.35) as shown in Figure 2 and Table 4. In addition, the chlorogenic acid, EGR and EGA showed the dark spot at the same distance (R_f = 0.1).

According to the results from TLC, caffeine was found in all extracts, whereas chlorogenic acid could be found only in the green coffee bean extracts due to the low

amount in roasted coffee bean extracts. These results are related to the previous study which stated that caffeine was found in both green and roasted coffee beans. The previous study also indicated that chlorogenic acid was found in a higher amount in green coffee bean than roasted coffee bean. This may be due to its degradation by heat (Farah, 2012). It could be assumed that caffeine and chlorogenic acid are key compounds in coffee bean that serve as antioxidant and anti-tyrosinase ingredient.

The ethanolic extracts were evaluated by HPLC using caffeine and chlorogenic acid as reference standards. The retention time of caffeine reference was 8.514 min, while retention time of chlorogenic acid was 9.450 min. The HPLC chromatogram of ERR and ERA showed a peak of caffeine, whereas EGR and EGA presented

Table 4. Retardation factors of extracts and standards.

Samples		R_f (cm)
Ethanolic extract	Green Robusta (EGR)	0.1, 0.35
	Green Arabica (EGA)	0.1, 0.35
	Roasted Robusta (ERR)	0.35
	Roasted Arabica (ERA)	0.35
Standard	Chlorogenic acid	0.1
	Caffeine	0.35

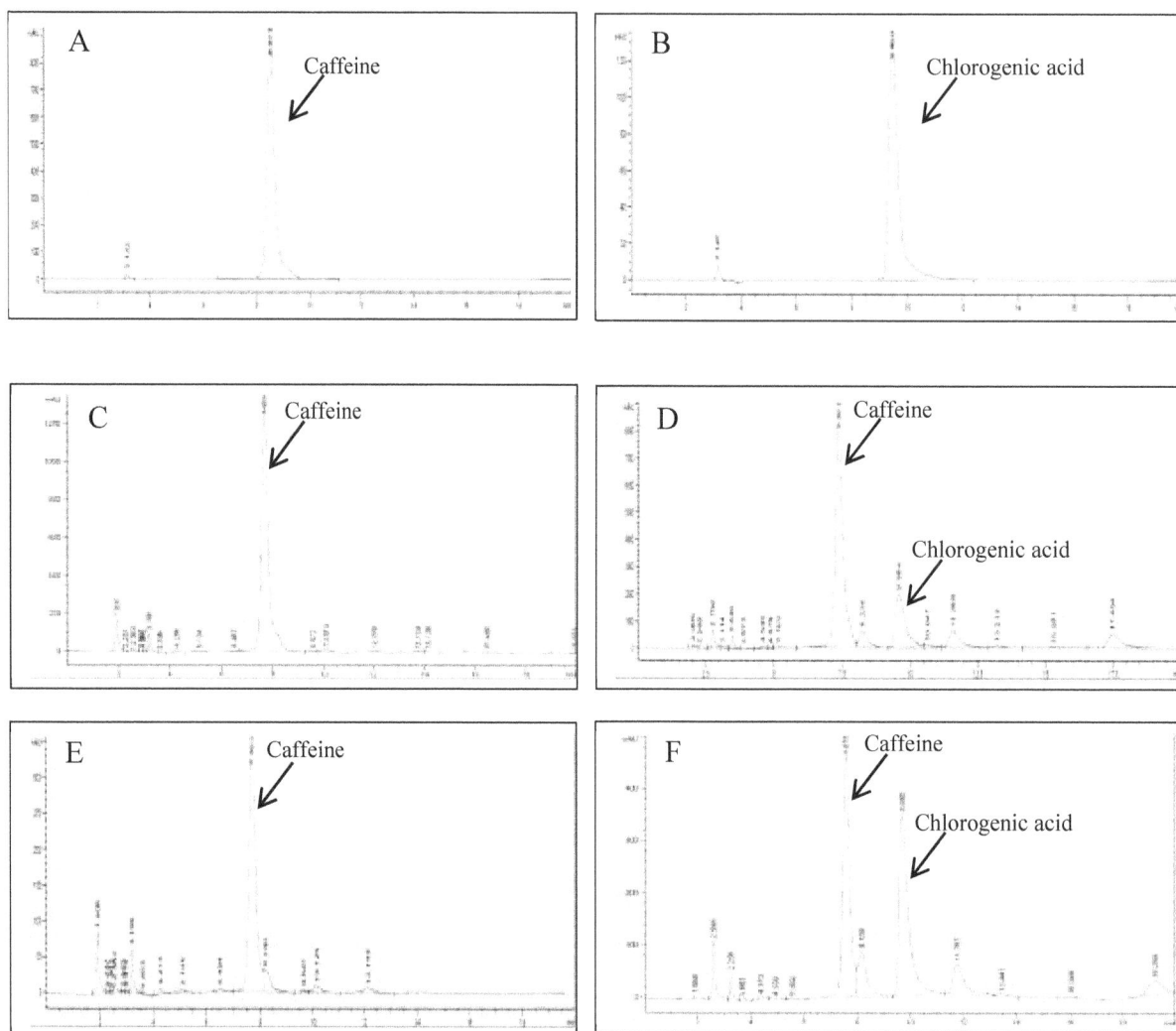

Figure 3. HPLC chromatograms of caffeine (A), chlorogenic acid (B), ERR (C), EGR (D), ERA (E) and EGA (F).

both peaks of caffeine and chlorogenic acid as shown in Figure 3. The HPLC chromatograms are related to the results from TLC chromatogram. The roasted coffee bean extract loss of chlorogenic acid may be due to high temperature during the roasting process.

The stability of coffee bean extracts

The ethanolic extracts were kept in various storage conditions: room temperature (RT), the room temperature in the dark condition (DRT), 4 and 45°C for 3 months

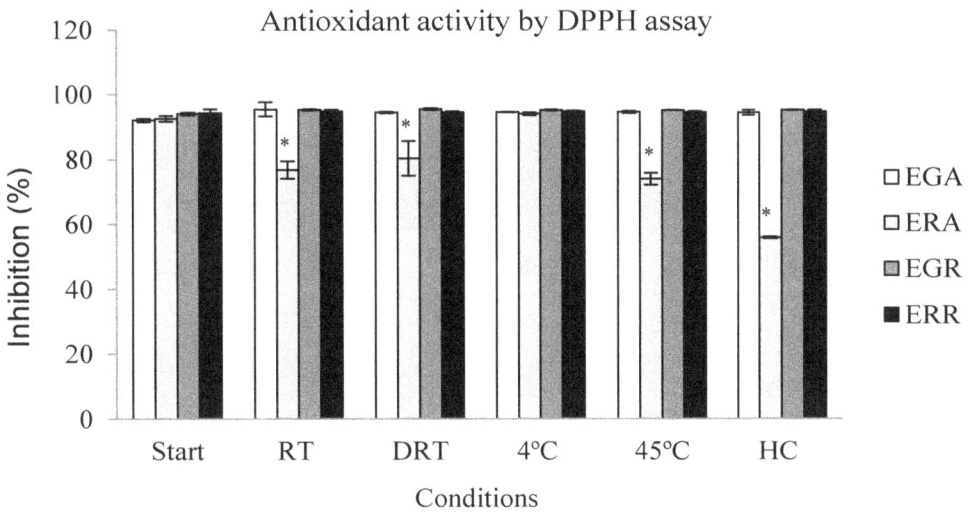

Figure 4. Percentage inhibition of coffee bean extracts by DPPH assay before and after the stability test (*=significant at P<0.05 compared between different conditions of each extract).

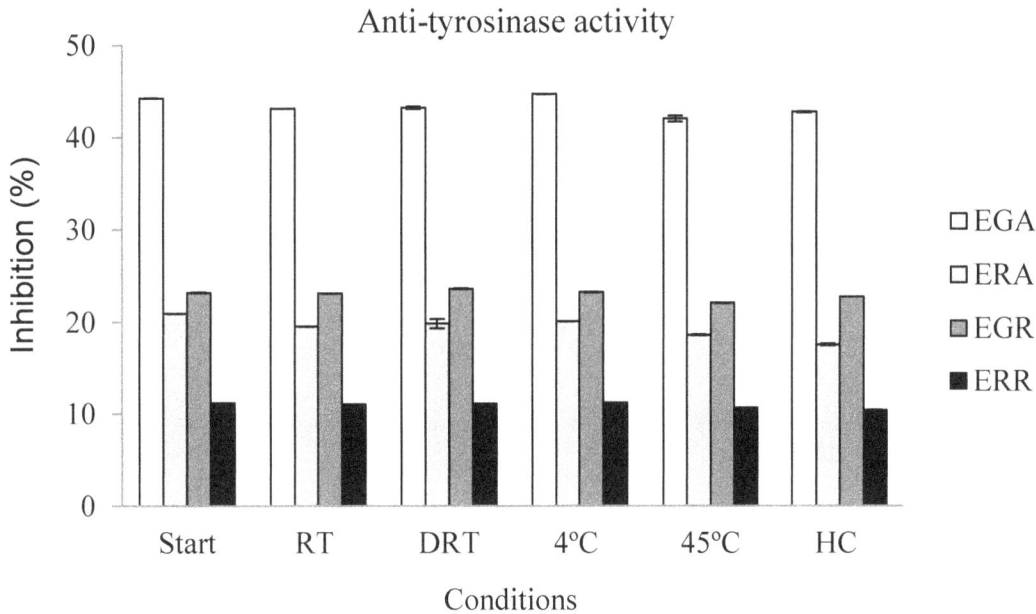

Figure 5. Percentage inhibition of coffee bean extracts by mushroom tyrosinase inhibition activity assay before and after stability test (*=significant at P<0.05 compared between different conditions of each extract).

and heating-cooling (HC) for 6 cycles. After stability test, the extracts were analyzed by DPPH assays and mushroom tyrosinase inhibition activity assay. The results are shown in Figures 4 and 5. The percentage of inhibition of green Arabica (EGA), green Robusta (EGR) and roasted Robusta (ERR) extracts did not change after being stored in all conditions. Whereas, roasted Arabica (ERA) extract showed a significant decrease in the percentage of inhibition (P<0.05) after being stored at all conditions except 4°C. In contrast, the results from the

mushroom tyrosinase inhibition activity assay showed that the percentage of inhibition did not change after being stored at various conditions. The results are related to their chemical compositions. Previous report indicated that Arabica coffee beans consist of coffee oil (cafestol and kahweol), triglycerides, fatty acids and tocopherol that are sensitive to heat, light and oxygen (Farah, 2012). Therefore, these compounds degrade after a stability test leading to a decrease in the antioxidant activity.

Therefore, the extracts should be kept to avoid light

and heat to protect the degradation of active compounds.

Conclusion

In this study, the green and roasted coffee bean extracts from Arabica and Robusta beans were extracted with hexane and then followed by ethanol with maceration. The hexane extracts showed higher percentage of yields than in the ethanolic extracts; this may be due to high lipid contents. However, the ethanolic extracts possessed higher total phenolic contents and an enhanced level of antioxidant activity than in the hexane extracts. All the extracts except HRR could inhibit tyrosinase activity when using L-tyrosine as a substrate, whereas the hexane extracts showed anti-tyrosinase activity when L-dopa was used as a substrate. Antioxidant and anti-tyrosinase activities of extracts are related to the amount of caffeine and polyphenol contents. The higher caffeine and polyphenol contents generated higher biological activities. The ethanolic extracts that indicated good biological activities and non-toxicity were chosen for a further study. From TLC and HPLC chromatograms, the selected ethanolic extracts consisted of caffeine, while chlorogenic acid was found only in the green coffee bean extracts. The extracts also possessed good activities after being stored at various conditions for 3 months. Therefore, the ethanolic coffee beans are a promising source of natural antioxidant and anti-tyrosinase agent, and should be further developed into cosmeceutical products such as anti-aging or brightening products.

ACKNOWLEDGEMENTS

The authors are grateful to Chiang Mai University, Chiang Mai, Thailand for financial support. They also thank the Faculty of Pharmacy, Chiang Mai University for all the facilities.

REFERENCES

Adham AN (2015). Simultaneous estimation of caffeic and chlorogenic acid content in *Ammi Majus* seed by TLC and HPLC. Int. J. Pharm. Pharm. Sci. 7(6):263-267.

Almeida AAP, Naghetini CC, Santos VR, Antonio AG, Farah A, Gloria MBA (2012). Influence of natural coffee compounds, coffee extracts and increased levels of caffeine on the inhibition of *Streptococcus mutans*. Food Res. Int. 49: 459-461.

Antonio AG, Iorio NLP, Pierro VSS, Candreva MS, Farah A, Santos KRN, Maia LC (2011). Inhibitory properties of Coffea canephora extract against oral bacteria and its effect on demineralisation of deciduous teeth. Arch. Oral Biol. 56:556-564.

Ayelign A, Sabally K (2013). Determination of Chlorogenic Acids (CGA) in Coffee Beans using HPLC. Am. J. Res. Commun. 1(2):78-91.

Brem B, Seger C, Pacher T, Hart M, Hadacek F, Hofer O, Vajrodaya S, Greger H (2004). Antioxidant dehydrotocopherols as a new chemical character of Stemona species. Phytochemistry 65:2719-2729.

Campa C, Mondolot L, Rakotondravao A, Bidel LPR, Gargadennec A, Couturon E, Fisca PL, Rakotomalala J, Jay-Allemand C, Davis AP (2012). A survey of mangiferin and hydroxycinnamic acid ester accumulation in coffee (Coffea) leaves: biological implications and uses. Ann. Bot. 1-19.

Cano-Marquina A, Tarin JJ, Cano A (2013). The impact of coffee on health. Maturitas 75:7-21.

Chandra S, Chatterjee P, Dey P, Bhattachary S (2012). Evaluation of in vitro anti-inflammatory activity of coffee against the denaturation of protein. Asian Pac. J. Trop. Biomed. pp. 178-180.

Chang TS (2009). An Updated Review of Tyrosinase Inhibitors. Int. J. Mol. Sci. 10:440-2475.

Charrier A, Berthaud J (2012). Botanical classification of coffee; in Clifford MN, ed., *Coffee botany, biochemistry and production of beans and beverage*. The AVI Publishing Company Inc., Westport, Connecticut. pp. 13-47.

Cheong MW, Tong KH, Ong JJM, Liu SQ, Curran P, Yu B (2013). Volatile composition and antioxidant capacity of Arabica coffee. Food Res. Int. 51:388-396.

Chu YF, Chen Y, Black RM, Brown PH, Lyle BJ, Liu RH, Ou B (2011). Type 2 diabetes-related bioactivities of coffee: Assessment of antioxidant activity, NF-KB inhibition, and stimulation of glucose uptake. Food Chem. 124: 914-920.

Chuakul W, Saralamp P, Paonil W, Temsiririrkkul R, Clayton T (1997). *Medical plants in Thailand*, Siambook and Publications Co., Ltd. Bangkok.

Devasagayam TPA, Tilak JC, Boloor KK, Sane KS, Ghaskadbi SS, Lele RD (2004). Free radicals and antioxidants in human health: current status and future prospects. J. Assoc. Physicians India. 52:794-804.

Farage MA, Miller KW, Elsner P, Maibach HI (2008). Intrinsic and extrinsic factors in skin ageing: a review. Int. J. Cosmet. Sci. 30:87-95.

Farah A (2012). Coffee constituents; in Chu YF. ed., *Coffee: Emerging Health Effects and Disease Prevention*. John Wiley & Sons, Inc. pp. 21-58.

Garzón GA, Riedl KM, Schwartz SJ (2009). Determination of anthocyanins, total phenolic content, and antioxidant activity in Andes Berry (Rubus glaucus Benth). J. Food Sci. 74(3):227-232.

Johnson CE, Oladeinde FO, Kinyua AM, Michelin R, Makinde JM, Jaiyesimi AA, Mbiti WN, Kamau GN, Kofi-Tsekpo WM, Pramanik S, Williams A, Kennedy A, Bronner Y, Clarke K, Fofonoff P, Nemerson D (2008). Comparative assessment of total phenolic content in selected medicinal plants. Niger. J. Nat. Prod. Med. 12:40-42.

Liang N, Lu X, Hu Y, Kitts DD (2016). Application of Attenuated Total Reflectance−Fourier Transformed Infrared (ATR-FTIR) Spectroscopy To Determine the Chlorogenic Acid Isomer Profile and Antioxidant Capacity of Coffee Beans. J. Agric. Food Chem. 64:681-689.

Liu Y, Kitts DD (2011). Confirmation that the maillard reaction is the principle contributor to the antioxidant capacity of coffee brews. Food Res. Int. 44: 2418-2424.

Moreira MEC, Pereira RGFA, Dias DF, Gontijo VS, Vilela FC, Moraes GOI, Giusti-Paiva A, Santos MH (2013). Anti-inflammatory effect of aqueous extracts of roasted and green Coffea arabica L. J. Funct Foods 5:466-474.

Mueller M, Hobiger S, Jungbauer A (2010). Anti-inflammatory activity of extracts from fruits, herbs and spices. Food Chem. 122(4):987-996.

O'Keefe JH, Bhatti SK, Patil HR, DiNicolantonio JJ, Lucan SC, Lavie C (2013). Effects of habitual coffee consumption on cardiometabolic disease, cardiovascular health, and all-cause mortality. J. Am. Coll. Cardiol. 62(12):1043-1051.

Pham-Huy LA, He H, Pham-Huy C (2008). Free radicals, antioxidants in disease and health. Int. J. Biomed. Sci. 4(2):89-96.

Poljsak B, Dahmane RG, Godic A (2012). Intrinsic skin aging: The role of oxidative stress. ACTA dermatovenerol APA. 21:33-36.

Pomerantz SH (1963). Separation, purification and properties of two tyrosinases from hamster melanoma. J. Biol. Chem. 238:2351-2357.

Prieto MA, Vázquez JA (2014). *In vitro* determination of the lipophilic and hydrophilic antioxidant capacity of unroasted coffee bean extracts and their synergistic and antagonistic effects. Food Res.

Int. 62:1183-1196.

Sendra ME (2009). Total phenolic content and antioxidant activity of myrtle (Myrtus communis) extracts. Nat. Prod. Commun. 4:819-824.

Tang SY, Whiteman M, Peng ZF, Jenner A, Yong EL, Halliwell B (2004). Characterization of antioxidant and antiglycation properties and isolation of active ingredients from traditional chinese medicines. Free Radic. Biol. Med. 36(12):1575-1587.

Vignoli JA, Bassoli DG, Benassi MT (2011). Antioxidant activity, polyphenols, caffeine and melanoidins in soluble coffee: The influence of processing conditions and raw material. Food Chem.

124:863-868.

Wagemaker TAL, Carvalho CRL, Maia NB, Baggio SR, Filho OG (2011). Sun protection factor, content and composition of lipid fraction of green coffee beans. Ind. Crops Prod. 33:469-473.

Yashin A, Yashin Y, Wang JY, Nemzer B (2013). Antioxidant and Antiradical Activity of Coffee. Antioxidants 2:230-245.

## 15

Phytochemical profile of stem bark extracts of *Khaya senegalensis* by Gas Chromatography-Mass Spectrometry (GC-MS) analysis

Celestine Uzoma Aguoru, Christopher Gbokaiji Bashayi and Innocent Okonkwo Ogbonna*

Department of Biological Sciences, University of Agriculture, Makurdi, Benue State, Nigeria.

The phytochemical constituents of stem bark extracts of *Khaya senegalensis* were isolated and analyzed using Gas Chromatography-Mass Spectrometry (GC-MS). A shade-dried stem bark of *K. senegalensis* was extracted using methanol and water as solvents. The main chemical compositions of the extracts were analyzed by GC-MS and preliminary phytochemical analysis was performed to confirm the various classes of active chemical. The chemical composition of methanolic stem bark extract of *K. senegalensis* included: 4-Hepten-3-one, 2, 6-Pyridinedicarboxylic acid, 3-O-methyl-d-glucose, myristic acid, pentadecanoic acid, n-Hexadecanoic acid, 9, 12-Octadecadienoic acid, and 11-Octadecenoic acid. Others are 9–Hexadecenoic acid, Stearic acid, I, E-11, Z-13-Octadecatriene, Cyclododecyne, Hexadecanoic acid, Ricinoleic acid, 13-Decosenoic acid, and 9-Hexadecenal. The Chemical composition of aqueous stem bark extract of *K. senegalensis* included 1, 2, 3-benzenetriol, n-Hexadecanoic acid, oleic acid, (Z)6,(Z)9-pentadecadeien-1-ol, 1,E-11,Z-13-octadecatriene, and 1-flourodecane. Other chemical constituents of the aqueous extract included 9-octadecanal, E-9-tetradecanal, and 2-methyl-Z, Z-3, 13-octadecadienol. The molecular weight of these compounds ranged from low to high with carbon skeleton of between C_7 and C_{37}. Both aromatic and aliphatic compounds were identified. *K. senegalensis* contains alkaloid, saponin, tannins and flavonoids. A good number of bioactive compounds were present in the stem bark of *K. senegalensis*.

Key words: Aqueous extracts, metanolic extracts, GC-MS analysis, *Khaya senegalensis*, phytochemical profile.

INTRODUCTION

The use of traditional medicine is age long and inherent with prospects and challenges in many cultures in Africa. Even before the recorded history, medicinal plants had been used in the treatment of variety of ailments of mankind. These herbs had been very useful health remedies over the years and are currently in use in many parts of the world (Fabricant and Fansworth, 2001; Kumar et al., 2009; Al-Bayati et al., 2008). Some plant parts are used directly by these traditional medicine practitioners. Some are extracted before use or modified

*Corresponding author. Email: innocentia09@yahoo.com.

and combined before administration. In most cases, where they are extracted before application, crude extracts are used. Therefore one cardinal challenge to contend with is dosage and the other is cytotoxicity issue in traditional medicine cycle.

The use of medicinal plants in the treatment of ailments and diseases dates back to prehistory (Fabricant and Fansworth, 2001) and developing countries mostly rely on traditional medicines (Kumar et al., 2009). Traditional herbs as healers of diseases are important especially to local communities since they are easily accessible, easy to assemble and affordable to the people (Kumar et al., 2009). Various diseases including cancer and Alzheimer's disease had been reported to be treated with active compounds from plants (Kumar et al., 2009; Sheeja and Kuttan, 2007). Researches on phytochemical analyses of plant extracts in most cases correlate the chemical constituents of the plants with their pharmacological activity (Prachayasittikul et al., 2008; Costa et al., 2008; Al-Bayati and Al-Mola, 2008; Chen et al., 2008; Pesewu et al., 2008; Turker and Usta, 2008; Nyamai et al., 2016).

The therapeutic effects of medicinal plants are attributed to the phytochemicals in them including: flavonids, alkaloids, steroids, trepenoids, phenolic acids, tannins, saponins among others (Nyamai et al., 2016). These secondary metabolites exert antimicrobial activity through different mechanisms. Tannins have been found to form irreversible complexes with proline-rich protein (Shimada, 2006) resulting in the inhibition of cell protein synthesis. Herbs that have tannin as their main components are astringent in nature and hasten the healing of wounds and inflamed mucous membrane (Okwu and Okwu, 2004).

The biological function of flavonoid includes protection against allergies, inflammation, free radicals, platelet aggregation, microbes, ulcers, hepatotoxins and tumors (Okwu, 2004). These observations therefore support the use of K. senegalensis in herbal care remedies. The plant K. senegalensis, also contains alkaloids which are ranked the most efficient therapeutically significant plant substance. Pure isolated plant alkaloids and their synthetic derivatives are used as a basic medicinal agent for their analgesic, antispasmodic and bactericidal effects. Specifically, saponins have been reported to have an antimicrobial effect and could serve as precursors of steroidal substances with a wide range of physiological activities (Mahato et al., 1988).

Khaya senegalensis A. Juss (Meliaceae) is a popular medicinal plant among the Nupes and Yorubas in Nigeria. It belongs to the family Meliaceae (mahogany). The aqueous stem bark extract is traditionally used by these tribes in the treatment of malaria, jaundice, edema and headache (Aliyu, 2006; Makut et al., 2008). The Hausa and Fulani tribes in Northern Nigeria also use K. senegalensis as a remedy for several human and animal ailments (Aliyu, 2006). K. senegalensis is a large meliaceous tree native to the sub-Sahara savannah from Senegal to Uganda, and to some other parts of Africa. It is one of the most popular traditional medicines in Africa (Makut et al., 2008). It has medicinal properties for the effective management of several ailments including diarrhea (Kubmarawa et al., 2008).

Nigeria has a tropical climate and vegetation with a countless numbers of varieties of plant species. Most of these plants could have medicinal uses that are unexploited. Knowing the chemical composition of the compounds contained in the medicinal plant is a prerequisite to solving a major feat in traditional medicine operation. This could enable drug synthesis from such plants to take place. As a result, some problems relating to dosage, toxicities, and antagonisms could be solved. The aim of the present article therefore is to identify the phytochemical constituents of stem bark extracts of K. senegalensis used by the traditional people in the treatment of ailments, and to analyze the extracts using Gas Chromatography-Mass Spectrometry (GC-MS). To the best of our knowledge, researchers had used GC-MS to determine the chemistry of the active ingredients of stem bark extracts of K. senegalensis.

MATERIALS AND METHODS

Plant

Khaya senegalensis stem bark was collected from Manveh village, Ancho District of Akwanga Local Government of Nasarawa State, Nigeria. An initial quality evaluation of the plant material was carried out in the Department of Biological Sciences, Federal University of Agriculture, Makurdi by C. U. Aguoru (PhD) and further at the National Research Institute for Chemical Technology (NARICT) Zaria to validate its authenticity. Stem bark of the plants were air-dried under shade and pulverized into fine powder with mortar and piston and finally with a clean and dried grinding machine.

Extraction procedure

Maceration method was employed for the extraction of plant active constituents, and methanol (70%) and water were used as solvents for the extraction of the plant materials (Salisu and Garba, 1997). Fifty grams of each of the powdered plant materials was put into 500 ml conical flasks and 300 ml of methanol was poured over it and left to stand for 3 days with intermittent stirring using a spatula. The conical flasks were covered with foil paper. After 3 days, the extracts were filtered and evaporated to dryness using rotary evaporator (Brinkmann, R110) and then dispensed into labeled sample vials and stored in the refrigerator at 4°C for subsequent use.

Preliminary phytochemical determination

The extracts of K. senegalensis stem bark was subjected to preliminary phytochemical analysis to test for the presence/absence of the various classes of active chemical constituent such as saponins, flavonoids, tannins, alkaloids, oxalate, phytate and cyanogenic glycoside using standard laboratory techniques as reported by Sood et al. (2012) and Chhetri et al. (2008).

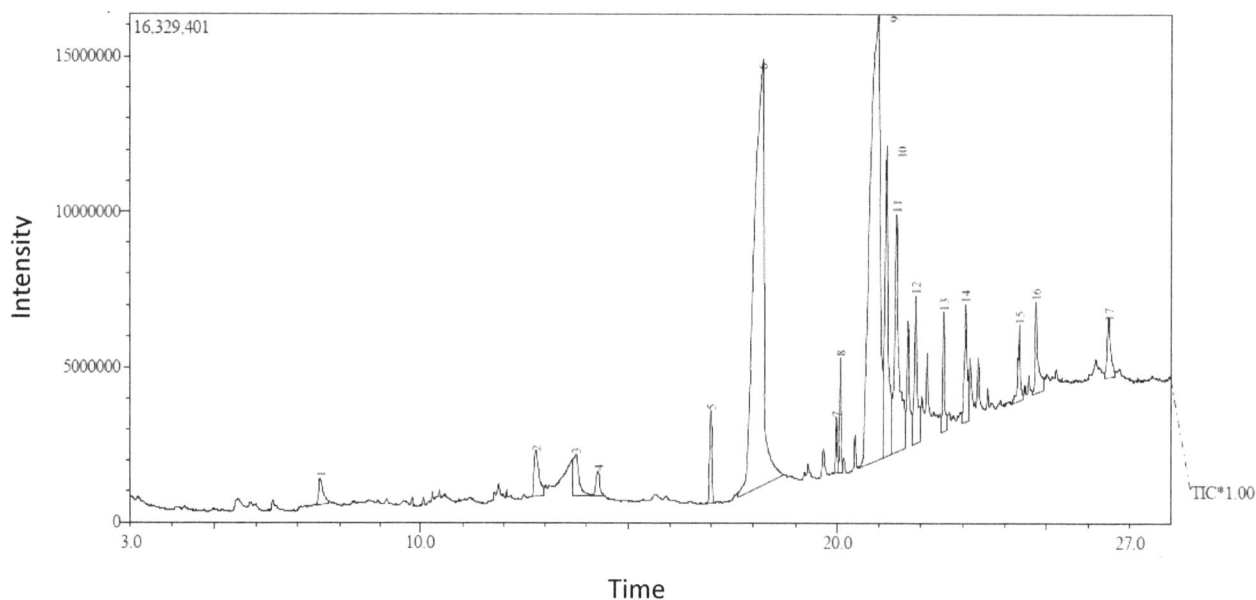

Figure 1. Total ion chromatogram of methanol extract of *K. senegalensis*.

Quantitative phytochemical analysis of *K. senegalensis* was also determined using standard biochemical techniques.

GC-MS analysis

The Chemical profiles of the extracts were determined by gas chromatography - mass spectrometry (GC-MS) model QP210 plus Shimadzu, Japan. The procedure for the analysis included the following details. Column temperature was set at 80°C, injection temperature at 250°C, pressure at 108.0 kPa, total flow was at 6.2 ml/min and linear velocity at 46.3 cm/s. The start time was 3.00 min and end time was 28.00 min. The compounds were identified using molecular weight and formula of the compounds and the retention time. Compound identification was obtained by comparing these values and the spectral data with those of authentic compounds from the library data of the corresponding compounds using automated Shimadzu software.

RESULTS

The total ion chromatogram of the methanol extract of *K. senegalensis* by GC-MS shows about seeenteen distinct peaks (Figure 1). Peak 6 and 9 show the highest percentage chemical composition. Each peak demonstrates a particular chemical compound. In Figure 2, the total ion chromatogram of aqueous extracts of *K. senegalensis* shows about 13 distinct peaks. Peak 3 had the highest percentage chemical water could extract. Peaks 4 and 2 were also high in terms of percentage composition.

Tables 1 and 2 present the GC-MS peak report of methanol and aqueous extracts of *K. senegalensis*, respectively. The Tables cover the percentage availability and the retention time of each of the eluted compound.

For the methanol extracts, the highest compound identified was n-Hexadecanoic acid (31.10 and 31.89% (Table 1) while the highest aqueous extracted compound was 3-O-methyl-d-glucose (45.57%) (Table 2). The chemical composition of methanolic stem bark extract of *K. senegalensis* included: 4-Hepten-3-one, 2, 6 Pyridinedicarboxylic acid, 3-O-methyl-d-glucose, Myristic acid, Pentadecanoic acid, n-Hexadecanoic acid, 9, 12 Octadecadienoic acid, and 11-Octadecenoic acid (Table 3). Others are 9 – Hexadecenoic acid, Stearic acid, I, E 11, Z-13-Octadecatriene, Cyclododecyne, Ricinoleic acid 13-Decosenoic acid, and 9-Hexadecenal. The molecular weight of these compounds ranged from low to high with carbon skeleton of between C_7 and C_{37}. Both aromatic and aliphatic compounds were identified. The chemical composition of aqueous stem bark extract of *K. senegalensis* included 1, 2, 3–Benzenetriol, n Hexadecanoic acid, Oleic acid, (Z) 6, (Z) 9 Pentadecadeien-1-ol, 1, E-11, Z-13-Octadecatriene, and 1-Flourodecane (Table 4). Other chemical constituents of the aqueous extract included 9-Octadecanal, E-9 Tetradecanal, and 2-methyl-Z, Z-3, 13-Octadecadienol.

Alkaloid, saponin, tannins and flavonoid were present in both of the extracts (Tables 5 and 6). In both the methanol and aqueous extracts, flavonoid was the highest (32.14 and 25.20%, respectively) occurring group of chemical.

DISCUSSION

The present study was designed to obtain the phytochemical profile of aqueous and methanolic extracts of *K. senegalensis* by GC-MS. The choice of the

Table 1. GC-MS peak report of methanol extract of *K. senegalensis.*

Peak No.	R. Time	Area%	Height%	A/H
1.	7.543	0.88	1.09	7.49
2.	12.783	1.66	1.88	8.20
3.	13.738	1.69	1.68	9.36
4.	14.284	0.71	1.03	6.36
5.	16.992	1.54	3.80	3.77
6.	18.229	31.10	17.52	16.52
7.	19.989	0.65	2.27	2.67
8.	20.080	1.36	4.74	2.67
9.	20.973	31.89	18.28	16.23
10	21.184	7.99	12.76	5.83
11.	21.414	8.07	9.78	7.68
12.	21.873	3.28	6.07	5.04
13.	22.538	1.71	4.91	3.24
14.	23.067	2.29	4.84	4.40
15	24.347	1.45	3.09	4.35
16.	24.739	2.05	3.75	5.08
17.	26.487	1.68	2.48	6.32

Table 2. GC-MS peak report of aqueous extract of *K. senegalensis.*

Peak	R. Time	Area%	Height%	A/H
1.	10.483	0.92	0.66	13.96
2.	17.993	17.40	16.25	10.78
3.	20.935	45.57	24.52	18.71
4.	21.137	11.90	18.44	6.49
5.	21.329	6.32	6.23	10.20
6.	21.788	4.52	7.34	6.20
7.	22.447	1.76	3.85	4.59
8.	22.974	1.38	2.24	6.18
9.	23.267	0.70	2.16	3.27
10.	24.265	2.92	6.86	4.28
11	24.656	1.15	2.63	4.41
12.	26.081	1.67	3.55	4.74
13.	26.396	3.79	5.25	7.27

extracting solvents (methanol and water) reflected how the local communities in the traditional treatments of ailments utilize the plants. The utilization of this plant for traditional medicine by the people also predicted that the plant could have some bioactive ingredients. The research of Kubmarawa et al. (2008) also supported the claim that extracts from the plant is used for the treatment of bacterial and fungal infections. This was one of the reasons that motivated our search for the actual chemical contained in the extracts.

Both the methanolic and aqueous extracts had many chemicals identified using retention time, relative percentage of the compound, molecular weight and molecular formula. The chemical compounds isolated from the methanolic extracts were mostly acidic including: 2, 6-Pyridinedicarboxylic acid, myristic acid, pentadecanoic acid, n-hexadecanoic acid, 9, 12-octadecadienoic acid, and 11-octadecenoic acid. Others were 9–hexadecenoic acid, stearic acid, hexadecanoic acid, ricinoleic acid and 13-decosenoic acid. The other classes of compounds isolated were 4-Hepten-3-one, 3-O-methyl-d-glucose, I, E-11, Z-13-Octadecatriene, Cyclododecyne, and 9-Hexadecenal. Some of these chemicals especially the acids have been demonstrated

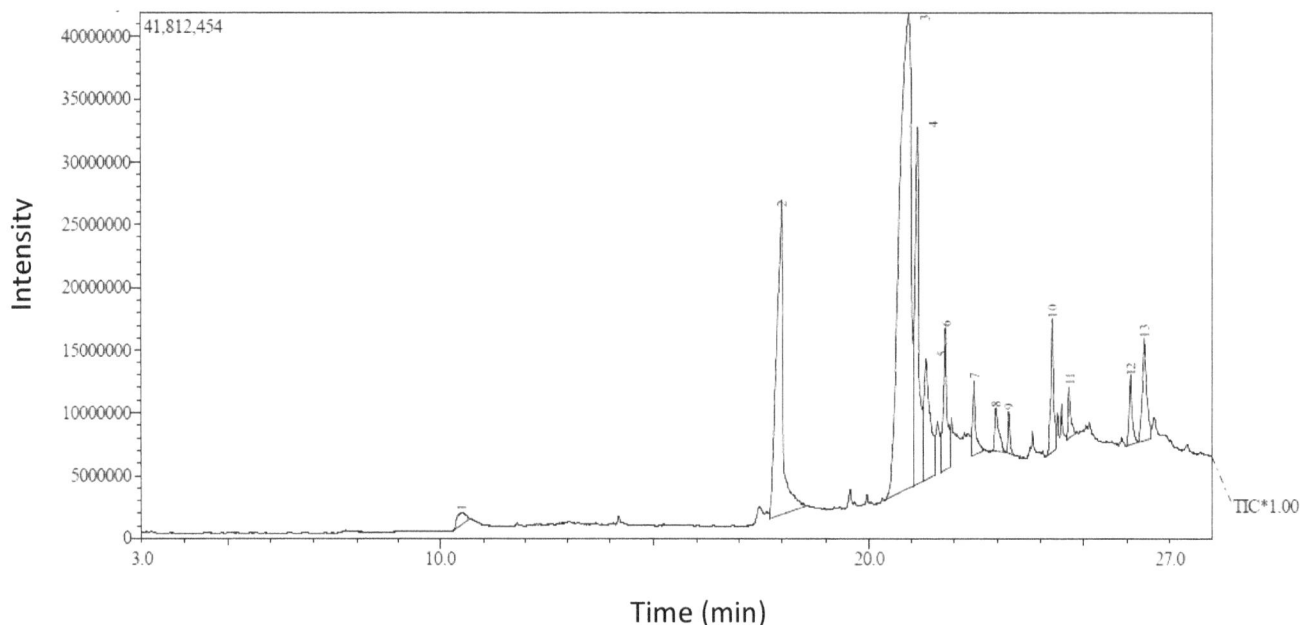

Figure 2. Total ion chromatogram of aqueous extract of *K. senegalensis.*

Table 3. Chemical composition of the methanol extract of *K. senegalensis* as identified by GC-MS.

Name	Mol. weight	Formula	Structure number*
4-Hepten-3-one	126	$C_8H_{14}O$	1
2, 6-Pyridinedicarboxylic acid	167	$C_7H_5NO_4$	2
3-O-methyl-d-glucose	194	$C_7H_{14}O_6$	3
Myristic acid	228	$C_{14}H_{28}O_2$	4
Pentadecanoic acid	270	$C_{17}H_{34}O_2$	5
n-Hexadecanoic acid	256	$C_{16}H_{32}O_2$	6
9, 12-Octadecadienoic acid	294	$C_{19}H_{32}O_2$	7
11- Octadecenoic acid	296	$C_{19}H_{36}O_2$	8
9 – Hexadecenoic acid	254	$C_{16}H_{30}O_2$	9
Stearic acid	284	$C_{18}H_{36}O_2$	10
I, E-11, Z-13-Octadecatriene	248	$C_{18}H_{32}$	11
Cyclododecyne	164	$C_{12}H_{20}$	12
Ricinoleic acid	298	$C_{18}H_{32}O_3$	13
13-Decosenoic acid	338	$C_{22}H_{42}O_2$	14
9-Hexadecenal	238	$C_{16}H_{30}O$	15

*As in Figure 3

to be bioactive (Shittu et al., 2007; Nyamai et al., 2016). The acidic organic chemical composition of aqueous stem bark extract of *K. senegalensis* included n-Hexadecanoic acid and Oleic acid. The alcoholic groupswere 2-methyl-Z, Z-3, 13-Octadecadienol, 1, 2, 3 – Benzenetriol, and (Z) 6, (Z) 9-Pentadecadeien-1-ol. Other chemical constituents of the aqueous extract included 9-Octadecanal, E -9-Tetradecanal, 1 E-11, Z-13-Octadecatriene and 1-Flourodecane. There are reports of phenols (Proestos et al., 2008) and carboxylic acids (Proestos et al., 2005) being responsible for the antimicrobial activity in medicinal plants.

In the present study, qualitative and quantitative phytochemical screenings of *K. senegalensis* for the various classes of compounds show the presence of alkaloid, saponin, tannins and flavonoid in both of the

Table 4. Chemical composition of the aqueous extract of *K. senegalensis* as identified by GC-MS.

Name	Mol. weight	Formula	Structure number*
1,2,3–Benzenetriol	126	$C_6H_6O_3$	16
n-Hexadecanoic acid	256	$C_{16}H_{32}O_2$	17
Oleic acid	282	$C_{18}H_{32}O_2$	18
(Z) 6, (Z) 9-Pentadecadeien-1-ol	224	$C_{15}H_{28}O$	19
1, E-11, Z-13-Octadecatriene	248	$C_{18}H_{32}$	11
1-Flourodecane	160	$C_{10}H_{21}F$	20
9-Octadecenal	266	$C_{18}H_{34}O$	21
E-9-Tetradecanal	210	$C_{14}H_{26}O$	22
2-methyl-Z, Z-3, 13-Octadecadienol	280	$C_{19}H_{36}O$	23

*As in Figure 3

Table 5. Qualitative phytochemical screening of *K. senegalensis.*

S/No	Phytochemical composition from qualitative Screening	*K. senegalensis*
1	Tannin	+
2	Oxalate	−
3	Phytate	−
4	Saponin	+
5	Glycoside	−
6	Alkaloid	+
7	Trypsin	−
8	Flavonoid	+

Key: + Present, - Absent.

Table 6. Quantitative phytochemical analysis of *K. senegalensis.*

Constituents	Methanol	Aqueous
Tannin (mg/100 g)	+ (0.55)	+ (0.53)
Oxalate (100 mg/100 g)	-	-
Phytate (mg/100 g)	-	-
Saponin (%)	+ (20.06)	+ (10.02)
Cynogenic	-	-
Glycoside (mg/100 g)	-	-
Alkaloid (%)	+ (22.28)	+ (8.45)
Trypsin (Tul/mg)	-	-
Flavonoid (%)	+ (32.14)	+ (25.20)

Key: + Present, - Absent.

extracts. Olmo et al. (1997) and Kubmarawa et al. (2008) also reported the presence of alkaloid, saponin and tannin in the stem bark extracts of *K. senegalensis* although they did not determine the individual chemicals as we have done in the present study using GC-MS. Some of the metabolites of the stem bark extracts of *K. senegalensis* have been reported to be responsible for antimicrobial activity Kumar et al. (2009).

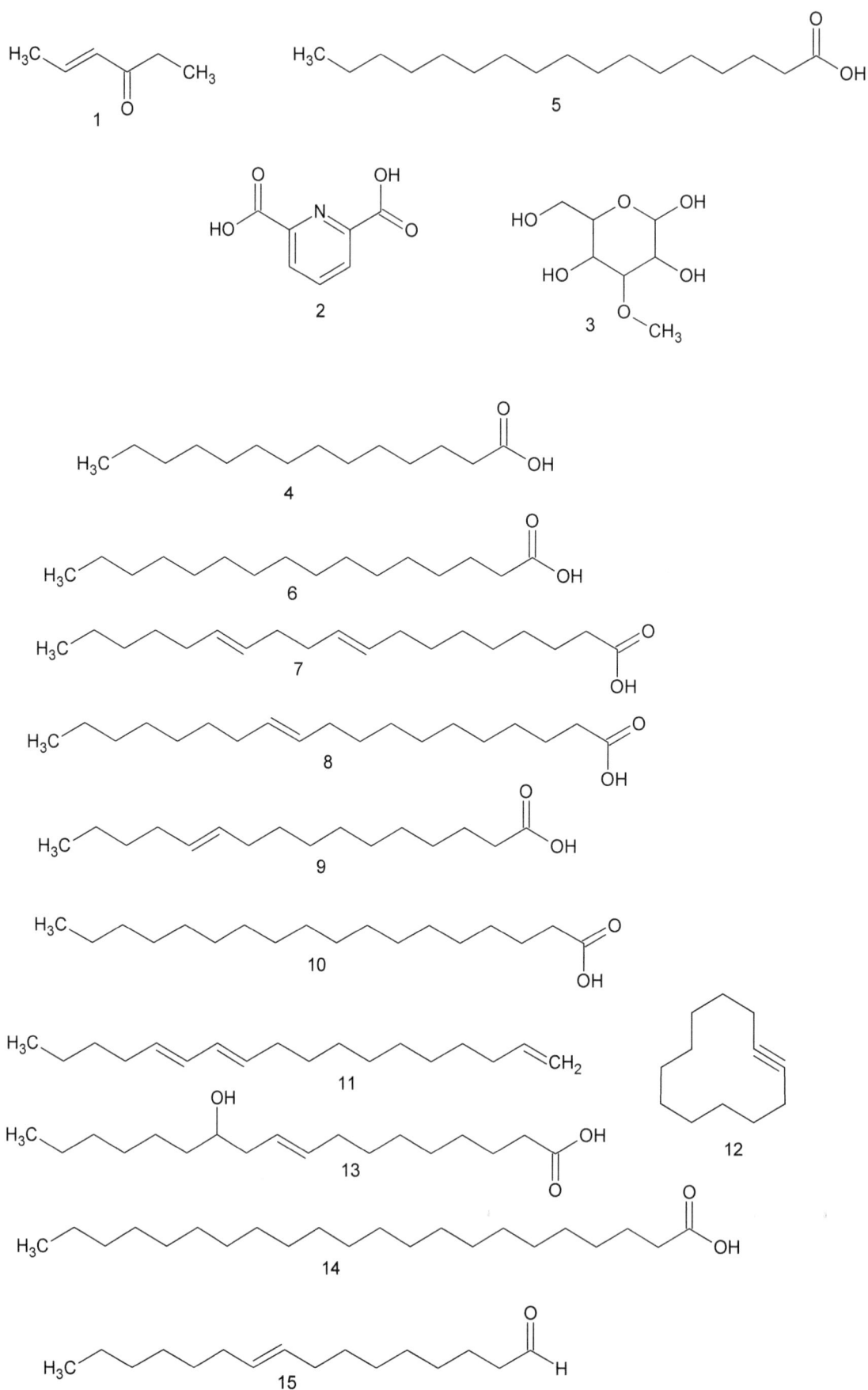

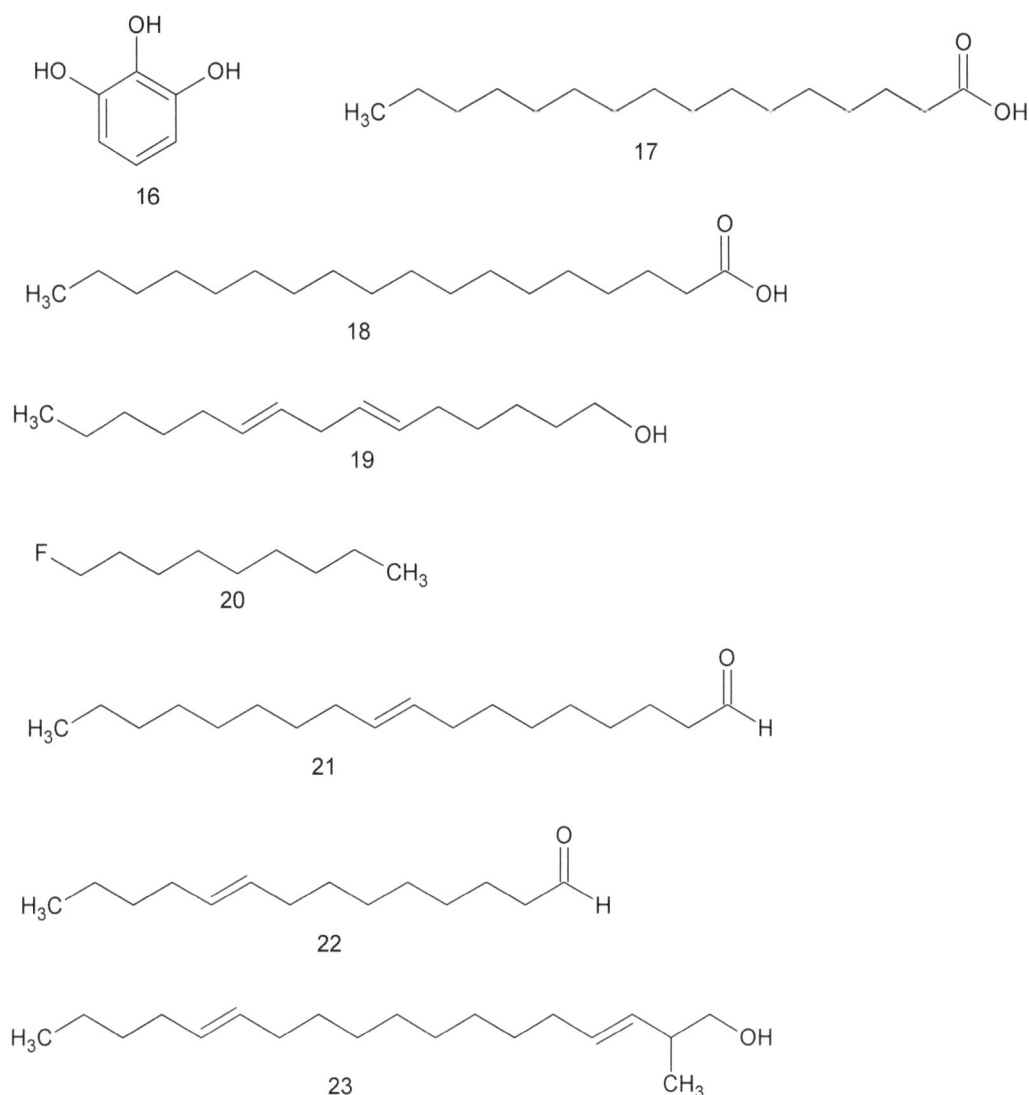

Figure 3. Chemical structures of extracts of *K. senegalensis* as identified by GC-MS.

Conclusion

Our present study shows that a good number of organic compounds are present in the stem bark of *K. senegalensis* and that these compounds account to a great extent for the claimed and reported ethno medicinal and bioactive potentials of the plant.

REFERENCES

Al-Bayati FA, Al-Mola HF (2008). Antibacterial and antifungal activity of different parts of *Trubulus terrestris* L. growing in Iraq. J. Zhejiang UnivSci. B. 2(9):154-159.

Aliyu BS (2006). Common ethnomedicinal plants of the Semarids Region of West Africa, their description and phytochemicals. Triumph Publishing Company Limited Kano, Nigeria. pp. 199-200.

Chen IN, Chang CC, Wang CY, Shyu YT, Chang TL (2008). Antioxidant and antimicrobial activity of Zingiberaceae plants in Taiwan. Plant Foods Human Nutr. 63:15-20.

Chhetri HP, Yogol NS, Sherchan J, Anupa KC, Mansoor S, Thapa P (2008). Phytochemical and antimicrobial evaluations of some medicinal plants of Nepal. Kathmandu University J. Sci. Eng. Technol. 1:49-54.

Costa ES, Hiruma-Lima CA, Limo EO, Sucupira GC, Bertolin AO, Lolis SF, Andrade FD, Vilegas W, Souza-Brito AR (2008). Antimicrobial activity of some medicinal plants of Cerrado, Brazil. Phytother. Res. 22:705-707.

Fabricant DS, Fansworth NR (2001). The value of plants used in traditional medicine for drug discovery. Environ. Health Perspect. 109:69-75.

Kubmarawa D, Khan ME, Punah AM, Hassan M (2008). Phytochemical screening and antimicrobial efficacy of extracts from *Khaya senegalensis* against human pathogenic bacteria. Afr. J. Biotechnol. 7(24):23-25.

Kumar A, Ilavarasan R, Jayachandran T, Decaraman M, Aravindhan P, Padmanabhan N, Krishman MRV (2009). Phytochemicals investigation on a tropical plant, *Syzgium cumini* from Kattuppalayam, Erode District, Tamil Nadu, South India. Pakistan J. Nutri. 8(1):83-85.

Mahato SB, Nandy AK, Roy G (1988). Triterpenoid saponins. Phytochem 27:3037-3067.

Makut MD, Gyar GP, Pennap AP (2008). Phytochemical screening and antimicrobial activity of the ethanolic and methanolic eatracts of the leaf and barks of Khaya senegalensis. Afr. J. Biotechnol. 7:1216-1219.

Nyamai DW, Arika W, Ogola PE, Njagi ENN, Ngugi MP (2016). Medicinally important phytochemicals: An updated research avenue. Research and Reviews: J. Pharmacogn. Phytochem. 4(1):35-49.

Okwu DE (2004). Phytochemicals and vitamins content of indigenous spices of South Eastern Nigeria. J. Sustain. Agric. Environ. 6:30-34.

Okwu DE, Okwu ME (2004). Chemical composition of Spondias mombia Linn plant parts. J. Sustain. Agric. Environ. 6:140-147.

Olmo LR, Da Silva MF, Das GF, Fo ER, Vieria PC, Fernandes JB, Pinheiro AL, Vilela EF (1997). Limonoids from leaves of Khaya senegalensis. Phytochemistry 44:1157-1165.

Pesewu GA, Cutler RR, Humber DP (2008). Antibacterial activity of plants used in traditional medicine of Ghana, with particular reference to MRSA. J. Ethnopharmacol. 116:102-111.

Prachayasittikul S, Buraparuangsang P, Worachartcheewan A, Isarankura-Na-Ayudhya C, Ruchirawat S, Prachayasittikul V (2008). Antimicrobial and antioxidant activity of bioreactive constituents from Hydnophytum formicarum Jack. Molecules 13:904-921.

Proestos C, Boziaris IS, Kapsokefalou M, Komaitis M (2008). Natural antioxidant constituents from selected aromatic plants and their antimicrobial activity against selected pathogenic microorganisms. Food Technol. Biotechnol. 46:151-156.

Proestos C, Chorianopoulos N, Nychas GJ, Komaitis M (2005). RPHPLC analysis of the phenolic compounds of plant extracts. Investigation of their antioxidant capacity and antimicrobial activity. J. Agric. Food Chem. 53:1190-1195.

Salisu L, Garba S (1997). Phytochemical screening and insecticida activity of Hyptis sauveolens and Striga hermonthica. Best J 5(1):160-163.

Sheeja K, Kuttan G (2007). Activation of cytotoxic T lymphocyte responses and attenuation of tumor growth in vivo by Andrographispaniculata extract and andrographolide. Immunopharma-co Immunotoxicol. 29:81-93.

Shimada T (2006). Salivary proteins as a defense against dietary tannins. J. Chem. Ecol. 32(6):1149-1163.

Shittu LAJ, Bankole MA, Ahmed T, Bankole MN, Shittu RK, Saalu CL Ashiru OA (2007). Antibacterial and antifungal activities of essentia oils of crude extracts of Sesame radiatum against some commor pathogenic microorganisms. Iran J. Pharmacol. Ther. 6:165-170.

Sood A, Kaur P, Gupta R (2012). Phytochemical screening anc antimicrobial assay of various seeds extract of Cucurbitaceae family Int. J. Appl. Bio. Pharm. Technol. 3(3):401-409.

Turker AU, Usta C (2008). Biological screening of some Turkish medicinal plants for antimicrobial and toxicity studies. Nat. Prod 22:136-146.

## 16

Evaluation of some biological activities of *Trigonella hamosa* aerial parts

Sameer H. Qari[1] and Nayer M. Fahmy[2*]

[1]Biology Department, Aljamom University College, Umm Al-Qura University Saudi Arabia.
[2]National Institute of Oceanography and Fisheries, Egypt.

The antimicrobial activity of *T. hamosa* aerial parts extract against *Bacillus subtilis, Staphylococcus aureus, Enterococcus fecalis, Escherichia coli, Pseudomonas auregenosa, Candida albicans, Fusarium* sp. and *Aspergilus niger* was evaluated by disc diffusion method. The minimum inhibitory concentrations (MICs) for susceptible test microorganisms were further determined. Also the antioxidant and α-amylase inhibition activities were investigated. The extract exhibited antimicrobial activity against *C. albican, B. subtilis* and *E. fecalis;* the MICs were 5.5, 7 and 8.5 mg/ml, respectively. Antioxidant and α-amylase inhibition activities of the extract were concentration dependent and the IC_{50} values were 0.19 and 35 mg/ml, respectively. Thin layer chromatography (TLC) bioautography was used to detect the bioactive fractions of the extract. It revealed that three different fractions of different polarities exhibited antimicrobial, α-amylase inhibition and antioxidant activities. The toxicity of the extract to brine shrimp (*Artemia salina*) larvae was assessed and the LC_{50} was found to be 2.3 mg/ml. This study suggests that the extract of *T. hamosa* aerial parts could be a source of bioactive compounds of different biological activities and is safe in terms of toxicity level.

Key words: *Trigonella hamosa,* antimicrobial, antioxidant, α-amylase, toxicity.

INTRODUCTION

Medicinal plants have been the subject of concern as a source of important therapeutic drugs useful for the treatment of various diseases. The interest in drugs derived from plants is primarily attributed to the belief that green medicine is safe and dependable compared to their synthetic counterparts. A wide range of substances that can be useful for the treatment of chronic as well as infectious diseases have been obtained from plants used in traditional medicine (Harish et al., 2010; Srinivas et al., 2011). It has been frequently shown that, different parts of medicinal plants which include stems roots, leaves, flowers, seeds, etc contain bioactive compounds (Bibi et al., 2005; Rai et al., 2007; Sindhu et al., 2013). The bioactive compounds derived from plants have broad spectrum of biological activities such as antimicrobial, antiviral, antioxidant, antitumor, enzyme inhibitors, etc. (Srinivas et al., 2011; Alagesan et al., 2012; Chikezie et al., 2015). Currently, it is well known that, the indistinctive

*Corresponding author. E-mail: nmfahmy6@yahoo.com.

use of antibiotics either for the treatment of human infectious diseases or for overprotection of animal farms has led to the emergence of antibiotic resistance phenomenon among pathogenic microbes (Khan et al., 2003; Hopwood, 2007). The high incidence of multidrug resistant pathogens has threatened the effectiveness of existing antibiotics and necessitated the urgent need for the discovery of novel antimicrobial compounds possessing unique mode of action to combat these resistant microbes (Westh et al., 2004; Penner et al., 2005; Barbosa et al., 2009; Hazni et al., 2008; Kumar et al., 2008; 2010; Rawat and Upadhyaya, 2013). Antimicrobial compounds derived from plants are effective candidates for the treatment of many infectious diseases with less side effects compared to their synthetic counterparts (Mukherjee and Wahile, 2006; Mehrotra et al., 2010).

The high level of blood glucose associated with diabetes mellitus is mainly due to either the secretion of inadequate amount of insulin by pancreas or the decreased ability to respond to insulin by cells. Inhibition of enzymes involved in hydrolysis of complex carbohydrates such as α- amylase is one of the important therapeutic strategies to treat diabetes (Nair et al., 2013). Medicinal herbs contain chemical constituents with α-amylase inhibition activity and could be potential drugs for the treatment of type II diabetes (Dastjerdi et al., 2015). It has been elucidated that, the onset and progression of complications associated with diabetes may be mediated by the generation of high level of free radicals not balanced by the antioxidative defense system as in healthy individuals (Salehi et al., 2013). Therefore, antioxidants play an important role in maintenance of the antioxidant level in the body and minimize the long term complications as well (Iwai, 2008). Bioactive compounds of medicinal plants have been studied for their antioxidant activity as alternative to synthetic ones (Parejo et al., 2002).

The genus *Trigonella* L. comprises about 135 species and is extremely important from medicinal point of view as they are famous for their steroidal Saponins contents. Most of the work has been carried out on T. *foenum-graecum* to discover the wealth bioactive compounds present in different parts of the plant and few reports are available on bioactivity of *Trigonella hamosa* L. (Hamed, 2007; Salah-Eldin et al., 2007; Yadav and Baquer, 2014). The present work was done to evaluate the antimicrobial, antioxidant and α-amylase inhibition activities as well as cytotoxicity of the aerial parts extract of T. *hamosa*

MATERIALS AND METHODS

Plant material

The aerial parts of T. *hamosa* L. were collected in spring of 2014 from Sohag Governorate, Egypt. The plant was identified by using a voucher specimen (T-119) deposited in the herbarium in Botany Dept., Faculty of Science, Sohag University, Sohag, Egypt.

Extraction and separation

The air-dried and powdered plant (1 Kg) was extracted exhaustivel with CH_2Cl_2-MeOH (1:1) at room temperature. The solvent wa distilled under reduced pressure, furnishing a gummy residue (2 g). The residue was kept in sterile glass vials and stored at 4°C unt use.

Antimicrobial activity

Microbial strains

The microbial strains used during this study included: *Bacillu subtilis* ATCC 6633, *Staphylococcus aureus* ATTC 25923 *Enterococcus fecalis* ATCC 29212, *Escherichia coli* ATCC 8739 *Pseudomonas auregenosa* ATCC 4027, *Candida albicans* ATCC 10231, *Fusarium* sp. and *Aspergilus niger*. These microbial strain were kindly provided by staff members of microbiology lab. National Institute of Oceanography and fisheries, Alexandria, Egypt

Preparation of inoculum

To prepare the inoculum of bacterial strains, cells were grown i nutrient broth and incubated for 24 h at 32°C. Cultures wer centrifuged at 7000 rpm, washed with sterile saline and adjusted t 0.1 O.D at 600 nm and stored at 4°C until use (Cwala et al., 2011) Fungal inoculum was prepared according to Wayne (2002) an culture suspension was standardized to 0.1 O.D at 530 nm.

Disc diffusion assay

Preliminary assessment of antimicrobial activity of T. *hamosa* extract was carried out by disc diffusion method. Nutrient agar (NA and potato dextrose agar (PDA) plates were spread with 50 μL o different bacterial and fungal cultures standardized to O.D 0. respectively. Sterile filter paper discs, 6 mm in diameter, wer impregnated with 50 μL of T. *hamosa* aerial parts extract (100 mg/ml) or methanol, dried and placed on the NA or PDA plate previously seeded with the respective microorganism. Afte incubation for 24 h for bacteria and 48 h for fungi, the presence o sterile zone around each paper disc indicative of antimicrobia activity was observed (Rajauria et al., 2012; Abdel-Shakour et al. 2015).

Determination of minimum inhibitory concentration (MIC)

The MICs for susceptible microbial indicators, as indicated by dis diffusion assay, were determined. Nutrient broth medium wa prepared in test tubes and sterilized by autoclaving. Water stoc solutions of T. *hamosa* aerial parts extract were aseptically adde to sterile nutrient broth medium to give a final concentration of 0. to 8.5 mg/ml. Each tube was inoculated with 10 μL of standardize inoculum of the respective test organism. Individual blanks wer done for each tube which contain the growth media and extrac without the inoculum. All tubes were incubated aerobically at 37°C for 24 h. The concentration at which no growth was observed i comparison with the blank tube was determined (Akinyemi et al. 2006).

α-amylase inhibition activity

To assess the α-amylase inhibition activity, α-amylase solution (0. mg/ml) and starch solution (10 mg/ml) were prepared in 0.02 M

Table 1. Antimicrobial activity of aerial parts extract of *T. hamosa*.

Test microorganism	*Mean diameter of growth inhibition zone (mm)
Bacteria	
Bacillus subtilis	14±0.6
Staphylococcus aureus	0
Pseudomonas aureginosa	0
Enterococcus fecalis	13±0.5
Escherichia coli	0
Fungi	
Candida albicans	16±1
Aspergillus niger	0
Fusarium sp.	0

* Values are presented in mean ± SD (n =3).

sodium phosphate buffer (pH 6.9) containing 0.006 M sodium chloride. The color reagent (dinitrosalicylic acid reagent) was prepared according to Miller (1959). In a test tube, 500 µL of enzyme solution was mixed with 500 µL of extract of different concentrations (20-55 mg/ml) prepared in deionized water and incubated for 10 min at 25°C. After pre- incubation, 500 µl of starch solution was added to each tube and further incubated at 25°C for 10 min. To stop the reaction, 1 ml of dinitrosalicylic acid reagent was added. The tubes were then incubated in boiling water bath for 5 min, cooled to room temperature and diluted with 10 ml of distilled water. To correct the background absorbance, individual blanks were made in which the starch solution was added after addition of the color reagent and boiling and the method was followed as described above (Suthindhiran et al., 2009; Dastjerdi et al., 2015). The inhibition activity of α-amylase was calculated as follows:

$$\text{Inhibition (\%)} = \frac{Abs\ control - Abs\ sample}{Abs\ control} \times 100$$

Antioxidant activity

The antioxidant activity of *T. hamosa* extract was evaluated by DPPH (1, 1-Diphenyl-2-picrylhydrazyl) radical scavenging activity. DPPH solution (20 µcg/ ml) and *T. hamosa* extract of different concentrations (0.125-0.75 mg/ml) were prepared in methanol. In a test tube equal volumes of DPPH solution and extract were mixed and incubated in the dark at room temperature for 30 min. The absorbance of each concentration and the control (containing equal volumes of DPPH and methanol) was measured at 517 nm (Khalaf et al., 2008; Ravikumar et al., 2008). Radical scavenging activity was calculated according to the following equation:

$$\text{Radical Scavenging Activity (\%)} = \frac{Abs\ control - Abs\ sample}{Abs\ control} \times 100$$

Thin layer chromatography (TLC) bioautography for bioactivity screening

Plant extract was separated using silica gel plates (GF254, Merck, Darmstadt, Germany) and developed in ethyl acetate: hexane (2:5 v/v) or ethyl acetate: hexane: methanol (3:1:1 v/v) as mobile system. After development in mobile phase, the plates were allowed to dry on air. To evaluate the antimicrobial activity of

separated compound, dried TLC plate was placed on nutrient agar medium previously seeded with *Candida albicans* and incubated for 2h at 4°C. The TLC plate was removed and the culture was incubated at 37°C for 24 h. The presence of sterile zone on the media indicated the presence of active component possessing antimicrobial activity (Moncheva et al., 2002). For α-amylase inhibition activity, dry developed TLC plate was put on sterile nutrient agar medium supplemented with 0.1% starch and kept at 4°C for 2h to allow diffusion of crude extract components to the nutrient agar medium. The TLC plate was removed and the plates were sprayed with α-amylase solution (0.5 mg/ml in 0.02 M sodium phosphate buffer pH 6.9). After incubation at 37°C for 12 h, the plate was flooded with iodine solution and examined for the presence of blue colored zone indicating the presence of active component possessing α-amylase inhibition activity (Fahmy, 2016). To detect compounds with antioxidant activity, plates were sprayed with 2.54 M DPPH solution in methanol. After drying, bands exhibiting antioxidant properties appeared in yellow color on purple background (Rajauria and Abu-Ghannam, 2013). The R_f (retention factor) value of the bioactive components was calculated.

Evaluation of the toxic effect

The toxicity of *T. hamosa* aerial parts extract was assessed by brine shrimp (Artemia *salina*) larvae assay. Eggs were hatched in natural sea water at 25°C under constant aeration for 48 h. The container was continuously illuminated by normal light along the hatching experiment. Different concentrations of the extract (1to 5 mg/ml) were made in sea water and incubated with 15-30 brine shrimp larvae. After 24 h, the nauplii were examined and the mortality was determined (El-Maghraby and Shebany, 2014).

RESULTS AND DISCUSSION

Antimicrobial activity

The extract of *T. hamosa* aerial parts was screened for antimicrobial activity by disc diffusion method. The results obtained for the antimicrobial activity of the extract are presented in Table 1 and expressed as inhibition zone in (mm). The extract exhibited antimicrobial activity against *Bacillus subtilis*, *Enterococcus fecalis* and *Candida albicans* but no activity was observed against

Table 2. MIC values of aerial parts extract of T. *hamosa*.

Test microorganism	MIC (mg/ml)
Candida albicans	5.5
Bacillus subtilis	7
Enterococcus fecalis	8.5

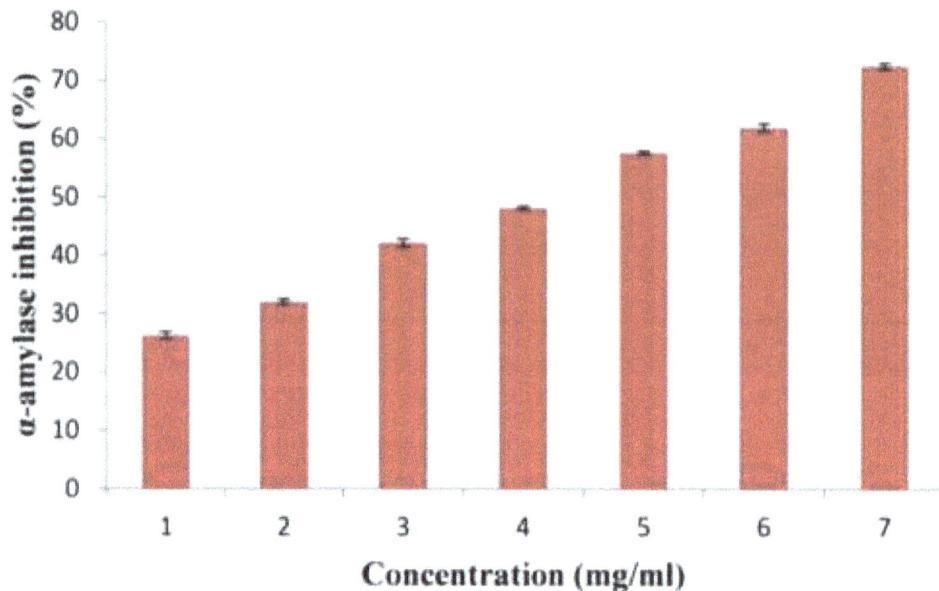

Figure 1. α- amylase inhibition activity of aerial parts extract of T. *hamosa*. Values are presented in mean ± SD (n =3).

Escherichia coli, Pseudomonas aurigenosa, Staphylococcus aureus, Aspergillus niger or *Fusarium* sp. These results suggest that the aerial parts of *T. hamosa* aerial parts possess antimicrobial activity against selected members of Gram negative bacteria, Gram positive bacteria and fungi. These results could suggest the presence of bioactive compound with broad spectrum antimicrobial activity (Aboud, 2015). Plants have been frequently reported as promising source of antimicrobial agents (Rabe and Staden, 1997; Njume et al., 2011). However, Kuete et al. (2013) studied the antibacterial activities of methanolic extract of the aerial parts of T. *hamosa* collected from Tanhat protected area (Saudi Arabia) against eight bacterial strains belonging to four species of Gram negative bacteria. They reported that the extract possesses no activity against the tested bacterial species. The production and accumulation of primary and secondary metabolites by plants is greatly affected by the environmental factors. Moreover, secondary metabolites biosynthesis by plants is the result of chemical interaction between plants and their environment, and variations in the plant metabolic profiles seem to be a direct response to changes in conditions of the plant surrounding environment (Sampaio et al., 2016). Therefore, the difference in environmental

conditions could account for variation in the metabolic profile of the same plant species collected from different geographical locations.

The minimum inhibitory concentrations of T. *hamosa* aerial parts extract for susceptible microorganisms tested are shown in Table 2. The MIC values against *Candida albicans, Bacillus subtilis* and *Enterococcus fecalis* were 5.5, 7 and 8.5 mg/ml, respectively.

α-amylase inhibition activity

The inhibitory effect of *T. hamosa* aerial parts extract against α- amylase enzyme was investigated. The inhibitory activity of the extract was observed at 20, 25, 30, 35, 40, 45 and 50 mg/ml. The extract showed a significant α- amylase inhibition activity under *in vitro* conditions. The inhibition activity showed a concentration-dependent manner. The highest concentration (50 mg/ml) of the extract tested showed a maximum inhibition of 72.64% on the activity of α-amylase and the lowest concentration (20 mg/ml) exhibited minimum inhibition percent of 25.9% (Figure 1). The IC50 was calculated as 35 mg/ml. Bioactive compounds exhibiting α-amylase inhibition activity constitute one of the most important

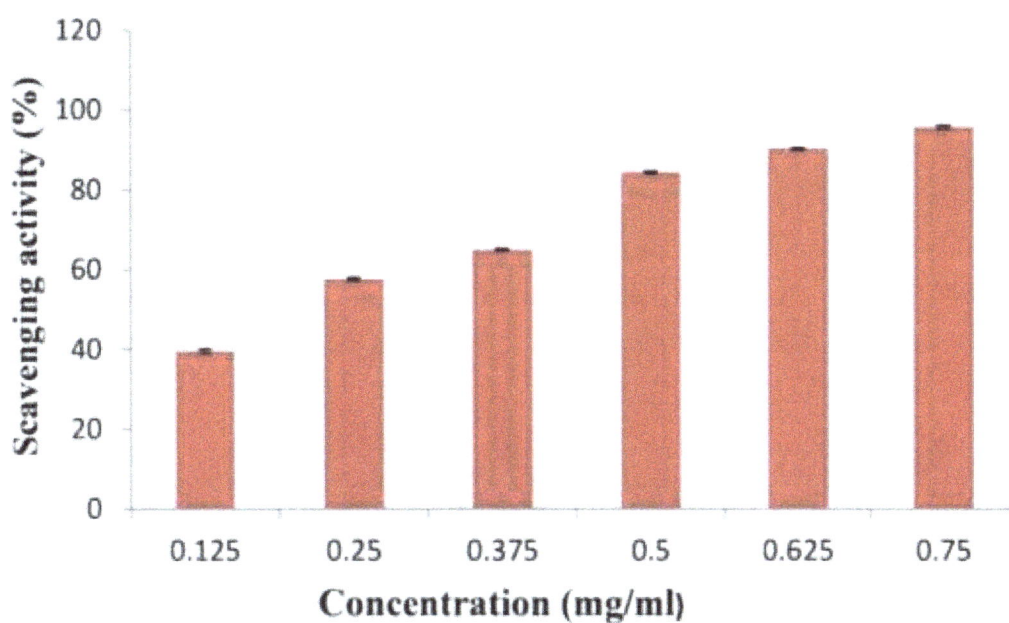

Figure 2. DPPH scavenging activity of aerial parts extract of *T. hamosa.* Values are presented in mean ± SD (n =3).

families of compounds with anti-diabetic activity. These compounds have great advantage and useful for the treatment of noninsulin diabetes mellitus (Cheng and Fantus, 2005; Upadhyay and Ahmad, 2011). Synthetic α-amylase inhibitors such as acarbose and miglitol induce gastrointestinal side effects; therefore, α-amylase inhibitors derived from medicinal herbs could be safer than their synthetic counterparts with lower negative effects (Dastjerdi et al., 2015). More than 1,200 plant species of plants used in traditional medicine have been reported to possess antidibetic activity. The search for novel bioactive compounds from these herbs could lead to potent inhibitors for enzymes involved in the development of diabetes (Narkhede, 2012).

Antioxidant activity

The antioxidant activity of *T. hamosa* aerial parts extract was examined by DPPH scavenging activity at 0.125, 0.250, 0.375, 0.5, 0.625 and 0.750 mg/ml. It showed a concentration dependent DPPH scavenging activity. The gradual increase in extract concentration resulted in a linear increase in DPPH scavenging activity and exhibited 95.7% activity at 0.75 mg/ml (Figure 2). The IC_{50} was calculated as 0.19 mg/ml. It is evident from the results that the extract possesses promising antioxidant activity. The DPPH method is the most common for measuring the radical scavenging activity of plant extracts due to rapidness, simplicity and independence of sample polarity (Marinova and Batchvarov, 20110). In the presence of compounds capable of donating hydrogen

atoms, the violet color of DPPH molecule is lost and the absorbance at wavelengths around 520 nm is decreased (Molynex, 2004). The free radical scavenging activity of T. *hamosa* aerial parts extract indicates the presence of efficient antioxidant compound(s) in terms of hydrogen atom donating ability

TLC bioautography

For TLC bioautography of antimicrobial and α-amylase inhibition activities, the TLC plates developed with ethyl acetate: hexane (2:5 v/v) were placed on nutrient agar plates previously inoculated with *Candida albicans* and sterile nutrient agar plates supplemented with starch, respectively. The results showed that only one band (R_f= 0.3) exhibited antimicrobial activity (Figure 3a) and one band (R_f= 0.19) showed α-amylase inhibition activity (Figure 3b). Regarding the TLC bioautography for antioxidant activity, when the TLC plate was developed with ethyl acetate: hexane (2:5 v/v), the fraction exhibiting antioxidant activity failed to migrate (Figure 3c), whereas, when the plate was developed with ethyl acetate: hexane: methanol (3:1:1 v/v) the fraction exhibiting antioxidant activity was detected at R_f = 0.79 (Figure 3d.). The fraction exhibiting antioxidant activity is characterized by yellow color in purple background as the delocalized spare electron of the DPPH molecule which give its deep violet color is transferred to hydrogen proton donated by the antioxidant compound(s) present in the extract leaving the yellow color of the picryl group (Molyneux, 2004). DPPH has been frequently used to screen the

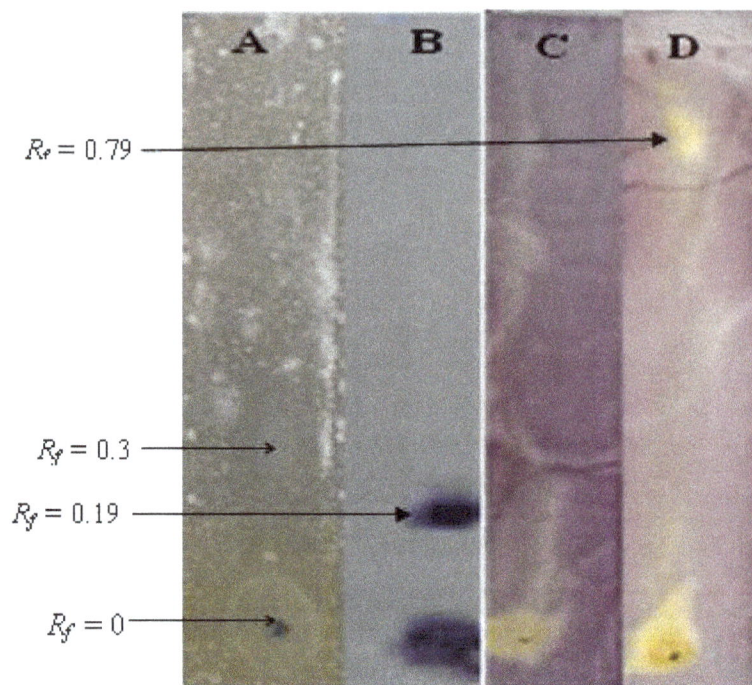

Figure 3. TLC bioautography for antimicrobial (A), α-amylase inhibition activity (B) and antioxidant activity (C and D).

antioxidant activity of plant extracts (Jaime et al., 2005; Gu et al., 2009; Bhagavathy et al., 2011). These results suggest that the bioactive compounds exhibiting antimicrobial, α-amylase inhibition and antioxidant activities have different polarities.

Toxic effect

Preliminary assessment of the toxological properties of *T. hamosa* extract was carried out by brine shrimp larvae assay. The percentage of mortality of brine shrimp larvae exposed to different concentrations of *T. hamosa* aerial parts extract is illustrated in Figure 4. At 1 mg/ml concentration, the extract displayed no toxicity, whereas, all the nauplii were killed at 5 mg/ml of the extract and the LC50 was 2.3 mg/ml.

Natural products from medicinal plants which have several pharmacological and biological activities could possess toxological properties as well. Therefore, toxicity assessment is important to achieve safe use of these products. Brine shrimp larvae assay is the most suitable for the evaluation of toxicity of plant extracts due to simplicity, rapidness and low requirements (Hamidi et al., 2014).

According to Meyer and Clarkson who proposed a toxicity indexes for the assessment of the toxicity of plant extracts and stated that, plant extracts with LC 50 greater than 1 mg/ml are considered nontoxic; *T. hamosa* aerial

parts extract is nontoxic to brine shrimp larvae (Meyer et al., 1982; Clarkson et al., 2004).

Moreover, it has been reported that brine shrimp larvae are more sensitive than cell culture and the toxic doses range from 10 to 100 greater than that of cell culture (Solis et al., 1993). This could suggest the safe use of *T. hamosa* aerial parts extracts for human use.

Conclusion

Our results indicated that the extract of *T. hamosa* aerial parts contains bioactive compounds of different biological activities such as antimicrobial, antioxidant and α-amylase inhibition activities which could be useful for pharmaceutical industries and is not toxic. Further studies are required for identification of these bioactive compounds.

ACKNOWLEDGEMENT

The authors are grateful to Prof. Kadry N. Abdel khalel (Botany Department, Faculty of Science, Sohag University) for the identification of the plant.

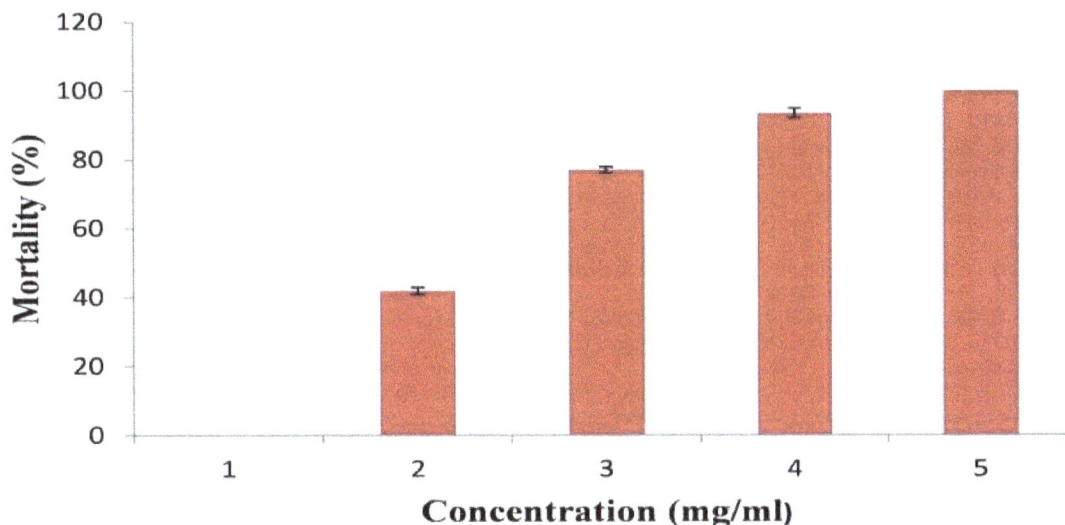

Figure 4. Percentage of mortality of brine larvae exposed to *T. hamosa* aerial parts extract. Values are presented in mean ± SD (n =3).

REFERENCES

Abdel-Shakour EH, Qari SHM, Beltagy EA, Abou El-Ela GM, Fahmy NM, Reffat BM (2015). Assessment of antimicrobial, antioxidant and enzyme inhibitory activities of *Streptomyces* sp. Nyr04 (KT074931) isolated from mangrove sediment in Red Sea (Egypt). Wulfenia 22(10):472-481.

Aboud AS (2015). Antimicrobial activities of aqueous and ethanolic extracts from *Nerium oleander* used in the treatment of burns infections isolates. J. Pharm. Chem. Biol. Sci. 2(4):248-258.

Akinyemi KO, Oluwa OK, Omomigbehin EO (2006). Antimicrobial activity of crude extracts of three medicinal plants used in south-west Nigerian folk medicine on some food borne bacterial pathogens. Afr. J. Trad. CAM 3(4):13-22.

Alagesan K, Raghupathi PK, Sankarnarayanan S (2012). Amylase inhibitors: Potential source of anti-diabetic drug discovery from medicinal plants. Int. J. Pharm. Life Sci. 3(2):1407-1412.

Barbosa LN, Rall VL, Fernandes AA, Ushimaru PI, da Silva Probst I, Fernandes AJ (2009). Essential oils against foodborne pathogens and spoilage bacteria in minced meat. Foodborne Pathog. Dis. 6:725-728.

Bhagavathy S, Sumathi P, Jancy S, Bell I (2011). Green algae *Chlorococcum humicola*-a new source of bioactive compounds with antimicrobial activity. Asian Pac. J. Trop. Biomed. 1(1):S1-S7.

Bibi SFB, Mehrangizk K, Hamid RS (2005). *In vitro* antibacterial activity of *Rheum ribes* extract obtained from various plant parts against clinical isolates of Gram negative pathogens. Iran. J. Pharm. Res. 2:87-91.

Cheng AYY, Fantus IG (2005). Oral antihyperglycemic therapy for type 2 diabetes Mellitus. Can. Med. Assoc. J. 172(2):213-226.

Chikezie PC, Ibegbulem CO, Mbagwu FN (2015). Bioactive principles from medicinal plants. Res. J. Phytochem. 9(3):88-115.

Clarkson C, Maharaj VJ, Crouch NR, Grace OM, Pillay P, Matsabisa MG, Bhagwandin N, Smith PJ, Folb PI (2004). *In vitro* antiplasmodial activity of medicinal plants native to or naturalized in South Africa. J. Ethnopharm. 92:177-191.

Cwala Z, Lgbinosa EO, Okoh AI (2011). Assessment of antibiotics production potentials in four actinomycetes isolated from aquatic environments of the Eastern Cape Province of South Africa. Afr. J. Pharm. Pharmacol. 5(2):118-124.

Dastjerdi ZM, Namjoyan F, Azemi ME (2015). Alpha Amylase Inhibition activity of some plants extract of *Teucrium* Species. Eur. J. Biol. Sci. 7(1):26-31.

El-Maghraby OMO, Shebany YM (2014). Detection of mycotoxin produce by endophytic fungi. Int. J. Life Sci. Res. 2(4):37-42.

Fahmy NM (2016). Microbiological studies on marine actinomycetes forming bioactive agents. Ph.D. Thesis, Al-Azhar univ., Cairo. P61.

Gu L, Wu T, Wang Z (2009). TLC bioautography-guided isolation of antioxidants from fruit of *Perilla frutescens var. acuta*. LWT— Food. Sci. Technol. 42(1):131-136.

Hamed AI (2007). Steroidal saponins from the seeds of *Trigonella hamosa* L. Nat. Prod. Commun. 2:143-146.

Hamidi MR, Jovanova B, Panovska TK (2014). Toxicological evaluation of the plant products using brine shrimp (*Artemia salina* L.) model. Maced. Pharm. Bull. 60(1):9-18.

Hazni H, Ahmad N, Hitotsuyanagi Y, Takeya K, Choo CY (2008). Phytochemical constituents from *Cassia alata* with inhibition against methicillin-resistant *Staphylococcus aureus* (MRSA). Plant Med. 74:1802-1805.

Hopwood DA (2007). *Streptomyces* in nature and medicine: the antibiotic makers. Oxford University Press, Oxford; New York.

Iwai K (2008). Antidiabetic and antioxidant effects of polyphenols in brown alga *Ecklonia stolonifera* in genetically diabetic KK-A(y) mice. Plant Foods Hum. Nutr. 63:163-169.

Jaime L, Mendiola JA, Herrero M (2005). Separation and characterization of antioxidants from *Spirulina platensis* microalga combining pressurized liquid extraction, TLC, and HPLC-DAD. J. Sep. Sci. 28(16):2111-2119.

Khalaf NA, Shakya AK, Al-Othman A, El-Agbar Z, Farah H (2008). Antioxidant activity of some common plants. Turk. J. Biol. 32:51-55.

Khan M, Kibm M, Oinoloso B (2003). Antimicrobial activity of the alkaloidal constituents of the root bark of *Eupomatia laurina*. Pharmaceut. Biol. 41:277-280.

Kuete V, Wiench B, Alsaid MS, Alyahya MA, Fankam AG, Shahat AA, Efferth T (2013). Cytotoxicity, mode of action and antibacterial activities of selected Saudi Arabian medicinal plants. BMC Complement. Altern. Med. 13(1):354.

Kumar H, Hullatti KK, Sharanappa P, Sharma P (2010). Comparative antimicrobial activity and TLC-bioautographic analysis of root and aerial parts of *Andrographis serpyllifolia*. Int. J. Pharm. Pharm. Sci. 2(1):52-54.

Kumar MS, Kirubanandan S, Sripriya R, Sehgal PK (2008). Triphala promotes healing of infected full-thickness dermal wound. J. Surg Res. 144:94-101.

Marinova G, Batchvarov V (2011). Evaluation of the methods for determination of the free radical scavenging activity by DPPH. Bulg.

J. Agric. Sci. 17 (1):11-24.

Mehrotra S, Srivastava AK, Nandi SP (2010). Comparative antimicrobial activities of neem, amla, aloe, assam tea and clove extracts against *Vibrio cholerae*, *Staphylococcus aureus* and *Pseudomonas aeruginosa*. J. Med. Plants Res. 4(18):2473-2478.

Meyer BN, Ferrigni NR, Putnam JE, Jacobsen LB, Nichols DE, McLaughlin JL (1982). Brine Shrimp: A convenient general bioassay for active plant constituents. Plant Med. 45:31-34.

Miller GL (1959). Use of dinitrosalicylic acid reagent for determination of reducing sugar. Anal. Chem. 31(3):426-428.

Molyneux P (2004). The use of the stable free radical diphenylpicrylhydrazyl (DPPH) for estimating antioxidant activity. Songklanakarin J. Sci. Technol. 26(2):211-219.

Moncheva P, Tishkov S, Dimitrova N, Chipeva V, Antonova-Nikolova S, Bogatzevska N (2002). Characteristics of soil actinomycetes From Antarctica. J. Cult. Collect. 3:3-14.

Mukherjee PK, Wahile A (2006). Integrated approaches towards drug development from Ayurveda and other Indian system of medicines. J. Ethnopharmacol.103:25-35.

Nair SS, Kavrekar V, Mishra A (2013). *In vitro* studies on alpha amylase and alpha glucosidase inhibitory activities of selected plant extracts. Eur. J. Exp. Biol. 3(1):128-132.

Narkhede MB (2012). Evaluation of alpha amylase inhibitory potential of four traditional culinary leaves. Asian J. Pharm. Clin. Res. 5(2):75-76.

Njume C, Afolayan AJ, Ndip RN (2011). Preliminary phytochemical screening and in vitro anti-*Helicobacter pylori* activity of acetone and aqueous extracts of the stem bark of *Sclerocarya birrea* (Anacardiaceae). Arch. Med. Res. 42:252-257.

Parejo I, Viladomat F, Bastida J, Rosas-Romero A, Flerlage N, Burillo J, Codina C (2002). Comparison between the radical scavenging activity and antioxidant activity of six distilled and nondistilled Mediterranean herbs and aromatic plants. J. Agric. Food Chem. 50:6882-6890.

Penner R, Fedorak RN, Madsen KL (2005). Probiotics and nutraceuticals: non-medicinal treatments of gastrointestinal diseases. Curr. Opin. Pharmacol. 5:596-603.

Rabe T, Van Staden J (1997). Antibacterial activity of South African plants used for medicinal purposes. J. Ethnopharmacol. 56:81-87.

Rai R (2007). Some traditional medicinal plants used for cold, cough and fever by tribal of Bastar (Chhattisgarh). J. Indian Bot. Soc. 86(1-2):27-36.

Rajauria G, Abu-Ghannam N (2013). Isolation and partial characterization of bioactive fucoxanthin from *Himanthalia elongata* brown seaweed: A TLC-based approach. Int. J. Anal. Chem. ID 802573.

Rajauria G, Jaiswal AK, Abu-Ghannam N, Gupta S (2012). Antimicrobial, antioxidant and free radical-scavenging capacity of brown seaweed *Himanthalia elongata* from western coast of Ireland. J. Food Biochem. 37:322-335.

Ravikumar YS, Mahadevan KM, Kumaraswamy MN, Vaidya VP, Manjunatha H, Kumar V, Satyanarayana ND (2008). Antioxidant, cytotoxic and genotoxic evaluation of alcoholic extract of *Polyalthia cerasoides* (roxb) Bedd. Environ. Toxicol. Pharmacol. 26:142-146.

Rawat V, Upadhyaya K (2013). Evaluation of antimicrobial activity and preliminary phytochemical screening of *Mesua ferrea* seeds extract. J. Nat. Prod. 6:17-26.

Salah-Eldin A, Mahalel UA, Hamed AI (2007). Protective Role of *Trigonella hamosa* saponins against diabetic perturbations and complications in rats. Nat. Prod. Commun. 2(8):811-816.

Salehi P, Asghari B, Esmaeili MA, Dehghan H, Ghazi I (2013). α-Glucosidase and α-amylase inhibitory effect and antioxidant activity of ten plant extracts traditionally used in Iran for diabetes. J. Med. Plants Res. 7(6):257-266.

Sampaio BL, Edrada-Ebe RA, Da Costa FB (2016). Effect of the environment on the secondary metabolic profile of *Tithonia diversifolia*: a model for environmental metabolomics of plants. Sci. Rep. 6:29265.

Solis PN, Wright CW, Anderson MM, Gupta MP, Phillipson JD (1993). A microwell cytotoxicity assay using *Artemia salina* (brine shrimp). Plant Med. 59:250-252.

Srinivas PV, Rao RU, Venkateshwarulu EL, Kumar AC (2011). Phytochemical screening and *in vitro* antimicrobial investigation of the methanolic extract of *Xanthium strumarium* leaf. Int. J. Drug. Dev. Res. 3:245-251.

Suthindhiran K, Jayasri MA, Kannabiran K (2009). α- glucosidase and α-amylase inhibitory activity of *Micromonospora* sp. VITSDK3 (EU551238). Int. J. integr. Boil. 6(3):115-120.

Upadhyay RK, Ahmad S (2011). Management strategies for control of stored grain insect pests in farmer stores and public ware houses. World J. Agric. Sci. 7(5):527-549.

Wayne PA (2002). National Committee for Clinical Laboratory Standards. Reference method for broth dilution antifungal susceptibility testing of filamentous fungi. Approved standard M38-2002.

Westh H, Zinn CS, Rosdahl VT (2004). An international multicenter study of antimicrobial consumption and resistance in *Staphylococcus aureus* isolates from 15 hospitals in 14 countries. Microb. Drug Resist.10:169-176.

Yadav UCS, Baquer NZ (2014). Pharmacological effects of *Trigonella foenum-graecum* L. in health and disease. Pharm. Biol. 52(2):243-254.

## 17

Antioxidant, hypolipidemic and preventive effect of Hawthorn (*Crataegus oxyacantha*) on alcoholic liver damage in rats

José Luis Martínez-Rodríguez[1], Claudia Araceli Reyes-Estrada[1], Rosalinda Gutiérrez-Hernández[1] and Jesús Adrián López[2]*

[1]Doctorado en Ciencias en la Especialidad en Farmacología Médica y Molecular de la Unidad Académica de Medicina Humana y Ciencias de la Salud de la Universidad Autónoma de Zacatecas. Campus Siglo XXI, Kilómetro 6, Ejido la Escondida, CP 98160. Zacatecas, Zac. México.
[2]Laboratorio de microRNAs de la Unidad Académica de Ciencias Biológicas de la Universidad Autónoma de Zacatecas. Av. Preparatoria S/N, Hidraulica, CP 98068 Zacatecas, Zac. México.

The use of alcoholic beverages is more common and accepted by our society despite the health risks. Alcohol catabolism produces free radicals that cause oxidative stress and damage in liver principally. Hawthorn (*Crataegus oxyacantha*) is a medicinal plant that has been shown to have wide variety of polyphenolic compounds with antioxidant and hypolipidemic effect. The objective of this study was the evaluation of Hawthorn methanol extract as preventive treatment in alcoholic damage. A rat model of chronic alcoholic intake was generated with the administration of 3 g/kg/day in two times with 35 % ethanol for twelve weeks to evaluate the protective effect of 50 mg/kg/day for twelve weeks of Hawthorn administration by the determination of aspartate aminotransferase (AST), alanine aminotransferase (ALT), γ-glutamyltranspeptidase (γ-GT), acid phosphatase (ACP), total bilirubin, liver glycogen, lipid peroxidation, serum total antioxidant capacity (TAC), total cholesterol, triglycerides, low density lipoproteins (LDL), and high density lipoproteins (HDL) levels in blood and hepatic tissues. Oxidative stress was evaluated by lipid peroxidation through MDA and TAC in the serum of animals. Lipid profile and glycogen was measured by LDL, HDL and glycogen concentration, respectively. Histological tissue cuts were visualized by hematoxylin eosin and Masson trichrome staining. Hawthorn treatment decreased AST, ALT, γ-GT and ACP activity in liver damage with a decrease of total bilirubin and an increase of liver glycogen stores in rats administrated with alcohol. Hawthorn showed an antioxidant and preventive effect decreasing liver lipid peroxidation levels and increasing serum TAC evidencing a hypolipidemic effect decreasing total cholesterol, triglycerides and LDL levels without affecting HDL levels. Our results indicate that Hawthorn exhibited a protective effect against liver damage in rats with chronic alcohol administration providing a possible alternative treatment for alcohol liver damage.

Key words: *Crataegus oxyacantha*, antioxidant, preventive treatment, hypolipidemic, alcoholic liver damage.

INTRODUCTION

Today the use of alcoholic beverages is more common and accepted by our society despite the health risks. Acute and chronic alcohol intakes have shown to be a big public health problem. Chronic alcohol consumption leads to various kinds of ailments as mainly liver and nervous system damage and other pathological conditions produced by these diseases such as hepatitis, steatosis, cirrhosis, brain atrophy, psychological and social problems, accidents, alcohol dependence, violence, among other conditions (De Rick et al., 2009). The alcohol is metabolized in liver principally by alcohol dehydrogenase (ADH), an enzyme that converts alcohol into acetaldehyde. Later acetaldehyde is oxidized into acetic acid by aldehyde dehydrogenase (ALDH). The alcohol abuse conduces to ADH saturation and it is metabolized by other routes as P450 cytochrome (CYP2E1) and catalase releasing high levels of free radicals (FR) producing oxidative stress generating an imbalance between oxidant and antioxidant agents affecting cellular processes (Haseba, 2014; Schattenberg and Czaja, 2014). When cells remain exposed to oxidative stress the cell structures are damaged, including lipids, proteins and nucleic acids depending on exposure time. FR can act as secondary messengers in intracellular signaling cascades and the most serious damage to cells is the alteration of genetic information causing mutations in DNA and/or activation of the cell death pathway like apoptosis and necrosis (Albano, 2008; Djordjević et al., 2008). The FR causes lipid peroxidation, a reaction between FR and structural lipid from cell membranes. The malondialdehyde (MDA) and 4-hydroxynonenal (4-HNE) are some of the principal products of lipid peroxidation (Long et al., 2006). The liver damage is very common during alcohol chronic consumption because liver is the principal organ responsible of metabolizing alcohol and it is one of the major organs affected for being in contact with FR production (Cederbaum et al., 2009).

Normally our organism can synthesize enzymatic antioxidants (e.g. superoxide dismutase [SOD], catalase, glutathione peroxidase and glutathione s-transferase) to neutralize FR and prevent oxidative stress generated in metabolic pathways. There are other antioxidants known as non-enzymatic antioxidants as glutathione and other functional antioxidant molecules (e.g. ubiquinol, uric acid and melatonin) (Hirst and Roessler, 2015; Michiels et al., 1994). Animals usually can get antioxidant compounds through daily diet to help their body to fight against oxidative stress fulfilling a function of "free radical scavengers" or exogenous antioxidants (e.g. vitamins A and E, β-carotene, phenolic acids, flavonoids and anthocyanidins) avoiding cellular oxidative damage in conjunction with endogenous antioxidants. The regulated endogenous antioxidants synthesis and exogenous antioxidant compounds intake balance are important to maintain homeostasis between oxidant and reducing agents. Plants are a major source of antioxidants and in many cases are related to its therapeutic effects from the

ethnopharmacological point of view. Hawthorn (Crataegus oxyacantha L, formerly known as Crataegus laevigata) is a fruit-bearing plant, member of Rosaceae family that grows mainly in Europe, Asia and North America. Hawthorn has proved be a potent antioxidant and medicinal plant because it has compounds as epicatechins, triterpene, saponins, oligomeric procyanidins, chlorogenic acid, flavonoids and flavon C glycosides (isoquerecitrin, hyperoside, orientin, isoorientin, quercetin, quercitrin, vitexin, isovitexin and rutin) (Konieczynski, 2015; Rigelsky and Sweet, 2002). Hawthorn has shown various therapeutic effects as mainly hypolipidemic, anti-inflammatory, immuno modulatory, digestive modulator, antimicrobial, anti-anxiety, antioxidant, cardiac stimulant and hypotensive agent (Benmalek et al., 2013; Elango and Devaraj, 2010; Vijayan et al., 2012). Most studies have focused on the use in cardiovascular diseases for their effectiveness in cardiac therapy. There are several studies that show a marked cardioprotective effect, reducing high blood pressure, lipid-lowering effect, cardiac arrhythmias, angina pectoris, myocardial infarction and an important use in congestive heart failure according to the New York Heart Association (Alp et al., 2015; Ammon and Händel 1981; Jalaly et al., 2015; Rastogi et al., 2015; Wang et al., 2013). In alcoholism process, hyperlipidemic, inflammatory, and oxidant effects are general. Taking in count that Hawthorn has shown to reverse these effects we analyzed the antioxidant capacity, hypolipidemic and preventive effect of Hawthorn on alcoholic liver damage in rats.

MATERIALS AND METHODS

Plant extract

The leaves of Hawthorn were collected from cultivated plants in Tlalnepantla, México City, and were authenticated by *Nutra-Herba de México Company*. Hawthorn extract was obtained by next procedure: Hawthorn´s leaves were washed and dried at room temperature and then crushed and pulverized by a mill. Next we macerated it taking 50 g of powder per 500 mL of methanol. Subsequently distillation reflux was performed at 62°C for 2 h. After that the mixture was filtered in vacuum and it was bleached with 12.5 g of activated carbon (5 g of activated carbon per 20 g of plant) and newly filtered to obtain a light brown liquid. This extract was subjected to evaporation in a rotary evaporator system (Yamato, RE-51, CA, USA) at 70°C in order to concentrate the sample. The concentrate was transferred to a beaker with ice triple distilled water (30 mL) causing precipitation of the extract. Vacuum filtration was applied to allow drying at room temperature obtaining a light yellow, fresh filtrate. The filtrate was lyophilized at 60°C/1,333 Pa (Virtis SP SCIENTIFIC Sentry 2.0., PA, U.S.A.) and this powder was suspended in distilled water to 100 mg/ml.

*Corresponding author. E-mail: jalopez@uaz.edu.mx.

Animals and experimental protocols

Male Wistar rats (n= 20) weighing 200 ± 10 g were randomly assigned to four groups of five rats each (control, liver damage, biosecurity and prevention group). Animals were treated for twelve weeks in a stable environment with controlled temperature (22± 2°C), humidity and light (12 h light: Dark cycle) with free access to food (Harlan Teklad Global Diets) and water. All the experiments reported here are in accordance to university regulations on the care and handling of experimental animals and environment care (NOM-062-ZOO-1999 and NOM-087-ECOL-SSA1-2002 respectively). The control group was administrated orally with water. The liver damage group was administrated with a dose of 3 g/kg/day in two times (morning and night) with 35% ethanol. The biosafety group was administrated only with the Hawthorn extract in dose of 50 mg/kg/day; and finally the prevention group was administrated with ethanol (3 g/kg/day in two times) and Hawthorn extract in dose of 50 mg/kg/day (in the afternoon). At the end of the experimental study, animals were weighted and sacrificed under anesthesia in ether atmosphere to obtain total blood and serum by cardiac puncture in order to evaluate enzymatic and metabolic indicators. The liver tissue was removed to analyze glycogen, lipid peroxidation level and histological indicators.

Liver damage evaluation

Liver damage was evaluated by measuring enzymatic and metabolic serum levels of alanine aminotransferase (ALT), aspartate aminotransferase (AST), γ-glutamyltranspeptidase (γ-GT), acid phosphatase (ACP) and bilirubin by *BioSystems* kits in a spectrophotometer (Beckman DU-65, CA, U.S.A.).

Measure of glycogen concentration

The Fong method (Fong et al., 1953) was used to perform liver glycogen concentration, which is based on the hydrolysis of glycogen to glucose units by potassium hydroxide in order to react with anthrone in sulfuric acid forming a green colored complex that is measured spectrophotometrically.

Lipid peroxidation

Damage of tissues by oxidative stress induces the formation of oxidation products as MDA. This lipid peroxidation product was determined by measurement of thiobarbituric acid reactive substances (TBARS) described by Mihara and Uchiyama (Mihara and Uchiyama, 1978). 1,1,3,3-tetramethoxypropane (Aldrich, MO, USA) calibration curve was used to quantify MDA concentration.

Total antioxidant capacity (TAC)

As an indicator of oxidative stress, we measured the total antioxidant capacity in the serum of animals. This indicator was analyzed by BioVision TAC colorimetric assay kit. For biological samples were taken 0.1 µL of homogenized and 99.9 µL of triple distilled water in each well of a microplate reader (STAT FAX 2100, FL, USA). A Tolox calibration curve was used to quantify TAC.

Lipidic profile

These indicators were analyzed by *Bio Systems kits*. Lipidic profile was evaluated by measuring total cholesterol, triglycerides, low density lipoproteins (LDL) and high density lipoproteins (HDL).

Histological indicator

Hematoxylin eosin (HE) and Masson trichrome staining (MTS) were used to identify cell damage with respect to the chronic administration of ethanol in liver tissue. Bencosme method was used to analyze this indicator (Bencosme, 1954) in a microscope Carl Zeiss Axiostar pluz model 440950 CP ACHROMAT coupled with digital camera (Olympus, model C'7070 Wide Zoom).

Statistical analysis

Data are presented as mean ± standard deviation and were analyzed statistically by one-way ANOVA followed by Tukey's multiple comparison. A discriminant classification analysis was made to observe the variability in the data obtained with respect to the measured indicators. We used STATGRAPHICS Centurion XV software for Windows. Differences were considered statistically significant at $p < 0.05$.

RESULTS

Hawthorn decreases liver damage in rats with alcohol administration

Rats with chronic alcohol administration were treated with 50 mg/kg/day of Hawthorn extract to evaluate its preventive effect in alcoholic liver damage. In present study several enzymatic indicators in liver damage as AST, ALT, γ-GT and ACP were analyzed. In case of ALT and AST, they are cytosolic enzymes. Their high serum levels indicate cell death as liver necrosis principally. In this study (Table 1), the liver damage group with administration of ethanol showed increases of 60.0% (1.74 µkat/L) and 72.3% (1.12 µkat/L) in AST and ALT respectively, compared to the average control value (0.65 and 1.09 µkat/L respectively). Biosecurity groups proved no statistically significant differences compared to control groups, while treatment with Hawthorn evidenced a reduction of 18.4 and 7.0% in AST and ALT compared with liver damage group (1.42 and 1.04 µkat/L respectively). The γ-GT and ACP enzymatic activity was analyzed too. The γ-GT is a membrane-bound enzyme in cells that have a secretory function as in liver and other secretory organs and ACP is a metabolic enzyme localized in high concentrations in liver, prostate, spleen and kidney lysosomes principally. The high serum levels of γ-GT and ACP can indicate damage in secretory organs as liver principally, therefore, enzymatic activity was analyzed in this work. The group of damage proved an increase of 82.1% (425.11 nkat/L) and 29.3% (525.88 nkat/L) in γ-GT and ACP respectively over the control group value (233.43 and 406.83 nkat/L respectively). In the case of prevention groups with Hawthorn administration, the groups evidenced a decrease of 38.5% (261.25 nkat/L) and 9.3% (477.1 nkat/L) in γ-GT and ACP respectively, compared with liver damage group. Biosecurity groups showed no statistically significant difference compared to control groups (Table 1). Glycogen is a polysaccharide formed in liver

Table 1. Hawthorn treatment diminishes enzymatic activity levels of AST, ALT, γ-GT and ACP in serum of rats with alcohol administration.

Groups	ALT (µkat/L)	AST (µkat/L)	γ-GT (nkat/L)	ACP (nkat/L)
Control	0.65±0.11[b]	1.09±0.12[b]	233.43±40.31[b]	406.83±23.29[b]
Liver damage	1.12±0.08[a]	1.74±0.10[a]	425.11±75.53[a]	525.88±73.62[a]
Biosecurity	0.71±0.11[b]	1.12±0.09[b]	156.13±33.42[b]	397.46±36.06[b]
Prevention	1.04±0.14[a]	1.42±0.10[a,b]	261.25±44.87[b]	477.14±50.09

[a]P<0.05 vs. control group; [b]P<0.05 vs. liver damage group. All data are expressed as mean ± standard deviation (n=5 rats per group; experiment repeated three times). One way analysis of variance and least significant difference multiple-range test were used to determine the differences of means.

principally as glucose store and when there is liver damage these glycogen levels get low being an effective damage indicator. In this test (Figure 1A and C), the control group gave an average value of 5.4 µg of glycogen per gram of liver tissue. The liver damage group for chronic ethanol administration showed a decrease in glycogen storage of 64.8% (1.9 µg/g) compared to control group. Biosecurity group did not show significant difference compared to control group. With respect to prevention group with Hawthorn, it evidenced a decrease of 18.5% (4.4 µg/g) compared to control group. Another indicator of liver injury is total serum bilirubin because the liver is responsible of its elimination and when there is damage in liver tissue, bilirubin uptake is low and accumulates in serum. Total bilirubin levels in control group showed an average value of 0.29 mg/dL, while liver damage group showed an increase of more than twice the value of the control group (0.68 mg/dL, that is, 2.3 times the control value). Biosecurity group proved no statistically significant difference compared to control group. The group administered with Hawthorn treatment reached a bilirubin increase of 55.2% (0.45 mg/dL) compared to control group (Figure 1B and C).

Hawthorn shows an antioxidant effect

In order to evidence Hawthorn antioxidant property over oxidative stress produced by alcoholic liver damage in this model, we evaluated liver lipid peroxidation level and serum TAC. In these experiments (Figure 2A and C), the control group showed an average value of 13.0 µmol/L, while liver damage group proved an increase of 90.1% (24.8 µmol/L) compared to control group. The biosecurity group showed no statistically significant difference. Using Hawthorn as treatment, preventive group evidenced a decrease of 14.2% (11.1 µmol/L) compared to control group. Furthermore, TAC is a test where we can evaluate samples antioxidant level given by reducing compounds obtained for feeding or/and administration of antioxidant treatments. The levels of TAC in the control group serum showed an average value of 5.37 nmol Trolox equivalent, while the group of damage showed a decrease of 19.2%

(4.34 nmol Trolox equivalent) with respect to control group. The biosecurity group with Hawthorn showed a high TAC value (11.6 nmol Trolox equivalent, that is, 2.2 times the control value). With respect to prevention treatment groups, Hawthorn proved an increase of 53.6% (8.26 nmol Trolox equivalent) compared to control group (Figure 2B and C).

Lipid levels in liver damage induced by chronic alcohol administration are regulated by Hawthorn treatment

One characteristic of alcoholic liver damage is the hyperlipidemia and steatosis for problems in metabolism and serum lipids uptake problems. Therefore we evaluated triglycerides, total cholesterol, LDL and HDL in serum samples. Triglycerides levels in control group showed an average value of 47.1 mg/dL, while liver damage group proved an increase of 54.5% (72.8 mg/dL). Biosecurity group gave values very similar to control group, while prevention group with Hawthorn evidenced a decrease in triglycerides of 38.0% (45.1 mg/dL) compared to liver damage group, normalizing triglyceride levels to normal value (Figure 3A and E).

The control gave an average value of 35.0 mg/dL of total cholesterol (Figure 3B and E) and liver damage group proved an increase of 67.3% (58.6 mg/dL) over the average control value. Biosecurity group average value did not show a significant difference compared to control value (42 mg/dL), while group of prevention with Hawthorn evidenced a slight increase in this indicator of 14.3% (40.0 mg/dL) compared to control group.

LDL indicator was analyzed (Figure 3C and E) and gave an average value of 33.1 mg/dL in control group, while the liver damage group showed a value of 54.1 mg/dL, that is, an increase of 63.4% compared to the control value. In biosecurity group, it proved a value of 36.5 mg/dL, while prevention group with Hawthorn evidenced an increase of 21.1% (40.1 mg/dL) compared to control group.

In HDL indicator (Figure 3D), control group showed an average value of 20.9 mg/dL, while liver damage group

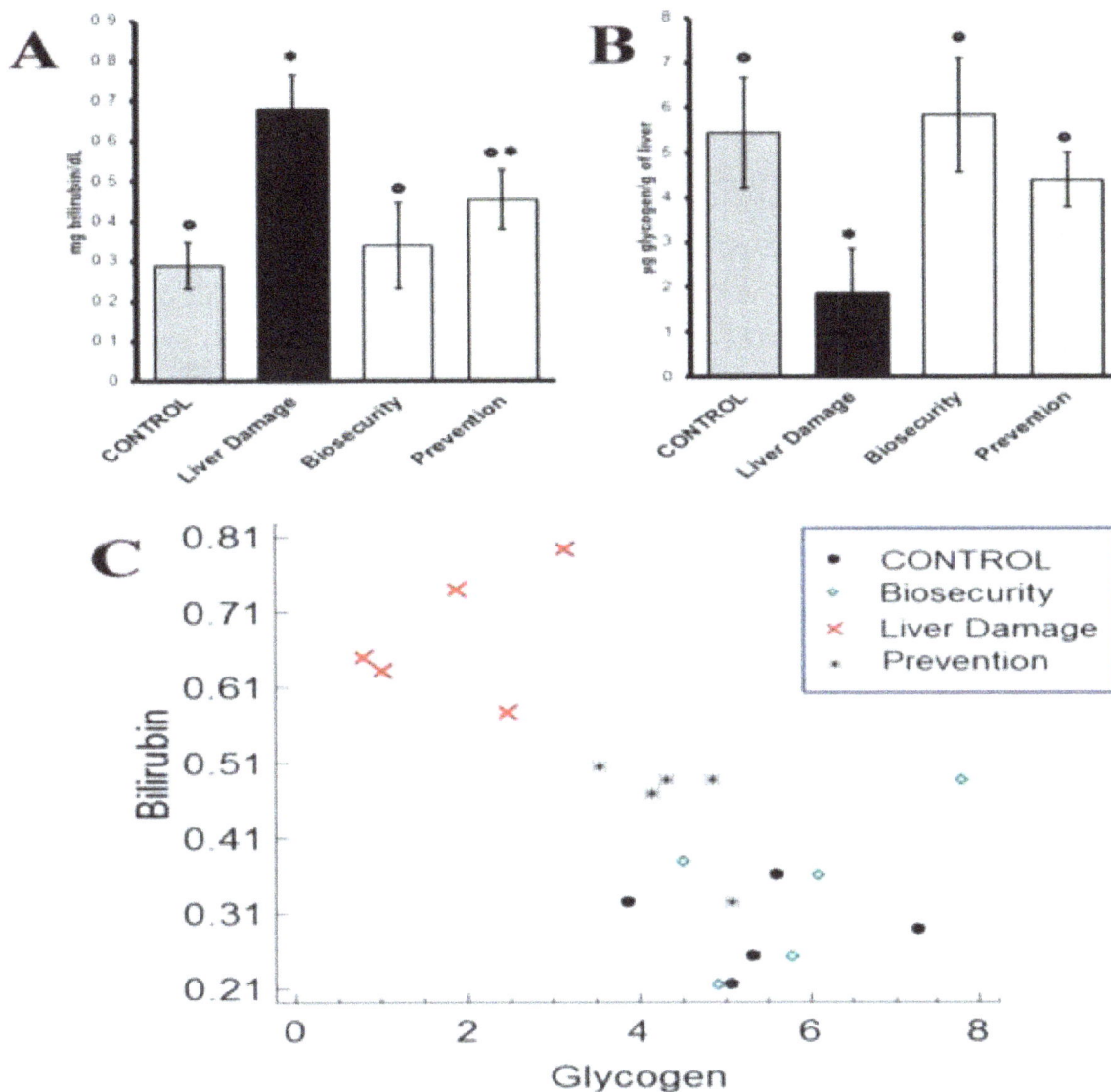

Figure 1. Hawthorn treatment increases liver glycogen stores and diminishes serum bilirubin levels in rats with alcohol administration. We analyzed liver glycogen concentrations and serum total bilirubin to evaluate liver cell damage and hawthorn preventive effect. (A) Liver damage group showed glycogen stores levels decrease of 64.8% while prevention group showed a decrease of 18.5% compared to control group. (B) Liver damage group showed high levels of serum total bilirubin compared to control group (2.3 times the control value) while co-administration of hawthorn as preventive treatment showed an increase of 55.2%. All biosecurity groups showed no statistically significant difference. (C) By a scatter diagram using a discriminant analysis we can see the relation between both indicators. Liver damage group shows isolated values compared to control and biosecurity group values indicating high levels of serum bilirubin and low glycogen levels in liver tissue demonstrating liver damage for chronic alcohol administration. Prevention group showed a dispersion of data values different to liver damage group data indicating an increase of liver glycogen and a decrease in serum total bilirubin compared to liver damage group demonstrating a preventive effect for the hawthorn co-administration. One way ANOVA and least significant difference multiple-range test were used to determine the differences of means. *$P<0.05$ vs. control group; °$P<0.05$ vs. liver damage group. All data are expressed as mean ± standard deviation (n=5 rats per group).

gave an increase of 14.4% (23.9 mg/dL) compared to control group. Biosecurity group with Hawthorn showed a value of 22.4 mg/dL, while prevention group evidenced a value of 21.7 mg/dL, that is, an increase of 3.8% compared to control group (Figure 3).

Hawthorn prevents pathologic changes in liver tissue of rats with alcoholism

Figure 4 shows the liver structures in each experimental group. Control group (Figure 4A and B) showed a normal

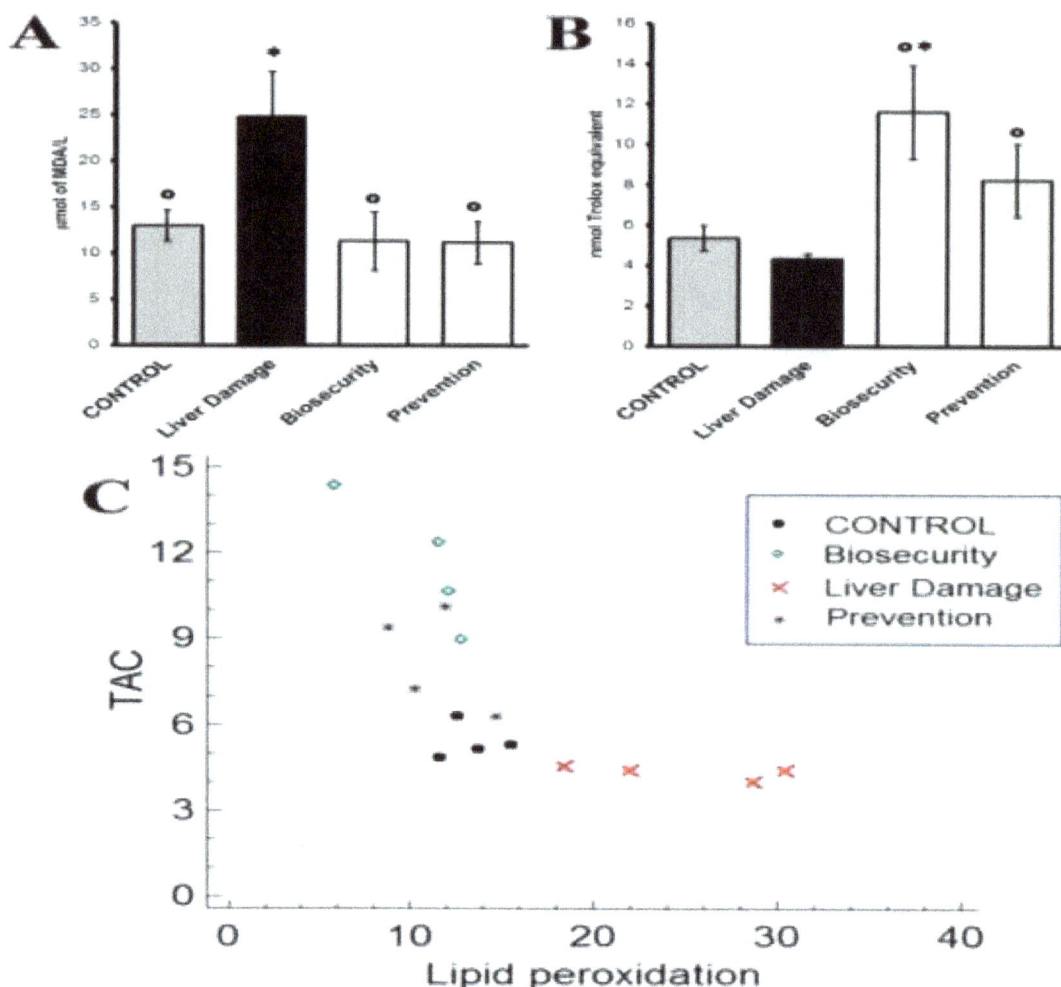

Figure 2. Hawthorn treatment diminishes liver lipid peroxidation level and increases serum TAC in rats with alcohol administration. We analyzed lipid peroxidation levels in liver tissue and TAC levels in serum to evaluate Hawthorn antioxidant property. (A) Hawthorn treatment showed a decrease of 55.1% in liver lipid peroxidation level compared to damage liver group. Hawthorn prevented oxidative stress caused by alcohol administration. (B) In TAC test, we can see an elevation of serum TAC when Hawthorn extract was administrated. Liver damage group showed a decrease of 19.2% compared to control group while prevention group showed an increase of 53.8%. In biosecurity group we can see a high elevation of TAC levels in more of two times control TAC value, indicating an efficient antioxidant effect. (C) Scatter diagram using a discriminant analysis shows the variability of each data in lipid peroxidation levels and serum TAC levels in the models. Graph shows a defined dispersion of each of the experimental groups. Liver damage group showed high oxidative damage and a low decrease of serum TAC compared to control group while prevention group indicates low oxidative damage (similar to control group) and high serum TAC levels. The results in lipid peroxidation levels were supported by TAC test. One way ANOVA and least significant difference multiple-range test were used to determine the differences of means. *$P<0.05$ vs. control group; °$P<0.05$ vs. liver damage group. All data are expressed as mean ± standard deviation (n=5 rats per group in lipid peroxidation indicator; n=4 rats per group in TAC test; discriminant analysis was done with n=4).

liver structure as it can be seen highly defined liver lobules around the central veins. The biosecurity group does not show pathologic changes in liver tissue indicating that hawthorn is a safe treatment to liver (Figure 4C and D). The liver damage group proved a loss of normal liver structure, cell congestion, cell necrosis, slight steatosis, liver fibrosis and sinusoidal distension (Figure 4E to I). Finally prevention group evidenced a liver

damage decrease. It proved slight cell congestion, necrosis and sinusoidal distension not showing fibrosis (Figure 4J to L).

DISCUSSION

Hawthorn is a medicinal plant that has therapeutic

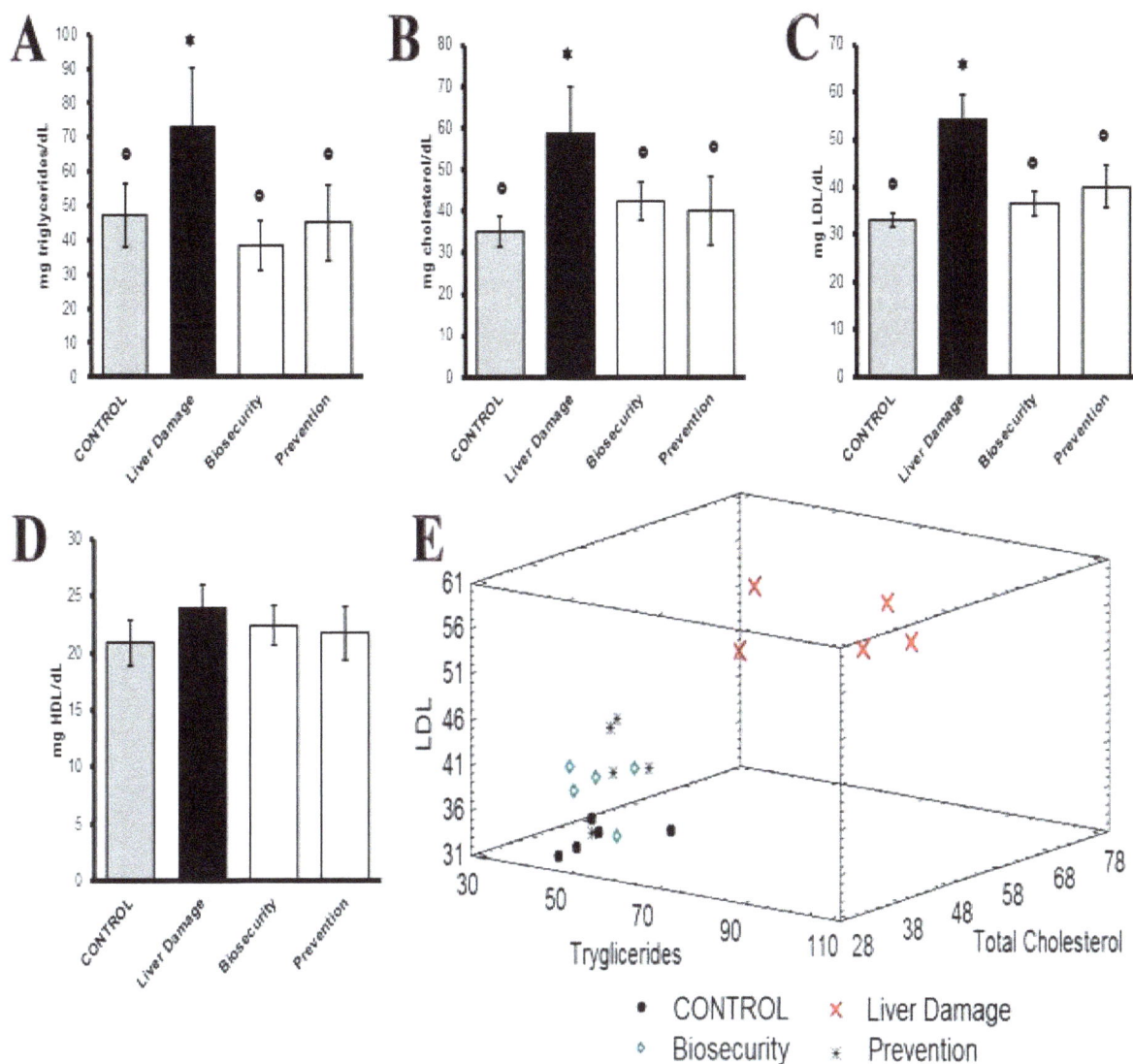

Figure 3. Hawthorn treatment shows a hypolipidemic effect in rats with alcohol administration. We analyzed serum lipid levels of triglycerides, cholesterol, LDL and HDL to evaluate liver damage and hawthorn preventive effect. (A) In triglycerides indicator, liver damage group showed an increase of 54.5% compared to control value while prevention group proved a decrease of 38.0% compared to liver damage group, normalizing to normal values. (B) Moreover high serum cholesterol levels were detected in liver damage group (increase of 67.3%) meanwhile prevention group showed a slight increase of 14.3%. (C) With respect to LDL indicator, liver damage group proved an increase of 63.4% compared to control value while prevention group showed an increase of 21.1%. (D) Finally in HDL indicator, the liver damage proved a no statistically significant difference of 14.4% compared to control group. Biosecurity and preventive groups did not show a significant change compared to control group HDL levels. (E) By a scatter diagram using a discriminant analysis it is shown the variability of each data in triglycerides, cholesterol and LDL levels in the models. Diagram shows that liver damage group has isolated values compared to control and biosecurity group data dispersion indicating high triglycerides, cholesterol and LDL serum lipid levels meanwhile preventive group proved similar values to control and biosecurity group. One way ANOVA and least significant difference multiple-range test were used to determine the differences of means. *$P<0.05$ vs. control group; °$P<0.05$ vs. liver damage group. All data are expressed as mean ± standard deviation (n=5 rats per group).

properties and over time it has become an important part of traditional herbal. Hawthorn has a variety of phenolic compounds that have shown various therapeutic effects as epicatechins, triterpenes, saponins, oligomeric procyanidins and big diversity of flavonoids. Phenolic compounds have attracted increasing attention from researchers. The antioxidants are necessary to maintain the balance between oxidant agents produced by metabolic pathways and antioxidants obtained in the diet and synthetized by our organism. The oxidative stress is

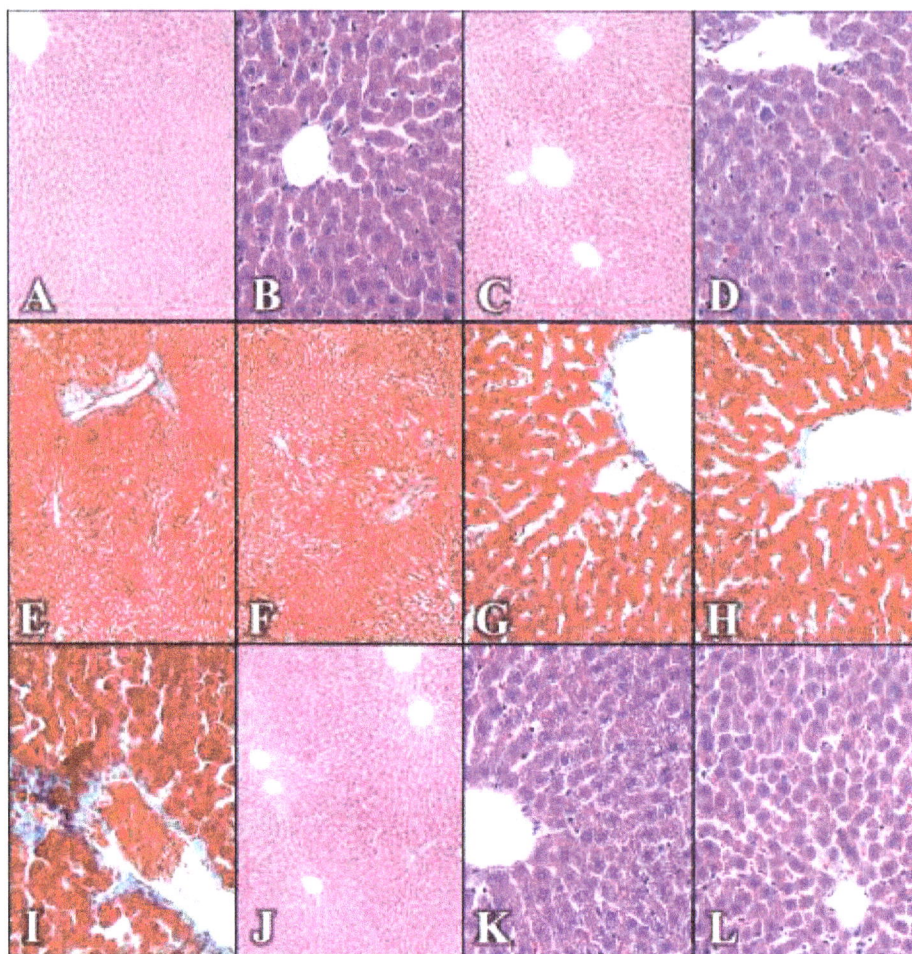

Figure 4. Hawthorn treatment diminishes tissue liver damage in rats with alcohol administration. We analyzed liver tissues to evaluate liver damage and hawthorn preventive effect. (A) Control group (10X, HE). Liver proved a normal structure with highly defined lobules around the central veins. (B) Control group (40X, HE). Histological image shows a normal liver structure with highly defined hepatocytes. (C) Biosecurity group (10X, HE). The Hawthorn administration does not show liver tissue damage. (D) Biosecurity group (40X, HE). Hawthorn treatment has proved a biosecure treatment for liver tissue showing a normal liver structure. (E and F) Liver damage group (10X, MTS). Liver proved cell congestion, fibrosis and high sinusoidal distension. (G, H and I) Liver damage group (40X, MTS). Liver showed a slight steatosis, necrosis and high sinusoidal distension. Moderate fibrosis was observed in certain areas of the liver lobule mainly near lobule central veins. J) Prevention group (10X, HE). Liver proved a normal lobule structure with slight congestion and sinusoidal distension. K and L) Prevention group (40X, MTS). Hawthorn reduces liver damage shown in liver damage group significantly. Liver proved in certain areas slight sinusoidal distension, cell congestion and necrosis not showing fibrosis.

a cell condition where there are high oxidant concentrations with respect to antioxidants promoting loss of cellular homeostasis and cell damage. The alcoholic liver damage is a pathology that presents FR formation by alcohol catabolism in the CYP2E1 route principally, generating oxidative stress and concluding to lipid peroxidation, inflammation, fibrosis, cell death and loss of parenchyma function (Cederbaum, 2003). Oxidative stress induces necrosis and apoptosis with a decrease in antioxidants as GSH and Vitamin E principally

(Loguercio and Federico, 2003). Taking in count that Hawthorn possesses an antioxidant effect, therefore it neutralizes FR and oxidative stress improving cell stability and avoiding and/or decreasing tissue damage, its therapeutic effect was evaluated. The Hawthorn hypo-lipidemic, antihypertensive and antioxidant properties reported by other studies are positive therapeutic effects in alcoholic liver disease.

In the present study, Hawthorn administration evidenced liver damage decrease for chronic alcohol administration in a rat model. Hawthorn showed an AST and ALT serum activity reduction, indicating a cell preventive effect against oxidative stress, because normally aminotransferases levels are low on plasma and the presence of high ALT and AST levels in serum are related with cell damage, as in the case of liver and kidney damage principally. These aminotransferases are specific indicators to evaluate necrosis in various liver diseases (Gutierrez et al., 2010; Kozakova et al., 2012). The aminotransferases levels were corroborated with γ-GT serum activity test in order to analyze membrane stability. γ-GT is a membrane-bound enzyme preset primarily in cells that have a secretory or absorptive function as liver and other organs as pancreas, prostate, brain and heart. It has been shown that γ-GT is considerate a predictive biomarker of cellular antioxidant inadequacy and damage indicator in multiple diseases (Koenig and Seneff, 2015) similar to the present study. The injury produced by alcohol metabolism generates lipid peroxidation and cell lysis liberating in high concentrations this enzyme to plasma indicating cell damage. Hawthorn reduced γ-GT serum activity indicating a hepatoprotective effect. On the other hand, ACP is an enzyme localized mainly in lysosomes of prostate, kidney, spleen and liver and high concentration of ACP in serum indicates cell damage. Such effect could be related to cell destruction and entrance of cellular content to blood.

In this work it was shown an ACP level decrease demonstrating a preventive effect probably by inhibiting cell destruction. Interestingly, Hawthorn effect over AST, ALT, γ-GT an ACP serum activity levels were supported by liver function techniques as glycogen and bilirubin. As glycogen is a storage polysaccharide and it is in high concentration in liver its decrement is related to cell damage (Fong et al., 1953). Therefore, cell deaths or damaged cells have less glycogen levels in liver. Remarkably, the groups treated with Hawthorn showed normal glycogen level indicating a hepatoprotective effect of Hawthorn. Liver function improvement was also analyzed by measuring total bilirubin in serum. In this sense hyperbilirubinemia usually signifies severe parenchymal liver disease, anemia or renal failure and it could be used as prognostic indicator in cholestatic liver and hepatic failure. In contrast, other works suggest that high bilirubin levels are related with a significant antioxidant and preventive effect decreasing risk in diseases as hypertension by inactivating and inhibiting the synthesis of FR, (O'Malley et al., 2015; Wang and Bautista, 2015) but in the present investigation, taking in count the liver damage, a bilirubin antioxidant effect was not evidenced. Hawthorn shows a preventive effect in liver based on reduction of serum enzymatic activity indicators as the cytosolic enzymes as AST, ALT and ACP related with a decreased membrane-bound enzyme γ-GT indicating a reduction of cell lysis and cell death. These results could be related to a decrease of oxidative

stress by the Hawthorn antioxidant effect avoiding activation of cell death pathways. The antioxidant Hawthorn capacity was showed by liver MDA decrease and serum TAC increase. Hawthorn shows a variety of polyphenols, flavonol glycosides and C-glycosyl flavones which may relate to an antioxidant effect of this medicinal plant (Yang and Liu, 2012). However, Hawthorn could regulate gene expression, as it has being shown by the increase of mRNA and protein level of Nrf2-dependent genes as glutathione S-transferases (GSTA, GSTP, GSTM, GSTT), NAD(P)H:quinone oxidoreductase 1 (NQO1) and heme oxygenase-1 (HO-1) in THLE-2 cells showing an antioxidant and detoxifying effect (Krajka-Kuźniak et al., 2014). For these therapeutic properties Hawthorn could prevent cell oxidative stress improving cell stability and decreasing cell damage for alcohol intake. The use of Hawthorn as preventive treatment in alcoholic liver disease shows a decrease in the progression of damage avoiding a significant pathologic change in the normal liver structure, fibrosis and steatosis.

Normally the alcoholic liver disease is accompanied by steatosis because ADH and ALDH cause the reduction of NAD into NADH. Reduction of NAD promotes fat accumulation in liver tissue for inhibition of metabolic pathways as gluconeogenesis and fatty acid β-oxidation, meanwhile lipid synthesis promotes liver tissue fat accumulation (Saheki et al., 2005). Other consequence of chronic ingest of alcohol is the increase of serum lipids as triglycerides, cholesterol and LDL with a respective decrease in HDL (Mantena et al., 2008). Hawthorn evidenced a regulator effect in serum lipids levels, decreasing LDL, triglycerides and total cholesterol without affecting HDL levels. Several works have shown that Hawthorn has an effect over LDL-receptors activity of rat liver plasma membrane isolated from atherogenic diet fed rats (Rajendran et al., 1996; Shanthi et al., 1994). The results obtained in γ-GT during chronic alcohol intake evidenced cell plasma membrane damage and this injury could be related with damage in LDL lipoproteins receptors, increasing its levels in plasma accompanied by high levels of triglycerides and cholesterol. In this study, it was proved that Hawthorn maintains normal levels of HDL; but a low increase of HDL level in liver damage group was observed. There are investigations about the effect of moderate alcohol intake that show an increase in HDL cholesterol levels by increasing the transport rate of apolipoproteins A-I and A-II (Silva et al., 2000).

Conclusions

Hawthorn showed a preventive effect on liver damage caused by chronic ethanol intake. An antioxidant effect was detected, increasing serum TAC levels and decreasing lipid peroxidation in liver tissue, regulating glycogen levels and improving uptake and elimination of bilirubin. This extract presented a hepatoprotective effect decreasing cell damage indicators as AST, ALT, γ-GT and ACP and avoiding loss of normal hepatic tissue structure, reducing fibrosis, steatosis, necrosis, congestion and sinusoidal distension. Hawthorn proved to be a therapeutic regulator of serum lipids as triglycerides, total cholesterol and LDL in alcoholic liver damage, decreasing high levels of these lipids without altering the levels of serum HDL. Hawthorn extract proved to be a safe treatment for healthy animals based on the indicators that we measured.

ACKNOWLEDGEMENTS

The authors would like to thank Silvia Cortez for her technical support with sample preparation.

REFERENCES

Albano E (2008). Oxidative mechanisms in the pathogenesis of alcoholic liver disease. Mol. Aspects Med. 29:9-16.

Alp H, Soner BC, Baysal T, Şahin AS (2015). Protective effects of Hawthorn (*Crataegus oxyacantha*) extract against digoxin-induced arrhythmias in rats. Anatol. J. Cardiol. 15:970-975.

Ammon H, Händel M (1981). *Crataegus*, toxicology and pharmacology. Part III: Pharmacodynamics and pharmacokinetics. Planta Med. 43(4):313-322.

Bencosme SA (1954). A trichrome staining method for routine use. Am. J. Clin. Pathol. 24:1324-1328.

Benmalek Y, Yahia OA, Belkebir A, Fardeau ML (2013). Anti-microbial and anti-oxidant activities of Illicium verum, *Crataegus oxyacantha* ssp monogyna and Allium cepa red and white varieties. Bioengineered 4(4):244-248.

Cederbaum AI (2003). Iron and CYP2E1-dependent oxidative stress and toxicity. Alcohol 30(2):115-120.

Cederbaum AI, Lu Y, Wu D (2009). Role of oxidative stress in alcohol-induced liver injury. Arch. Toxicol. 83(6):519-548.

De Rick A, Vanheule S, Verhaeghe P (2009). Alcohol addiction and the attachment system: an empirical study of attachment style, alexithymia, and psychiatric disorders in alcoholic inpatients. Subst. Use Misuse. 44(1):99-114.

Djordjević V, Zvezdanović L, Cosić V (2008). Oxidative stress in human diseases. Srp. Arh. Celok. Lek. 136:158-165.

Silva ERDO, Foster D, Harper MM, Seidman CE, Smith JD, Breslow JL, Brinton EA (2000). Alcohol consumption raises HDL cholesterol levels by increasing the transport rate of apolipoproteins AI and A-II. Circulation 102(19):2347-2352.

Elango C, Devaraj SN (2010). Immunomodulatory effect of Hawthorn extract in an experimental stroke model. J. Neuroinflammation. 7:1.

Fong J, Schaffer FL, Kirk PL (1953). The ultramicrodetermination of glycogen in liver; a comparison of the anthrone and reducing-sugar methods. Arch. Biochem. Biophys. 45(2):319-326.

Gutierrez R, Alvarado JL, Presno M, Perez-Veyna O, Serrano CJ, Yahuaca P (2010). Oxidative stress modulation by *Rosmarinus officinalis* in CCl4-induced liver cirrhosis. Phytother. Res. 24(4):595-601.

Haseba T (2014). Molecular evidences of non-ADH pathway in alcohol metabolism and Class III alcohol dehydrogenase (ADH3). Nihon Arukoru Yakubutsu Igakkai zasshi. 49(3):159-168.

Hirst J, Roessler MM (2015). Energy conversion, redox catalysis and generation of reactive oxygen species by respiratory complex I. Biochim. Biophys. Acta 1857(7):872-883.

Jalaly L, Sharifi G, Faramarzi M, Nematollahi A, Rafieian-Kopaei M, Amiri M, Moattar F (2015). Comparison of the effects of Crataegus oxyacantha extract, aerobic exercise and their combination on the serum levels of ICAM-1 and E-Selectin in patients with stable angina pectoris. Daru 19:23-54.

Koenig G, Seneff S (2015). Gamma-Glutamyltransferase: A Predictive Biomarker of Cellular Antioxidant Inadequacy and Disease Risk. Dis Markers. 2015:818570.

Konieczynski P (2015). Electrochemical fingerprint studies of selected medicinal plants rich in flavonoids. Acta Pol. Pharm. 72(4):655-661.

Kozakova M, Palombo C, Paterni Eng M, Dekker J, Flyvbjerg A, Mitrakou A, Gastaldelli A, Ferrannini E (2012). Fatty liver index gamma-glutamyltransferase, and early carotid plaques. Hepatology 55(5):1406-1415.

Krajka-Kuźniak V, Paluszczak J, Oszmiański J, Baer-Dubowska W (2014). Hawthorn (*Crataegus oxyacantha* L.) Bark Extract Regulates Antioxidant Response Element (ARE)-Mediated Enzyme Expression Via Nrf2 Pathway Activation in Normal Hepatocyte Cell Line. Phytother. Res. 28(4):593-602.

Loguercio C, Federico A (2003). Oxidative stress in viral and alcoholic hepatitis. Free Radic. Biol. Med. 34(1):1-10.

Long J, Wang X, Gao H, Liu Z, Liu C, Miao M, Liu J (2006). Malonaldehyde acts as a mitochondrial toxin: Inhibitory effects on respiratory function and enzyme activities in isolated rat liver mitochondria. Life Sci. 79(15):1466-1472.

Mantena SK, King AL, Andringa KK, Eccleston HB, Bailey SM (2008). Mitochondrial dysfunction and oxidative stress in the pathogenesis of alcohol-and obesity-induced fatty liver diseases. Free Radic. Biol. Med. 44(7):1259-1272.

Michiels C, Raes M, Toussaint O, Remacle J (1994). Importance of Se-glutathione peroxidase, catalase, and Cu/Zn-SOD for cell survival against oxidative stress. Free Radic. Biol. Med. 17(3):235-246.

Mihara M, Uchiyama M (1978). Determination of malonaldehyde precursor in tissues by thiobarbituric acid test. Anal. Biochem. 86(1):271-278.

O'Malley SS, Gueorguieva R, Wu R, Jatlow PI (2015). Acute alcohol consumption elevates serum bilirubin: an endogenous antioxidant. Drug Alcohol Depend. 149:87-92.

Rajendran S, Deepalakshmi P, Parasakthy K, Devaraj H, Devaraj SN (1996). Effect of tincture of Crataegus on the LDL-receptor activity of hepatic plasma membrane of rats fed an atherogenic diet. Atherosclerosis 123(1-2):235-241.

Rastogi S, Pandey MM, Rawat A (2015). Traditional herbs: a remedy for cardiovascular disorders. Phytomedicine. 23(11):1082-1089.

Rigelsky JM, Sweet BV (2002). Hawthorn: pharmacology and therapeutic uses. Am. J. Health Syst. Pharm. 59(5):417-422.

Saheki T, Kobayashi K, Iijima M, Moriyama M, Yazaki M, Takei Y, Ikeda S (2005). Metabolic derangements in deficiency of citrin, a liver-type mitochondrial aspartate–glutamate carrier. Hepatol. Res. 33(2):181-184.

Schattenberg JM, Czaja MJ (2014). Regulation of the effects of CYP2E1-induced oxidative stress by JNK signaling. Redox Biol. 3:7-15.

Shanthi S, Parasakthy K, Deepalakshmi P, Devaraj SN (1994). Hypolipidemic activity of tincture of Crataegus in rats. Indian J. Biochem. Biophys. 31(2):143-146.

Vijayan NA, Thiruchenduran M, Devaraj SN (2012). Anti-inflammatory and anti-apoptotic effects of Crataegus oxyacantha on isoproterenol-induced myocardial damage. Mol. Cell. Biochem. 367(1-2):1-8.

Wang J, Xiong X, Feng B (2013). Effect of Crataegus usage in cardiovascular disease prevention: an evidence-based approach. Evid. Based Complement. Altern. Med. 2013:149363.

Wang L, Bautista LE (2015). Serum bilirubin and the risk of hypertension. Int. J. Epidemiol. 44(1):142-152.

Yang B, Liu P (2012). Composition and health effects of phenolic compounds in hawthorn (Crataegus spp.) of different origins. J. Sci. Food Agric. 92(8):1578-1590.

## 18

Amaranthus viridis modulates anti-hyperglycemic pathways in hemi-diaphragm and improves glycogenesis liver function in rats

Shihab Uddin[1], Md. Mahmodul Islam[2]*, Md. Mynul Hassan[3], Amrita Bhowmik[4] and Begum Rokeya[5]

[1]Department of Biochemistry and Molecular Biology, Jahangirnagar University, Savar, Bangladesh.
[2]Department of Pharmacy, Dhaka International University, Banani, Dhaka, Bangladesh.
[3]Dept of Biotechnology and Genetic Engineering, Khulna University, Khulna, Bangladesh.
[4]Department of Applied Laboratory Sciences, Bangladesh University of Health Sciences, Dhaka, Bangladesh.
[5]Department of Pharmacology, Bangladesh University of Health Sciences, Dhaka, Bangladesh.

Amaranthus viridis **is an ecumenical species in the botanical family of Amaranthaceae, which has been traditionally used to treat several skin diseases along with some antilipidemic activities. The present study was carried out to investigate the anti-hyperglycemic effect of 75% ethanolic extract of** *A. viridis* **in Neonatal streptozotocin (N-STZ) induced rats' hemi-diaphragm, including screening for secondary plant metabolites. Qualitative phytochemical studies were done by various conventional methods for the possible secondary metabolites. For antidiabetic assay via hemi-diaphragm, Long-Evan rats were used in the study. Type 2 diabetes was induced by a single** *ip* **injection of streptozotocin to 48 h old pups (N-STZ) and after 3 months, rats were confirmed by an oral glucose tolerance test and further selected for the experiment. Studies to evaluate the glucose utilization capacity of** *A. viridis* **in isolated rat hemi-diaphragm were done. The data were analyzed by appropriate statistical analysis.** *In vitro* **glucose uptake by hemi-diaphragm study showed glucose uptake increased significantly in left diaphragm of type 2 diabetes mellitus with insulin alone treated and** *A. viridis* **alone treated group, where** *A. viridis* **alone treated group showed very highly significance (p=0.000). Treatment with both insulin and** *A. viridis* **increased the glucose uptake also very significantly (p=0.004).** *A. viridis* **extract acted more significantly compared to insulin in T2DM rats. In the normal rats at left hemi diaphragm,** *A. viridis* **extract also increased glucose uptake more significantly (p=0.009) compared to insulin (p=0.013). At the right diaphragm, glucose uptake increased in all treated groups compared to control group but not significantly. This plant may contain potential anti-hyperglycemic agents which possibly act through some extra pancreatic mechanism that include glucose uptake by diaphragm and increased glycogenesis by liver.**

Key words: *Amaranthus viridis,* **antidiabetic, hemi-diaphragm, streptozotocin, glucose, Long-Evan rats.**

INTRODUCTION

It is staggering to consider the threat that diabetes poses to our current healthcare system. Recent technological and therapeutical advancement in the management of diabetes mellitus includes pancreas regeneration, islet transplantation, pancreas transplantation, glucose monitoring at continuous basis, uninterrupted subcutaneous insulin infusion and assorted medication (George, 2009). For mortals with T2DM mellitus (T2DM), an assortment of treatments is available. Most of the pharmacological aid schemes for T2DM are typically grounded on efficacy. Hence, prosperous responses to such therapeutics are frequently variable and unmanageable to predict. In this circumstances, delineation of drug reaction is expected to considerably heighten our ability to provide patients with the most effective treatment strategy given their individual backgrounds. Hence pharmacogenetic analysis of medications against diabetes is still in its early stage. Up to date, major pharmacogenetic acquisitions have focused on biguanides, TZDs and sulfonylureas (Distefano et al., 2010). Most recently researchers have focused on the management diabetes and its associated complications. A variety of approaches have been taken for this purpose.

The plant is usually known as green amaranth or slender amaranth. Possible origin is South America, although widely distributed in tropical weed, foreign to hot-temperate regions and distributed in the tropical and subtropical regions of the world. It is an annual herb with erect or ascending habit, growing to 1 m tall. Leaves are light green and the fruit are obviously wrinkled. It has prominent axillary spines and its leaves can have an obvious reddish or purplish tinge (Stanley et al., 1984). *A. viridis* is found to be a very common garden weed. Also it is found in areas such as roadsides, parks, pastures and other disturbed sites, but seldom cropped, often flattened and prostrate, vacant lots, sometimes crevices of sidewalks and edge of asphalt strips, etc. (Stone, 1970), casual in croplands and waste places too (Whistler, 1988).

The *A. viridis* is a good source of vitamins B and C, taken as vegetables (Sayed et al., 2007). Leaves and seeds are also edible. Previous experiments ascertained it to be a superior source of protein (Macharla et al., 2011). Traditionally it is used to cure eczema, psoriasis and rashes including antinociceptive and antipyretic properties, reported by Kumar (Kumar et al., 2009). Besides these, it is reported by Krishnamurthy that *A. viridis* has anti-inflammatory, antihyperglycemic, hypolipidemic activity as well as acne and skin cleansing property (Krishnamurthy et al., 2011). It has a wide application over diuresis, for snake bites, scorpion stings, dysentery, constipation, eczema, bronchitis, anemia, leprosy and stomach problems like many incidences (Pandhare et al., 2012; Macharla et al., 2011). According to Syed et al. it is quite beneficial to pregnant women to subside labor pains and diabetes (Syed et al., 2007). Its pharmacological study also reveals that it is antiviral (Obi et al., 2006). Meanwhile, its anti-allergenicity is claimed by Sayed et al. (2007). According to Kumar, *A. viridis* is

a potent hepatoprotective and antioxidant plant (Kumar et al., 2011). Studies also claimed that it is a good source of anthelmintic and isoproterenol-induced cardiac toxicity inhibitory plant (Ashok et al., 2011; Kumar et al., 2012).

Plants that exhibit activity against hyperglycemia are mainly owing to their ability to bushel the function of pancreatic tissues by causing an alleviation in insulin output or conquer the intestinal assimilation of glucose or aid of metabolites in insulin subordinate processes. Most plants contain cartenoids, terpenoids, glycosides, flavonoids, alkaloids etc. that are usually entailed as having antidiabetic effect (Jung et al., 2006). Type 2 diabetes represents a progressing decline in beta-cell function. Regarding the restrictions of being therapies in fixing the quality of life to normal as well as reducing the risk of chronic diabetic complications by maintaining normal blood glucose level, the search for alternating sources of oral hypoglycemic agents is a requirement. Due to the limitation of recent therapies to control all the metabolic defects of diabetes as well as their possible pathological outcomes with the great expense, there is a clear need for the development of alternative strategies for diabetes treatment.

There has been a possibility of anti-hyperglycemic potentialities of *A. viridis* reported by Krishnamurthy et al. (2011). However, so far hemi-diaphragm pathways of *A. viridis* on Long Evan rats against the hypoglycemic activities, has not been done. So in this study, an attempt was made to evaluate the anti-hyperglycemic activity of ethanolic extract of *A. viridis* plant and also to find out the chemical factors present therein causative for the biological activity. The pharmacological study was carried out on streptozotocin induced type 2 Neonatal model in Long Evan rats. Glucose utilization capacity of bioactivity guided fractions of *A. viridis* in isolated rat hemi-diaphragm in both normal and N-STZ rats was performed and the observed activity was identified, characterized and quantified.

MATERIALS AND METHODS

Chemicals and reagents

Ethanol (PubChem CID: 702), Ferric chloride (PubChem CID: 24380), potassium ferrocyanide (PubChem CID: 11963580), Chloroform (PubChem CID: 6212), sulphuric acid (PubChem CID: 1118), sodium dihydrogen phosphate (PubChem CID: 23672064) were purchased from Sigma-Aldrich Co (St. Louis, MO, USA). 4,6-Ethylidene glucose streptozotocin (PubChem CID: 3081692) were purchased from Merck (Darmstadt, Germany) and Human insulin (PubChem CID: 16131099) from Sanofi Bangladesh (Bangladesh). All other chemicals used were from the laboratory stock of the Department of Pharmacology, Bangladesh University of Health Sciences, Dhaka, Bangladesh and were of the highest grade

*Corresponding author. E-mail: mmislam44@gmail.com.

available.

Plant mate rial collection and identification

In this study, whole plant part of *A. viridis* (family: amaranthaceae, local name: Notey shak) was used. The plants were collected from Pabna, Bangladesh (Geographic coordinates: Latitude: 24°00'23" N, Longitude: 89°14'13" E and elevation above sea level: 19 m = 62 ft) availablesources from the field in the month of June, 2015. The plant was identified by the Bangladesh National Herbarium, Dhaka (Accession No: DACB-38568).

Preparation of ethanol extracts of *Amaranthus viridis*

Mature and fresh whole plants were washed thoroughly after collection and air dried. The weights of plants before and after dry were recorded. After then, the whole plants were grinded and again weighed. Finally, these grind portions were extracted by using 75% ethanolic solvent. The ethanolic extract was prepared by using Soxhlet (Beijing Getty glassware Co. Ltd. maintained at 70°C) and following the completion of extraction was concentrated by using water evaporator (Fujian Snowman Co. Ltd. 5 Litters, asserted at 80°C). The ethanolic extracts at semi dried state were encouraged to dry in a freeze drier (HETOSICC, Heto Lab Equipment, Denmark) at -55°C temperature and preserved in a reagent bottle at -8°C in a freezer for analysis.

Preparation of animals for treatment

Adult Long Evans rats weighting 160 to 220 g were included in the study. The animals were bred at Bangladesh Institute of Research and Rehabilitation for Diabetes, Endocrine and Metabolic Disorders (BIRDEM) animal house, Dhaka, Bangladesh, maintained at a constant room temperature of 22±5°C with humidity of 40 to 70% and the natural 12 h day-night cycle. Animal housing and handling were performed in accordance with Good Laboratory Practice (GLP) mentioned in US guidelines (NIH publication # 85-23, revised in 1985). The experimental protocols were critiqued and sanctioned by the Institutional Animal Ethics Committee prior to initiation of the experiment. The rats were fed upon a stock lab pellet diet and water supplied *ad libitum*. Standard rat diet contained wheat (40%), wheat bran (20%), fish meal (10%), germ (3.9%), oil cake (10%), milk (3.8%), pulses (3.9%), soyabean oil (1.5%), rice polishing (5%), molasses (0.95%) and salt (0.95%). Embavit GS (vitamin mixture) 250 g was added per 100 kg of rat food. The influence of circadian rhythm was avoided by starting all experiments at 7:30 am. The experiments were conducted according to the ethical guidelines approved by Bangladesh Association for Laboratory Animal Science.

Preparation of type 2 diabetes model rats

Type 2 diabetes was hastened by a single *ip* injection of streptozotocin (STZ) dissolved in citrate buffer (10 ml), at a dose of 90 mg/kg of body weight into the rat pups (48 h old, average weight 7 g) as described by Weir and Bonner-Weir et al. (2013). Following 3 months of STZ injection, rats were examined by oral glucose tolerance test (OGTT) for their blood glucose level. Diabetic model rats with blood glucose level >7.00 mmol/L, at fasting condition were selected for studying the effects of *A. viridis* extracts.

Phytochemical screening of *A. viridis*

Three (3) g of *A. viridis* 75% ethanolic extract was boiled with 30 ml

distilled water for 5 min in a water bath and was filtered while hot. The extract sample or filtrate was taken for the experiments wherever applicable using standard protocols (Sharmistha et al., 2012) to test the presence of bioactive compounds.

In vitro glucose uptake study of *A. viridis* by isolated rat hemi-diaphragm

Glucose uptake by rat hemi-diaphragm was estimated by the methods described elsewhere (Walaas and Walaas, 1952; Chattopadhyay et al., 1992) with some modifications. 32 male and female Long Evans normal and Type 2 rats were weighed and rats weighing between 170 to 210 g were used in the study. The weight of the rats were measured before and after fasting. Four sets containing graduated test tubes (n=4) for each hemi-diaphragm were taken. Group I served as a control which contained 2 ml of Tyrode (NaCl (8 gm/L), KCl (0.20 gm/L), CaCl$_2$ (0.20 gm/L), MgCl$_2$ (0.10 gm/L), NaH$_2$PO$_4$ (0.05 gm/L), NaHCO$_3$ (1 gm/L), Glucose (1 gm/L) having pH 6.5) solution with 2% glucose, Group II contained 2 ml Tyrode solution with 2% glucose and regular insulin (Novo Nordisk) 0.62 ml of 0.4 units per ml solution. Group III contained 2 ml Tyrode solution with 2% glucose and 1.38 ml of *A. viridis* extract (30 mg extract dissolved in 3 ml H$_2$O and adjust PH to 7.4) and the Group IV contained 2 ml Tyrode solution with 2% glucose and regular insulin 0.62 ml of 0.4 units per ml solution and 1.38 ml of *A. viridis* extract. The volumes of all the test tubes were made up to 4 ml with distilled water to match the volume of the test tubes of Group IV. Long Evans rats were tested overnight and killed by decapitation. The diaphragms were dissected out quickly with minimal trauma and divided into two halves. Two diaphragms from the same animal were not used for the same set of experiment. Four numbers of diaphragms were used for each group. The hemi-diaphragms were placed in test tubes and incubated for 30 min at 37°C in an atmosphere of 100% oxygen with shaking at 140 cycles/min. Glucose uptake per gram of tissue was calculated as the difference between the initial and final glucose content in the incubated medium.

Estimation of glucose level

The glucose oxidase (GOD-PAP) test was performed using the established method published by Trinder (Trinder, 1969) without modification.

Statistical analysis

Data from the experiments were analyzed using the Statistical Package for Social Science (SPSS) software for windows version 21 (SPSS Inc., Chicago, Illinois, USA). All the data were expressed as Mean ± SD or as Median (Range) as appropriate. Statistical analysis of the results was performed by using the student's t-test (paired and unpaired), ANOVA (analysis of variance) followed by Bonferroni and Dunnett post hoc test and Mann Whitney (u) test. GraphPad Prism (Version 5) software was used for all statistical analysis and P<0.05 was considered as significance.

RESULTS

Phytochemical screening of 75% ethanolic extract of *A. viridis*

The present investigation was carried out to assess the

Table 1. Phytochemical screening for the possible secondary metabolites of the *A. viridis* extract.

Serial no	Phytochemicals	Results
1	Tannin	++
2	Saponin	++
3	Alkaloid	++
4	Flavonoid	++
5	Phenol	++
6	Steroid	-
7	Terpenoid	+
8	Carbohydrate	-

++ = Presence; + = trace; - = absence.

qualitative phytochemical analysis of 75% ethanolic extract of *A. viridis*. The phytochemical screening reveals the presence of various plants' secondary metabolites as shown in Table 1. Tannin, saponin, alkaloid, flavonoid and phenols were found in the extract of *A. viridis*. Terpenoid was in trace amount but carbohydrate and steroids were not found in our phytochemical studies.

Check values of STZ induced Type 2 diabetic rats in different groups

To generate a rat model mimicking human type 2 diabetes with impaired insulin secretion and insulin resistance, we used STZ injection (90 µg/kg, body weight) to 48 h old pulps. STZ injection to neonates led to the injury of the pancreas resulting in destruction of the functional β-cells. At the age of 3 months, when an oral glucose challenge (500 mg/kg, body weight) was done, the remaining β cell could not cope with the load, which reflected in the postprandial rise of serum glucose level at 30 min (Table 2). The rise was significant among all rats compared to baseline value. On the basis of this experiment these rats were selected and sorted into three distinct groups to carry out the experiments with feeding of different extracts.

Effect of *A viridis* extracts using glucose uptake by isolated rat-hemi (left) diaphragm on normal rats in vitro assay

In order to explore the mechanism underlying the anti-hyperglycemic activity of *A. viridis in vitro* glucose uptake study of rat hemi-diaphragm was done. The results of glucose uptake by the left hemi-diaphragm in normal rats are presented in Table 3 and Figure 1. The results showed that glucose uptake was enhanced by hemi-diaphragm when the normal rats were treated with insulin alone (glucose uptake m ± SD, mg/g/30 min, control 2.02 ± 0.62 vs insulin 6.59 ± 2.01; p=0.013). When hemi-diaphragm was treated with *A. viridis* extract, glucose

uptake was also increased significantly (glucose uptake m ± SD, mg/g/30 min, control 2.02 ± 0.62 vs plant extract 6.93 ± 0.62; p = 0.009). When the hemi-diaphragm of normal rats was exposed to both insulin and *A. viridis* extract, it did not increase glucose uptake significantly.

Effect of *A. viridis* extracts using glucose uptake by isolated rat-hemi (right) diaphragm on normal rats in vitro assay

The results of glucose uptake by rat right hemi diaphragm in normal rats is presented in Table 4 and Figure 2. The results showed that glucose uptake was enhanced by hemi-diaphragm when the normal rats were treated with insulin alone (glucose uptake m ± SD, mg/g/30 min, control 0.568 ± 0.350 vs insulin 2.684 ± 2.527; p = 0.148). When hemi-diaphragm was treated with *A. viridis* extract, glucose uptake was also increased but not-significantly (glucose uptake m ± SD, mg/g/30 min, control 0.568 ± 0.350 vs plant extract 1.893 ± 1.704 p = 0.178). When the hemi-diaphragm of normal rats was exposed to both insulin and *A. viridis* extract, it also did not increase glucose uptake significantly.

Effect of *A viridis* extracts using glucose uptake by isolated rat-hemi (left) diaphragm on STZ induced type 2 rats in vitro assay

The results of glucose uptake by rat left hemi-diaphragm in T2DM rats is presented in Table 5 and Figure 3. When the T2DM rats were treated with insulin alone the glucose uptake was significantly increased in compared to control (glucose uptake m ± SD, mg/g/30 min, control 2.55 ± 0.36 vs insulin 5.26 ± 1.21; p = 0.037). In the treatment with *A. viridis* extract, glucose uptake was significantly higher in comparison to control (glucose uptake m ± SD, mg/g/30 min, control 2.55 ± 0.36 vs plant extract 9.74 ± 0.87; p = 0.000) as well as insulin alone (glucose uptake m ± SD, mg/g/30 min, insulin 5.26 ± 1.21 vs plant extract 9.74 ± 0.87; p = 0.002), respectively.

Insulin with *A. viridis* extract was also exposed to a significant increased glucose uptake when it compared with control (glucose uptake m ± SD, mg/g/30 min, control 2.55 ± 0.36 vs insulin with plant extract 6.46 ± 0.93; p = 0.004) as well as plant extract alone (glucose uptake m ± SD, mg/g/30 min, plant extract 9.74 ± 0.87 vs insulin with plant extract 6.46 ± 0.93; p = 0.012), respectively.

Effect of *A. viridis* extracts using glucose uptake by isolated rat-hemi (right) diaphragm on STZ induced type 2 rats in vitro assay

The results of glucose uptake by rat right hemi diaphragm in T2DM rats is presented in Table 6 and

Table 2. Check values of STZ induced Type 2 diabetic rats in different groups.

Groups	Fasting (0 min)	After OGTT (30 min)
WC (n=6)	7.44±0.57 (100%)	14.62±1.92 (197%)
Glc (n=6)	7.71±0.55 (100%)	14.82±1.35 (192%)
AVEtE (n=6)	7.72±0.87 (100%)	14.73±1.39 (191%)

Paired samples T test	
Groups	0 min vs 30 min
WC (n=6)	0.000
Glc (n=6)	0.000
AVEtE(n=6)	0.000

Results are expressed as Mean ±SD. OGTT= Oral Glucose Tolerance Test, STZ= Streptozotocin; WC = Type 2 Water Control; Glc = Type 2 Glibenclamide treated group and AVEtE= 75% ethanol extract of *A. viridis*.

Table 3. Effect of *A. viridis* extracts using glucose uptake by isolated rat-hemi (Left) diaphragm on normal rats *in vitro* assay.

Group (G)	Treatment	Incubation medium	Glucose uptake (mg/g/30 min)	p value
G1	Control	Tyrode solution with Glucose (2%)	2.02±0.62 (100%)	-
G2	Insulin	Tyrode solution with Glucose and Insulin (Actrapid 40 u/ml)	6.59±2.01 (326%)	G1 Vs G2, p=0.013*
G3	Plant extract	Tyrode solution with Glucose and plant extract (30 mg/3 ml H_2O)	6.93±0.62 (343%)	G1 Vs G3, p=0.009**
G4	Insulin+ plant extract	Tyrode solution with Glucose, Insulin and plant extract	4.38±1.25 (211%)	G1 Vs G4, p= 0.021*

Results were expressed as Mean ±SD. Statistical analysis between group comparison was done by using one-way ANOVA with post hoc Bonferroni test. *= $p<0.05$; **=$p<0.01$.

Table 4. Effect of *A viridis* extracts using glucose uptake by isolated rat-hemi (Right) diaphragm on normal rats *in vitro* assay.

Group (G)	Treatment	Incubation medium	Glucose uptake (mg/g/30 min)	p value
G1	Control	Tyrode solution with Glucose (2%)	0.568±0.350 (100%)	
G2	Insulin	Tyrode solution with Glucose and Insulin (Actrapid 40 u/ml)	2.684±2.527 (471%)	G1 Vs G2, p=0.148
G3	Plant extract	Tyrode solution with Glucose and plant extract (30mg/3ml H_2O)	1.893±1.704 (333%)	G1 Vs G3, p=0.178
G4	Insulin+ plant extract	Tyrode solution with Glucose, Insulin and. plant extract	1.898±0.977 (334%)	G1 Vs G4, P=0.067

Results were expressed as Mean ±SD. Statistical analysis between group comparison was done by using one-way ANOVA with post hoc Bonferroni test. *= $p<0.05$; **=$p<0.01$.

Figure 4. When the T2DM rats were treated with insulin alone the glucose uptake was increased by 59% compared to control group but not significantly. In the treatment with *A. viridis* extract, glucose uptake was 84% higher in comparison to control group. Glucose uptake was found to be increased up to 119% in case of

Table 5. Effect of *A.viridis* extracts using glucose uptake by isolated rat-hemi (Left) diaphragm on STZ induced type 2 rats *in vitro* assay.

Group (G)	Treatment	Incubation medium	Glucose uptake (mg/g/30 min)	p value
G1	Control	Tyrode solution with Glucose (2%)	2.55±0.36 (100%)	
G2	Insulin	Tyrode solution with Glucose and Insulin (Actrapid 40 u/ml)	5.26±1.21 (206%)	G1 Vs G2, **p=0.037***
G3	Plant extract	Tyrode solution with Glucose and plant extract (30 mg/3 ml H_2O)	9.74±0.87 (381%)	G1 Vs G3, **p=0.000**, G2 Vs G3; p=0.002**
G4	Insulin+ plant extract	Tyrode solution with Glucose, Insulin and plant extract	6.46±0.93 (253%)	G1 Vs G4, **p=0.004**, G3 Vs G4, p=0.012***

Results were expressed as Mean ±SD. Statistical analysis between group comparison was done by using one-way ANOVA with post hoc Bonferroni test. *= p<0.05; **=p<0.01.

Table 6. Effect of *A viridis* extracts using glucose uptake by isolated rat-hemi (right) diaphragm on STZ induced type 2 rats *in vitro* assay.

Group (G)	Treatment	Incubation medium	Glucose uptake (mg/g/30 min)	p value
G1	Control	Tyrode solution with Glucose (2%)	1.385±0.980 (100%)	
G2	Insulin	Tyrode solution with Glucose and Insulin (Actrapid 40 u/ml)	2.195±1.293 (159%)	G1 Vs G2, p=0.359
G3	Plant Extract	Tyrode solution with Glucose and plant extract (30mg/3ml H_2O)	2.548±1.423 (184%)	G1 Vs G3, p=0.233
G4	Insulin+ Plant Extract	Tyrode solution with Glucose, Insulin and. plant extract	3.033±0.823 (219%)	G1 Vs G4, P=0.043*

Results were expressed as Mean ±SD. Statistical analysis between group comparison was done by using one-way ANOVA with post hoc Bonferroni test. *= p<0.05; **=p<0.01.

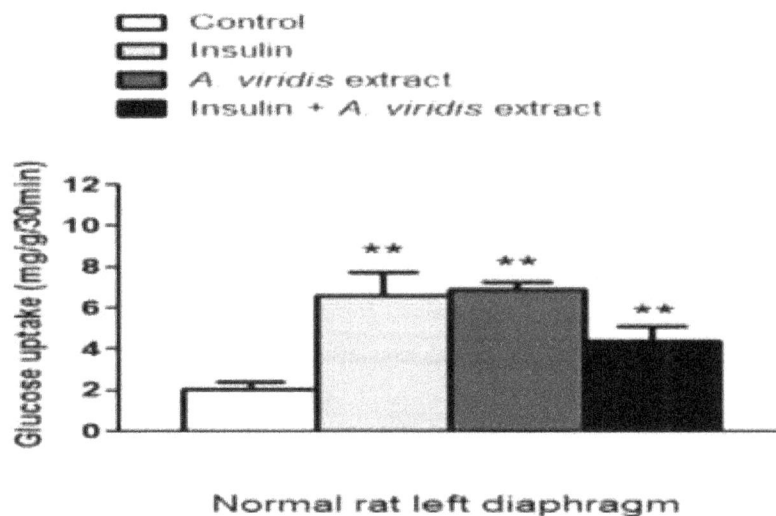

Figure 1. Effect of *A viridis* extracts using glucose uptake by isolated rat-hemi (Left) diaphragm on normal rats *in vitro* assay. *= p<0.05; **=p<0.01.

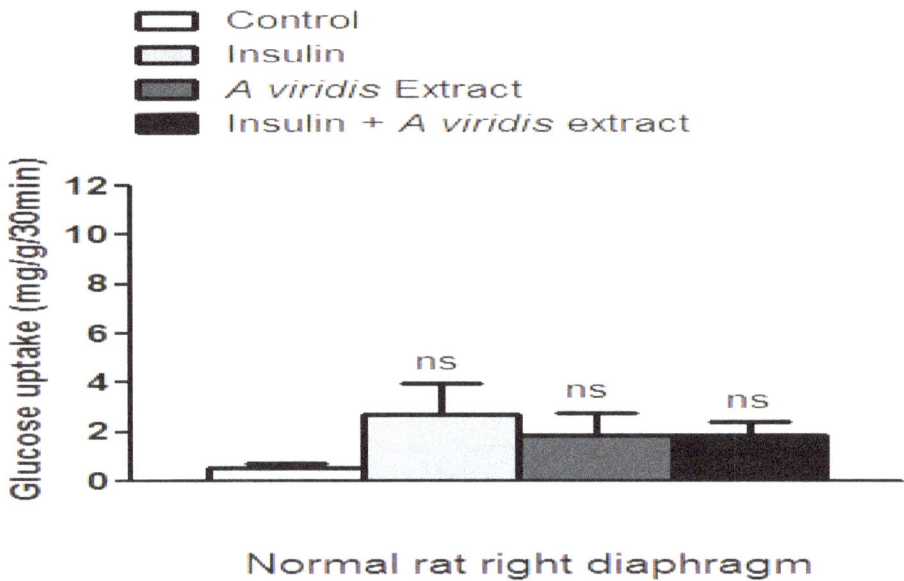

Figure 2. Effect of *A. viridis* extracts using glucose uptake by isolated rat-hemi (Right) diaphragm on normal rats *in vitro* assay. *= p<0.05; **=p<0.01 and ns= not significance.

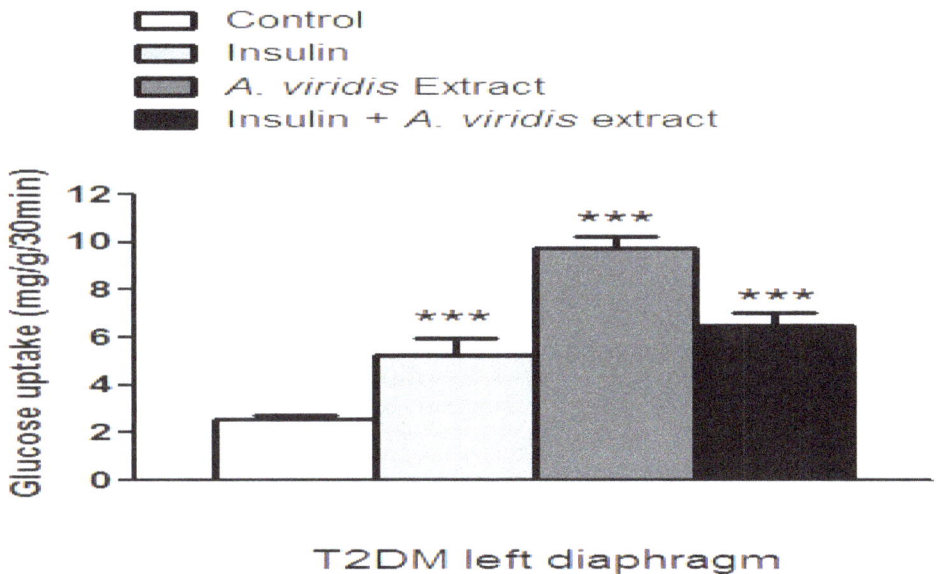

Figure 3. Effect of *A. viridis* extracts using glucose uptake by isolated rat-hemi (Left) diaphragm on STZ induced type 2 rats *in vitro* assay. *= p<0.05; **=p<0.01.

A. viridis extract with insulin, compared with control group as well as plant extract and insulin individually.

DISCUSSION

Previous studies have shown that antidiabetic plants possess the presence of alkaloids, glycosides and polyphenols like phytoconstituents (Sharmistha et al., 2012).

Therefore in the beginning of the study, preliminary phytochemical screening of the 75% ethanolic extract of whole plant for secondary plant metabolites was performed. The results revealed the presence of saponin, tannin, flavonoids, alkaloids, terpinoids, phenol (Table 1). The presence of a significant number of secondary plant

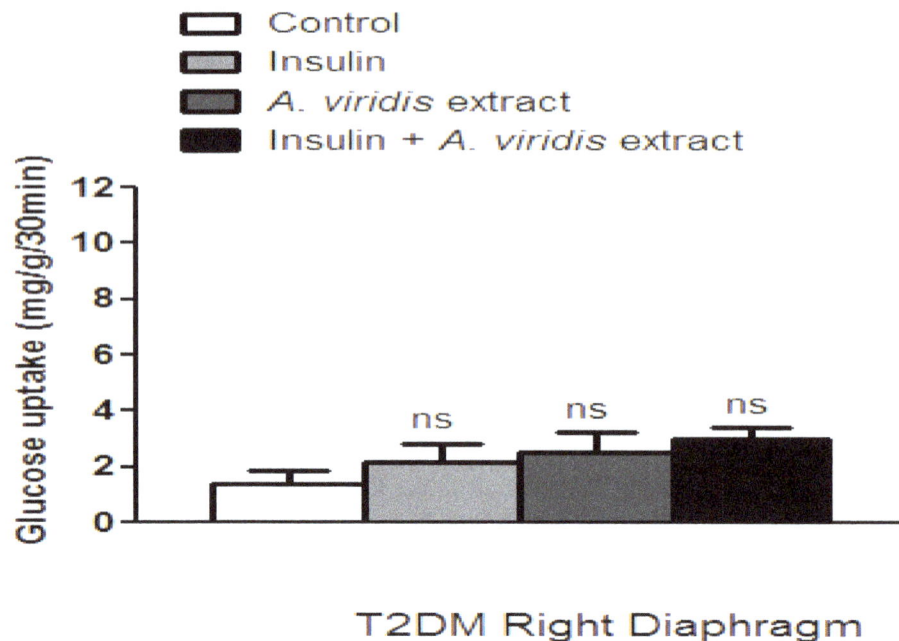

Figure 4. Effect of *A. viridis* extracts using glucose uptake by isolated rat-hemi (right) diaphragm on STZ induced type 2 rats *in vitro* assay. ns = not significance.

metabolites in *A. viridis* might be responsible for the biological activities observed later in this study.

Type 2 diabetes was developed by injecting STZ (a pancreatic β cell toxin) to 48 h old pups, which inside the β-cell dissociates into glucose and methylnitrogenase. The later alkaylates and modified biomolecules breakdown DNA and destroys β cell, thereby causing diabetes. Early injury of the β cells resulted in the partial recovery of β cell leading to type 2 diabetes as a result of insulin resistance in target tissues and impaired insulin secretion, accompanied by increased adiposity.

When at the age of 3 months these rats have been challenged with an oral glucose load, all of them could not cope with the glucose load due to the defective β cells. Although their fasting glucose values were a bit higher (ranging from 7.44 to 7.72), indicating the presence of some functioning β cells but their post challenge glucose values were significantly higher which proved that these rats have developed type 2 diabetes (Table 2).

Therefore, it may be assumed that the hypoglycemic activity of *A. viridis* in type 2 model rats at least, may be partly due to increased uptake of glucose for the formation of glycogen by enhanced glycogenesis. To put further insight regarding the mechanism of anti-hyperglycemic effect of *A. viridis* extract in both normal and T2DM rats *in vitro* glucose uptake by hemi-diaphragm was performed.

In this study, individual insulin ($p = 0.013$) and *A. viridis* ($p = 0.009$) treated group showed a significant increment in glucose uptake in normal rats at left diagram (Tables 3

and 4). Hence, in case of T2DM rats $p = 0.037$ with insulin alone and $p = 0.000$ with *A. viridis* extract (Table 5). Moreover, treatment with both insulin and *A. viridis* extract caused significantly much higher glucose uptake by rat left hemi-diaphragm ($p = 0.004$). Thus it can be concluded that *A. viridis* improves hyperglycemia by extrapancreatic mechanism as the left diaphragm improves glucose uptake more than right diaphragm.

Conclusion

The present study demonstrates that phytochemical screening of 75% ethanol extract contains a number of secondary plant metabolites including flavonoids, alkaloids which might be associated with the obtained antidiabetic properties of *A. viridis*. *In vitro* glucose consumption by hemi-diaphragm study exhibited increased state of the glucose by hemi-diaphragm in the presence of *A. viridis* extract. From the findings it can be concluded that different secondary metabolites of plant materials had some extra pancreatic mechanism like glucose consumption by peripheral tissues. Thus, the plant might be considered for further chemical studies and detailed toxicological studies for future drug development.

ACKNOWLEDGEMENTS

We gratefully acknowledge the logistic supports provided by the Asian Network of Research on Antidiabetic Plant (ANRAP) and the study was conducted in the Department of Pharmacology, Bangladesh University of Health Sciences, Dhaka Bangladesh; and the Department of Biochemistry and Molecular Biology, Jahangirnagar University, Dhaka, Bangladesh.

Abbreviations

N-STZ, Neonatal streptozotocin; **A. viridis,** Amaranthus viridis; **T2DM,** type 2 diabetes mellitus; **BIRDEM,** Bangladesh Institute of Research and Rehabilitation for Diabetes, Endocrine and Metabolic Disorders; **GLP,** good laboratory practice; **OGTT,** oral glucose tolerance test; **GOD-PAP,** glucose oxidase; **SPSS,** statistical package for social science; **ANOVA,** analysis of variance; **M±SD,** mean ± standard deviation.

REFERENCES

Chattopadhyay RR, Sarkar SK, Ganguly S, Banerjee RN, Basu TK (1992). Effect of leaves of vinca rosen linn on glucose utilization and glycogen deposition by isolated rat hemi-diaphragm. India. J. Physiol. Pharmacol. 36:137-138.

Distefano JK, Watanabe RM (2010). Pharmacogenetics of Anti-Diabetes Drugs. Pharmaceuticals 3(8):2610-2646.

George CM (2009). Future trends in diabetes management. Nephrol. Nurs. J. 36(5):477-483.

Jung M, Park M, Lee HC, Kang YH, Kang ES, Kim SK (2006). Anti-diabetic agents from medicinal plants. Curr. Med. Chem. 13(10):1203-1218.

Krishnamurthy G, Lakshman K, Pruthvi N, Chandrika PU (2011). Antihyperglycemic and hypolipidemic activity of methanolic extract of Amaranthus viridis leaves in experimental diabetes. Indian. J. Pharmacol. 43(4):450-454.

Kumar BSA, Lakshman K, Jayaveea KN, Shekar DS, Khan S, Thippeswamy BS (2012). Antidiabetic, antihyperlipidemic and antioxidant activities of methanolic extract of Amaranthus viridis Linn in alloxan induced diabetic rats. Exp. Toxicol. Pathol. 64:75-79.

Kumar BSA, Lakshman K, Swamy VBN, Kumar PAA, Shekar DS, Manoj B, Vishwantha GL (2011). Hepatoprotective and Antioxidant Activities of Amaranthus viridis Linn. Maced. J. Med. Sci. 4(2):125-130.

Kumar BSA, Lakshman K, Jayaveera KKN, Shekar DS, Muragan CSV, Manoj B (2009). Antinociceptive and Antipyretic Activities of Amaranthus Viridis Linn in Different Experimental Models. Avicenna. J. Med. Biotechnol. 1(3):167-171.

Macharla SP, Goli V, Bhasker KV, Devi PS, Dhanalakshmi C, Sanjusha C (2011). Effects of antiinflammatory activity of Amaranthus viridis Linn. Ann. Biol. Res. 2:435-438.

Obi RK, Iroagba II, Ojiako OA (2006). Virucidal potential of some edible Nigerian vegetables. Afr. J. Biotechnol. 5(19):1785-1788.

Pandhare R, Balakrishnan S, Popat M, Khanage S (2012). Antidiabetic and antihyperlipidaemic potential of Amaranthus viridis (L.) Merr. in streptozotocin induced diabetic rats. Asian Pacific J. Trop. Dis. 2:S180-S185.

Sayed MA, Rumi MAK, Ali L, Banu A, Hussain ZA, Azad AK (2007). Effect of socioeconomic risk factors on the difference in prevalance of diabetes between rural and urban population in Bangladesh. Biol. Med. Res. Council 33(1):1-12.

Sharmistha C, Chandra KJ (2012). Preliminary Phytochemical Screening and Acute Oral Toxicity Study of the Flower of Phlogacanthus thyrsiflorus Nees in Albino Mice. Int. Res. J. Pharm. 3(4):2230-8407.

Stanley TD, Ross EM (1984). Flora of South-eastern Queensland. Brittonia. 36(2): 205.

Stone BC (1970). The Flora of Guam: A Manual for the Identification of the Vascular Plants of the Island. Micronesica. 6(1/2): 1-659.

Trinder P (1969). Glucose: GOD-PAP method enzymatic colorimetric method. Ann. Clin. Biochem. 6:24-27.

Walaas E, Walaas O (1952). Effect of insulin on rat diaphragm under anaerobic conditions. J. Biol. Chem. 195:367-73.

Whistler WA (1988). Checklist of the weed flora of western Polynesia: an annotated list of the weed species of Samoa, Tonga, Niue, and Wallis and Futuna, along with the earliest dates of collection and the local names, South Pacific Commission, Noumea, New Caledonia. Technical Paper No. 194. ISBN 9822030959.

Weir GC, Bonner-Weir S (2013). Islet β cell mass in diabetes and how it relates to function, birth, and death. Ann. N. Y. Acad. Sci. 1281(1):92-105.

## 19

Determination of metabolites products by *Cassia angustifolia* and evaluate antimicobial activity

Ali Hussein Al-Marzoqi[1], Mohammed Yahya Hadi[2] and Imad Hadi Hameed[1]*

[1]Department of Biology, Babylon University, Hilla City, Iraq.
[2]College of Biotechnology, Al-Qasim Green University, Iraq.

Phytochemicals are chemical compounds often referred to as secondary metabolites. Forty four bioactive phytochemical compounds were identified in the methanolic leaves extract of *Cassia angustifolia*. The identification of phytochemical compounds is based on the peak area, retention time molecular weight and molecular formula. Gas chromatography-mass spectrometry (GC-MS) analysis of *C. angustifolia* revealed the existence of the 2,5-dimethyl-4-hydroxy-3(2H)-furanon, 2-propyl-tetrahydropyran-3-ol, estragole, benzene, 1-ethynyl-4-fluoro-, 5-hydroxymethylfurfural, anethole, 7-oxabicyclo[4.1.0]heptan-2-one,6-methyl-3-(1-methylethyl)-, 2-methoxy-4-vinylphenol, 1,2,2-trimethylcyclopentane-1,3-dicarboxylic acid, E-9-tetradecenoic acid, caryophyllene, cholestan-3-ol,2-methylene-, (3ß,5α)-, Benzene, 1-(1,5-dimethyl-4-hexenyl)-4-methyl-, ß-curcumene, 7-epi-cis-sesquisabinene hydrate, Cyclohexene, 3-(1,5-dimethyl-4-hexenyl)-6-methylene-,[S-(R*,S*)]-m, octahydrobenzo[b]pyran, 4a-acetoxy-5,5,8a,-trimethyl, dodecanoic acid, 3-hydroxy, tetraacetyl-d-xylonic nitrile, 1-ethenyl 3, trans(1,1-dimethylethyl)-4,cis-methoxycyclohexan-1-ol, phen-1,4-diol,2,3-dimethyl-5-trifluoromethyl, 5-benzofuranacetic acid, 6-ethenyl-2,4,5,6,7,7a-hexahydro-3,6-dime, 5-benzofuranacetic acid, 6-ethenyl-2,4,5,6,7,7a-hexahydro-3,6-dime, phytol, acetate, desulphosiniqrin, oxiraneundecanoic acid, 3-pentyl-,methyl ester, cis,Phytol, 9,12,15-Octadecatrienoic acid, 2-phenyl-1,3-dioxan-5-yl ester, butanoic acid, 1a,2,5,5a,6,9,10,10a-octahydro-5,5adihydroxy-4-(h), 9-Octadecenoic acid, 1,2,3-propanetriyl ester, (E,E,E) and Diisooctyl phthalate. *C. angustifolia* was highly active against *Aspergillus terreus* (6.01±0.27).

Key words: Antifungal, gas chromatography-mass spectrometry, fourier-transform infrared spectroscopy, phytochemicals, *Cassia angustifolia*.

INTRODUCTION

Medicinal plants are those plants which contain substances that can be used for the therapeutic purposes in one or more of its organ or substances which are precursors for the synthesis of useful drugs (Sofowora, 1982; Bako et al., 2005; Altameme et al., 2015a). The use of medicinal herbs to relieve and treat diseases is

*Corresponding author. E-mail: imad_dna@yahoo.com.

increasing because of their mild features and few side effects (Basgel and Erdemoglu, 2006). These plants are unlicensed and freely available, however, and there is no requirement to demonstrate efficacy, safety or quality (Ernst, 1998). The genus *Cassia* comprises 580 species of shrubs and trees which are widely distributed throughout the world, of which only twenty species are indigenous to India which belongs to the family Caesalpiniaceae, which generally consist of trees, shrubs and a few woody herbs. *Cassia angustifolia* Vahl (Family: Caesalpinaceae), popularly known as senna, is a valuable plant drug in Ayurvedic and modern system of medicine for the treatment of constipation. The pods and leaves of senna, as well as the pharmaceutical preparations containing sennosides A and B, are widely used in medicine because of their laxative properties. Senna is used in medicine as a cathartic; it is especially useful in habitual constipation. The laxative property of senna is based on two glycosides viz. sennoside A and sennoside B, whereas sennoside C and D have also been reported in the plant. Apart from sennoside, the pod and leaf also contain glycosides of anthraquinones rhein and chrysophenic acid, recently two naphthalene glycosides have also been isolated from leaves and pods (Gupta, 2010).

Antimicrobial activity has been reported in many plants by various workers (Sarin, 2005; Bansal et al., 2010; Chahal et al., 2010; Seth and Sarin, 2010; Malwal and Sarin, 2011; Hameed et al., 2015a). A new anthraquinone glycoside (emodin 8-0- sophorside) and seven known glycosides were isolated from the leaves of *C. angustifolia* and their structures were elucidated by spectral analysis (Kinjo et al., 1994). It has anti-inflammatory properties (Vanderperren et al., 2005), detoxification ability (Bournemouth, 1992) and also helps improve the function of the digestive system (Hoffmann, 1990). *Cassia senna* helps to reduce the nervous tension (Mills, 1993) and also helps in aiding the spleen and liver in production of blood and red blood cells (Spiller et al., 2003; Altameme et al., 2015b; Hamza et al., 2015). The present study was undertaken to investigate the antimicrobial activity and phytochemical analysis of *C. angustifolia*.

MATERIALS AND METHODS

Collection and preparation of plant material

C. angustifolia was purchased from local market in Hilla city, middle of Iraq. After thorough cleaning and removal of foreign materials, the seeds were stored in airtight container to avoid the effect of humidity and then stored at room temperature until further use (Hameed et al., 2015b; Jasim et al., 2015).

Preparation of sample

About fifteen grams of methanolic leaves extract of *C. angustifolia* powdered was soaked in 30 ml methanol for ten hours in a rotatory shaker. Whatman No.1 filter paper was used to separate the extract of plant. The filtrates were used for further phytochemical analysis. It was again filtered through sodium sulphate in order to remove the traces of moisture (Hussein et al., 2015; Hameed et al., 2015c).

Gas chromatography – mass spectrum analysis

The GC-MS analysis of the plant extract was made in a Agilent 7890 A instrument under computer control at 70 eV. About 1 µl of the methanol extract was injected into the GC-MS using a micro syringe and the scanning was done for 45 min. As the compounds were separated, they eluted from the column and entered a detector which was capable of creating an electronic signal whenever a compound was detected (Imad et al., 2014a; Kareem et al., 2015). The greater the concentration in the sample, the bigger was the signal obtained which was then processed by a computer. The time from when the injection was made (Initial time) to when elution occurred is referred to as the retention time (RT). While the instrument was run, the computer generated a graph from the signal called chromatogram. Each of the peaks in the chromatogram represented the signal created when a compound eluted from the gas chromatography column into the detector (Mohammed and Imad, 2013; Imad et al., 2014b). The X-axis showed the RT and the Y-axis measured the intensity of the signal to quantify the component in the sample injected. As individual compounds eluted from the gas chromatographic column, they entered the electron ionization (mass spectroscopy) detector, where they were bombarded with a stream of electrons causing, them to break apart into fragments. The fragments obtained were actually charged ions with a certain mass (Hameed et al., 2015d). The mass/charge (M/Z) ratio obtained was calibrated from the graph obtained, which was called the mass spectrum graph which is the fingerprint of a molecule. Before analyzing the extract using gas chromatography and mass spectroscopy, the temperature of the oven, the flow rate of the gas used and the electron gun were programmed initially. The temperature of the oven was maintained at 100°C. Helium gas was used as a carrier as well as an eluent. The flow rate of helium was set to 1 ml per minute. The electron gun of mass detector liberated electrons having energy of about 70eV. The column employed here for the separation of components was Elite 1 (100% dimethyl poly siloxane). The identity of the components in the extracts was assigned by the comparison of their retention indices and mass spectra fragmentation patterns with those stored on the computer library and also with published literatures (Imad et al., 2014c). Compounds were identified by comparing their spectra to those of the Wiley and NIST/EPA/NIH mass spectral libraries.

Determination of antifungal activity

Five-millimeter diameter wells were cut from the agar using a sterile cork-borer, and 50 µl of the samples solutions (*C. angustifolia*) was delivered into the wells. Antimicrobial activity was evaluated by measuring the zone of inhibition against the test microorganisms. Methanol was used as solvent control. Amphotericin B and fluconazole were used as reference antifungal agent (Hameed et al., 2015b). The tests were carried out in triplicate. The antifungal activity was evaluated by measuring the inhibition-zone diameter observed after 48 h of incubation.

Statistical analysis

Data were analyzed using analysis of variance (ANOVA), and differences among the means were determined for significance at P

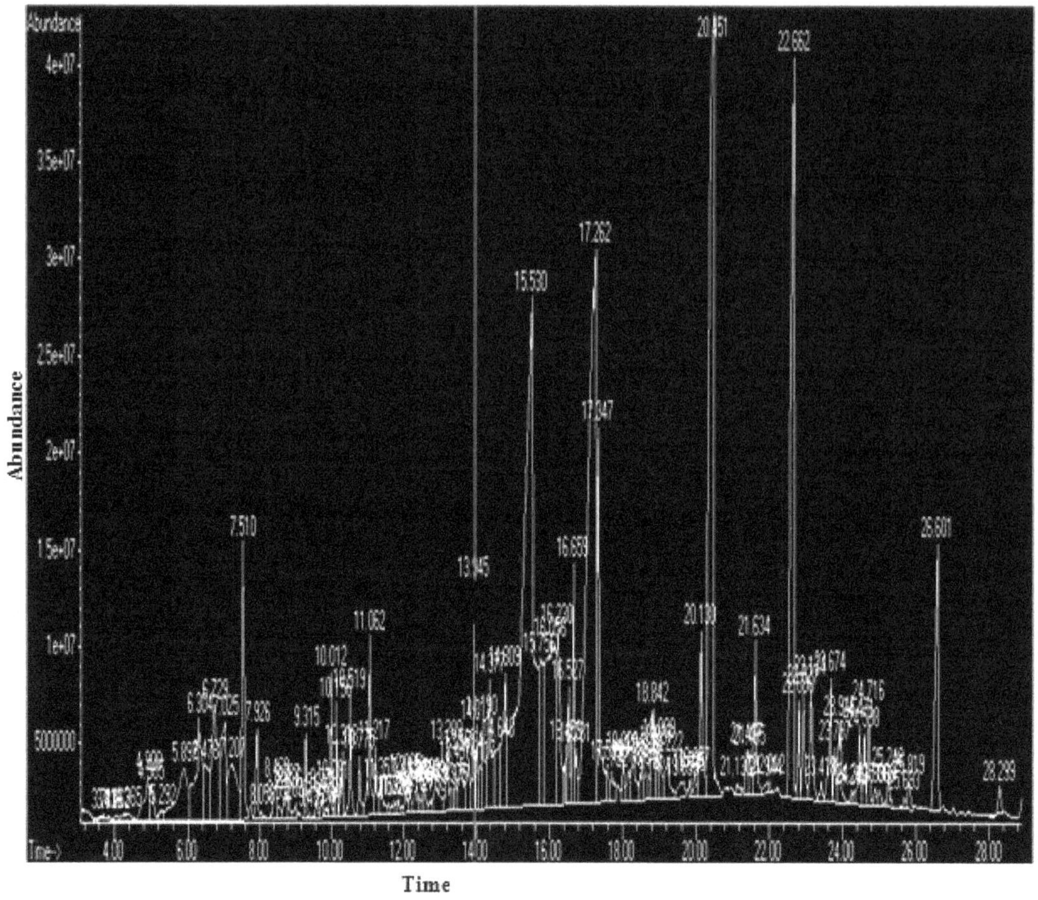

Figure 1. GC-MS chromatogram of methanolic extract of *Cassia angustifolia.*

< 0.05, using Duncan's multiple range test (by SPSS software) Version 9.1.

RESULTS AND DISCUSSION

Gas chromatography and mass spectroscopy analysis of compounds was carried out in methanolic extract of *C. angustifolia*, as shown in Table 1. The GC-MS chromatogram of the forty four peaks of the compounds detected was shown in Figure 1. Chromatogram GC-MS analysis of the methanol extract of *Althaea rosea* showed the presence of 44 major peaks and the components corresponding to the peaks were determined as follows. The first set up peaks were determined to be 2,5-dimethyl-4-hydroxy-3(2H)-furanon (Figure 2). The next peaks considered to be 2-Propyl-tetrahydropyran-3-ol, Estragole, Benzene, 1-ethynyl-4-fluoro-, 5-Hydroxymethylfurfural, Anethole, 7-Oxabicyclo[4.1.0]heptan-2-one,6-methyl-3-(1-methylethyl)-, 2-Methoxy-4-vinylphenol, 1,2,2-Trimethylcyclopentane-1,3-dicarboxylic acid, E-9-Tetradecenoic acid, Caryophyllene, Cholestan-3-ol,2-methylene-,(3ß,5α)-, Benzene, 1-(1,5-dimethyl-4-

hexenyl)-4-methyl-, ß-curcumene, 7-epi-cis sesquisabinene hydrate, Cyclohexene, 3-(1,5-dimethyl-4 hexenyl)-6-methylene-,[S-(R*,S*)]-m, Octahydrobenzo[b pyran,4a-acetoxy-5,5,8a,-trimethyl, Dodecanoic acid, 3 hydroxy, Tetraacetyl-d-xylonic nitrile, 1-Etheny 3,trans(1,1-dimethylethyl)-4,cis-methoxycyclohexan-1-ol, Phen-1,4-diol,2,3-dimethyl-5-trifluoromethyl, 5 Benzofuranacetic acid, 6-ethenyl-2,4,5,6,7,7a-hexahydro 3,6-dime, 5-Benzofuranacetic acid, 6-ethenyl 2,4,5,6,7,7a-hexahydro-3,6-dime, Phytol, acetate Desulphosiniqrin, Oxiraneundecanoic acid, 3-pentyl ,methyl ester,cis, Phytol, 9,12,15-Octadecatrienoic acid 2-phenyl-1,3-dioxan-5-yl ester, Butanoic acid 1a,2,5,5a,6,9,10,10a-octahydro-5,5adihydroxy-4-(h), 9 Octadecenoic acid, 1,2,3-propanetriyl ester, (E,E,E) and Diisooctyl phthalate (Figures 3 to 45). Methanolic extraction of plant showed notable antifungal activities against *Aspergillus niger*, *Aspergillus terreus*, *Aspergillus flavus*, and *Aspergillus fumigatus* (Table 2). *C angustifolia* was very highly active against *A. terreus* (6.01±0.27). *Aspergillus* was found to be sensitive to all test medicinal plants and mostly comparable to the standard reference antifungal drug amphotericin B and fluconazole to some extent.

Table 1. Major phytochemical compounds identified in *Cassia angustifolia*.

Serial No.	Phytochemical compound	RT (min)	Formula	Molecular weight	Exact mass	Chemical structure	MS Fragment- ions	Pharmacological actions
1	2,5-dimethyl-4-hydroxy-3(2H)-furanone	4.883	$C_6H_8O_3$	128	128.047344		57, 72, 85, 94, 109, 128	Antimicrobial effect
2	2-Propyl-tetrahydropyran-3-ol	5.908	$C_8H_{16}O_2$	144	144.115029		55, 73, 87, 101, 116, 144	Anti-infective agent in human microbial infections.
3	Estragole,	6.303	$C_{10}H_{12}O$	148	148.088815		51, 55, 63, 77, 91, 105, 121, 133, 148	Anti-inflammatory activity
4	Benzene, 1-ethynyl-4- fluoro	6.720	C_8H_5F	120	120.0375285		50, 63, 74, 81, 94, 100, 120	Antibacterial activity / Antifungal activity

Table 1. Cont'd

5	5-Hydroxymethylfurfural	7.247	$C_6H_6O_3$	126	126.0311694		53, 69, 81, 84, 97, 109, 126	Antioxidant and specific anti-cancer agents
6	Anethole	7.510	$C_{10}H_{12}O$	148	148.088815		51, 55, 63, 74, 77, 91, 105, 117, 133, 148	Antihyperglycemic effect
7	7-Oxabicyclo[4.1.0]heptan-2-one,6-methyl -3-(1-methylethyl)-	7.750	$C_{10}H_{16}O_2$	168	168.115029		55, 69, 83, 97, 111, 126, 139, 150, 168	New chemical compound
8	2-Methoxy-4-vinylphenol	7.933	$C_9H_{10}O_2$	150	150.06808		51, 77, 89, 107, 121, 135	Antioxidant, *anti* microbial and anti inflammatory

Table 1. Cont'd

#	Compound	RT	Formula	MW	Exact Mass	Structure	m/z fragments	Activity
9	1,2,2-Trimethylcyclopentane-1,3-dicarboxylic acid	8.431	$C_{10}H_{16}O_4$	200	200.104859		55, 68, 82, 109, 136, 154, 182	Anti- fungal
10	E-9-Tetradecenoic acid	8.746	$C_{14}H_{26}O_2$	226	226.19328		55, 69, 83, 97, 110, 166, 208	Analgesic and *anti*-inflammatory effect
11	Caryophyllene	9.301	$C_{15}H_{24}$	204	204.1878		79, 93, 105, 120, 133, 147, 161, 175, 189, 204	Anti-inflammatory, antibiotic, antioxidant, anticarcinogenic and local anaesthetic
12	Cholestan-3-ol,2-methylene-,(3ß,5α)-	9.616	$C_{28}H_{48}O$	400	400.370516		69, 81, 95, 175, 227, 260, 315, 400	Anti-oxidant
13	Benzene , 1-(1,5-dimethyl-4-hexenyl)-4-methyl-	10.010	$C_{15}H_{22}$	202	202.172151		55, 65, 69, 77, 83, 91, 95, 105, 119, 132, 145, 159, 187, 202	Antimicrobial and anti-inflammatory

Table 1. Cont'd

No.	Compound	RT	Formula	MW	Exact mass	m/z	Structure	Biological activity
14	ß-curcumene	10.165	$C_{15}H_{24}$	204	204.1878	55, 69, 77, 93, 105, 119, 133, 147, 161, 176, 189, 204		Anti-tumor, anti-cancer, anti-repellent, antitussive and anti-platelet
15	7-epi-cis-sesquisabinene hydrate	10.274	$C_{15}H_{26}O$	222	222.198365	55, 69, 82, 93, 105, 119, 161, 175, 204, 222		nti-cancer
16	Cyclohexene ,3-(1,5-dimethyl-4-hexenyl)-6-methylene-,[S-(R*,S*)]-	10.508	$C_{15}H_{24}$	204	204.1878	55, 69, 77, 93, 109, 133, 147, 161, 175, 189, 204		Anti-bacterial and antifungal
17	Octahydrobenzo[b]pyran,4a-acetoxy-5,5,8a,-trimethyl	10.771	$C_{14}H_{24}O_3$	240	240.1725445	55, 69, 97, 111, 124, 137, 151, 165, 180, 197, 240		Anti-Candida and anti-inflammatory
18	Dodecanoic acid , 3-hydroxy	11.218	$C_{12}H_{24}O_3$	216	216.1725445	55, 69, 83, 96, 112, 126, 138, 151, 180, 200, 215		Antifungal activity

Table 1. Cont'd

19	Tetraacetyl-d-xylonic nitrile	11.012	$C_{14}H_{17}NO_9$	343	343.090332		60, 73, 112, 133, 164, 197, 226, 270	Have anti-viral effects
20	1-Ethenyl 3,trans(1,1-dimethylethyl)-4,cis-methoxycyclohexan-1-ol	11.246	$C_{13}H_{22}O_2$	210	210.16198		57, 70, 79, 91, 104, 121, 137, 151, 163, 192, 210	Unknown
21	Phen-1,4-diol,2,3-dimethyl-5-trifluoromethyl	11.378	$C_9H_9F_3O_2$	206	206.055464		57, 69, 83, 91, 123, 149, 206	Antimicrobial effect
22	5-Benzofuranacetic acid,6-ethenyl -2,4,5,6,7,7a-hexahydro-3,6-dime	12.036	$C_{16}H_{20}O_4$	276	276.13616		53, 77, 91, 105, 121, 148, 176, 216, 244, 276	New chemical compound

Table 1. Cont.

No.	Compound	RT	Formula	MW	Exact Mass	Structure	Fragments (m/z)	Activity
23	2H-Benzo[f]oxireno[2,3-E]benzofuran-8(9H)-one,9-[[[2-(dimethylamin]]]	12.877	$C_{19}H_{32}N_2O_3$	336	336.241293		58, 71, 81, 91, 109, 123, 149, 166, 185, 204, 219, 233, 248	Antitumor, anti-inflammatory, antifungal, pesticidal and insecticidal
24	Phytol, acetate	13.953	$C_{22}H_{42}O_2$	338	338.318481		57, 68, 81, 95, 109, 123, 137, 151, 179, 208, 249, 278	Anti-inflammatory, antileishmanial and antitrypanosomal
25	Desulphosiniqrin	14.399	$C_{10}H_{17}NO_6S$	279	279.077658		60, 73, 85, 103, 127, 145, 163, 213, 262	New chemical compound
26	Oxiraneundecanoic acid ,3-pentyl-,methyl ester , cis	16.482	$C_{19}H_{36}O_3$	312	312.266445		55, 74, 87, 97, 111, 127, 155, 183, 199, 227, 264, 294	Anti-oxidant
27	Phytol	16.665	$C_{20}H_{40}O$	296	296.307917		57, 71, 81, 95, 111, 123, 137, 196, 221, 249, 278	Anti-cancer activities

Table 1. Cont'd

#	Name	RT	Formula	Mass	Exact Mass	Structure	m/z	Activity
28	9,12,15-Octadecatrienoic acid, 2-phenyl-1,3-dioxan-5-yl ester	18.296	$C_{28}H_{40}O_4$	440	440.29266		55, 67, 79, 105, 129, 165, 185, 219, 265, 334, 440	Antiviral and anti-obesity properties
29	Butanoic acid ,1a,2,5,5a,6,9,10,10a-octahydro-5,5adihydroxy-4-(h)	18.874	$C_{24}H_{34}O_6$	440	440.29266		71, 91, 107, 122, 135, 151, 177, 213, 241, 299, 387, 418	Unknown
30	9-Octadecenoic acid , 1,2,3-propanetriyl ester , (E,E,E)-	19.846	$C_{57}H_{104}O_6$	884	884.78329		55, 69, 83, 98, 220, 264, 282, 339, 356, 393, 449, 489	Anti-spasmodic and immune modulators
31	Diisooctyl phthalate	20.373	$C_{24}H_{38}O_4$	390	390.27701		57, 71, 83, 113, 132, 149, 167, 279, 390	Antimicrobial activity and Anti oxidant.
32	8,14-Seco -3,19-epoxyandrostane-8,14-dione,17-acetoxy-3ß-methoxy	21.449	$C_{24}H_{36}O_6$	420	420.251188		55, 69, 83, 96, 111, 149, 177, 209, 265, 304, 360, 420	New chemical compound

Table 1. Cont'd

#	Name	Retention time	Molecular formula	MW	Exact mass	Structure	Fragment ions	Use/Activity
33	Squalene	22.604	$C_{20}H_{50}$	410	410.391253		69, 81, 95, 121, 149, 175, 203, 231, 257, 285, 341, 367, 395	Widely used in the cosmetics industry as an *anti*-wrinkle agent
34	Cyclopropanebutanoic acid ,2-[[2-[[2-pentylcyclopropyl)methyl]cyclo	22.845	$C_{25}H_{42}O_2$	374	374.318481		74, 121, 227, 270, 298, 334	Used as a poultice as an *anti*-inflammatory
35	Cyclotriaconta-1,7,16,22,-tetraone	23.159	$C_{30}H_{52}O_4$	476	476.38656		55, 81, 125, 183, 239, 279, 321, 337, 379, 419, 458	New chemical compound
36	2-[4-methyl-6-(2,6,6-trimethylcyclohex-1-enyl)hexa-1,3,5-trienyl]cyclo	23.451	$C_{23}H_{32}O$	324	324.245316		555, 91, 135, 173, 187, 239, 324	Antimicrobials and anti-virals
37	Oxirane ,2,2-dimethyl-3-(3,7,12,16,20-pentamethyl-3,7,11,15,19,-hen	23.657	$C_{30}H_{50}O$	426	426.386166		69, 81, 95, 135, 203, 231, 271, 299, 357, 426	Anti-diarrhoeal activity
38	9,19-Cyclolanost-24-en-3-ol,acetate , (3β)-	23.686	$C_{32}H_{52}O_2$	468	468.39673		55, 69, 81, 95, 109, 135, 203, 217, 286, 311, 365, 408, 424	Anti mosquito larvicidal activity

Table 1. Cont'd

#	Name	RT	Formula	Mass	Exact mass	Structure	Fragments	Activity
39	9-Desoxo-9-x-acetoxy-3,8,12-tri-O-acetylingol	25.025	$C_{28}H_{40}O_{10}$	536	536.262146		55, 69, 122, 207, 236, 297357, 417, 477	Anti- inflammatory effects
40	γ-Tocopherol	25.236	$C_{28}H_{48}O_2$	416	416.365543		57, 107, 151, 191, 205, 246, 274, 303, 344, 373, 416	anti-oxidant activity
41	Olean-12-ene-3,15,16,21,22,28-hexol,(3ß,15α,16α,21ß,22α)-	25.683	$C_{30}H_{50}O_6$	506	506.360739		135, 190, 207, 231, 249, 280, 298, 334, 352, 384, 439, 506	Anti-tumourogenic properties
42	Vitamin E	26.581	$C_{29}H_{50}O_2$	430	430.38108		57, 69, 91, 121, 165, 205, 246, 274, 302, 330, 358, 386	Anti-oxidant activity
43	Campesterol	28.315	$C_{28}H_{80}O$	400	400.370516		55, 71, 81, 145, 161, 213, 255, 289, 315, 382, 400	Campesterol is a phytosterol whose chemical structure is similar to that of cholesterol. have *anti*-inflammatory effects.
44	Carbonic acid , (ethyl)(1,2,4-triazol-1-ylmethyl)diester	3.224	$C_6H_9N_3O_3$	171	171.064391		55, 70, 82, 98, 112, 171	Anti-inflammatory

Table 2. Zone of inhibition (mm) of *Aspergillus Spp.* test to *Cassia angustifolia* bioactive compounds and standard antibiotics.

Plant/ antibiotics	Aspergillus spp.			
	Aspergillus niger	*Aspergillus terreus*	*Aspergillus flavus*	*Aspergillus fumigatus*
Cassia angustifolia	3.08±0.10	6.01±0.27	5.00±0.16	4.03±0.20
Amphotericin B	2.01±0.20	2.99±0.16	4.05±0.10	4.90±0.30
Fluconazol	4.08±0.61	2.96±0.14	3.00±0.81	4.90±0.40
Control	0.00	0.00	0.00	0.00

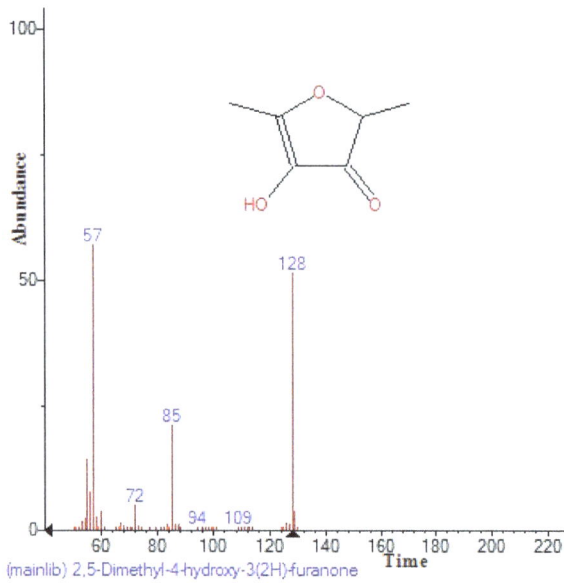

Figure 2. Structure of 2,5-dimethyl-4-hydroxy-3(2H)-furanone present in *Cassia angustifolia* with RT= 4.883 using GC-MS analysis.

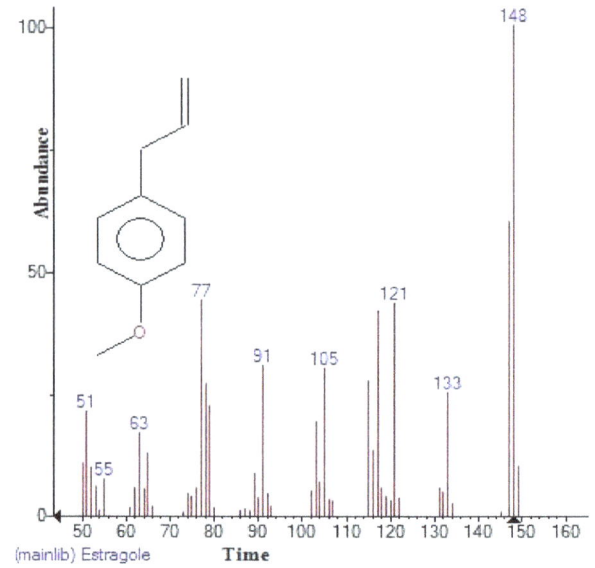

Figure 4. Structure of Estragole present in *Cassia angustifolia* with RT= 6.303 using GC-MS analysis.

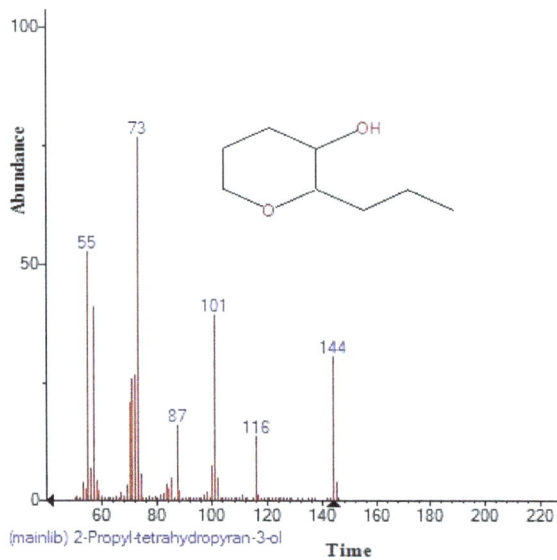

Figure 3. Structure of 2-Propyl-tetrahydropyran-3-ol present in *Cassia angustifolia* with RT= 5.908 using GC-MS analysis.

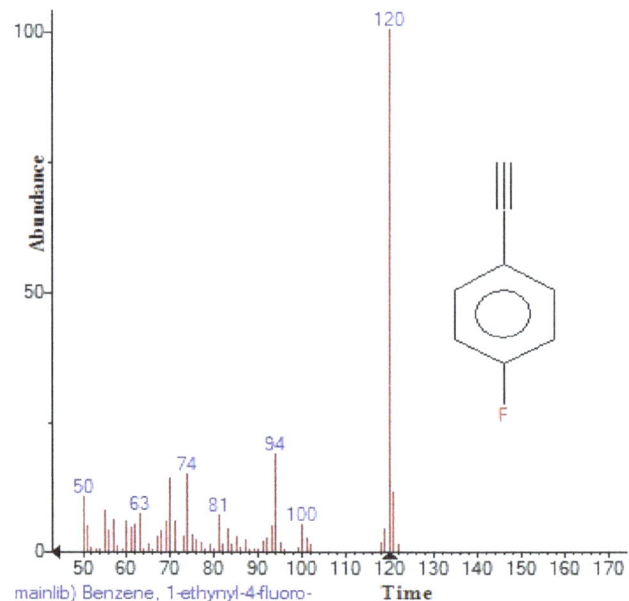

Figure 5. Structure of Benzene, 1-ethynyl-4- fluoro present in *Cassia angustifolia* with RT= 6.720 using GC-MS analysis.

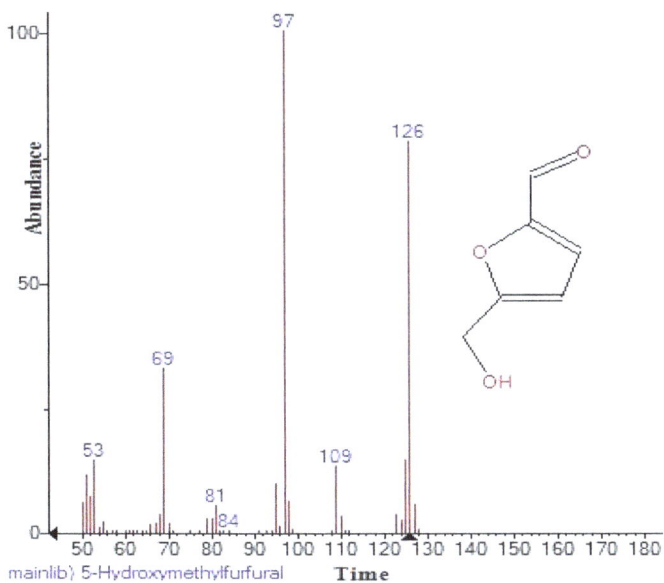

Figure 6. Structure of 5-Hydroxymethylfurfural present in *Cassia angustifolia* with RT= 7.247 using GC-MS analysis.

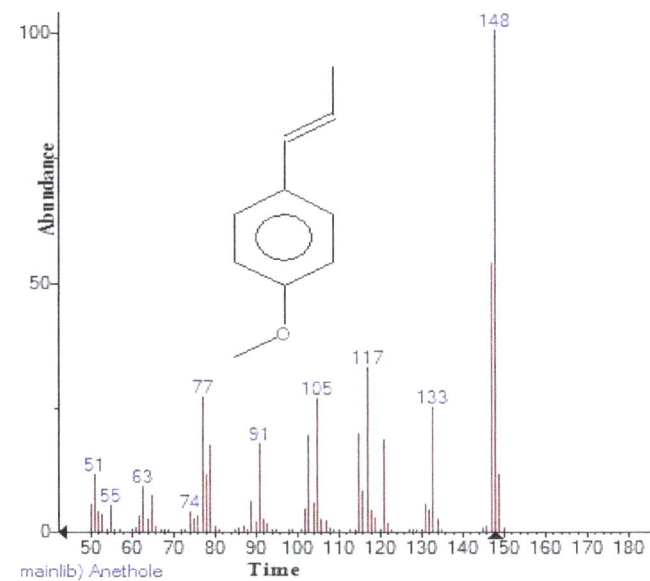

Figure 7. Structure of Anethole present in *Cassia angustifolia* with RT= 7.510 using GC-MS analysis.

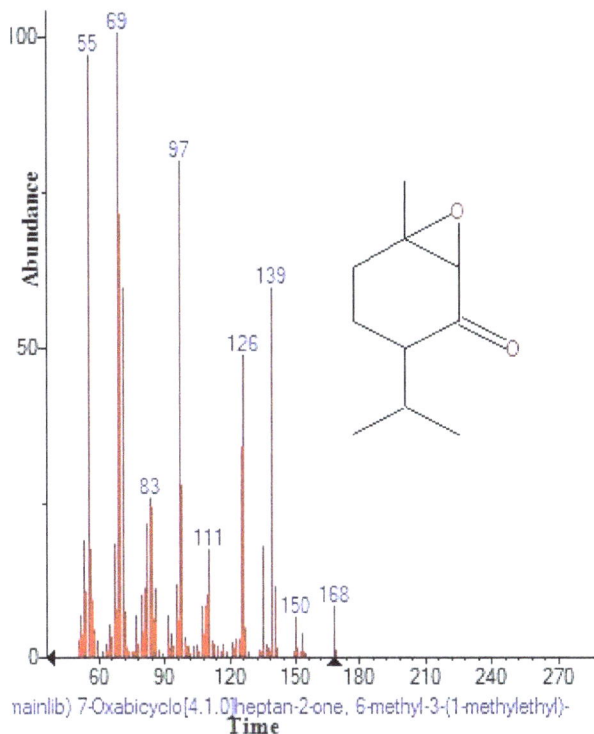

Figure 8. Structure of 7-Oxabicyclo[4.1.0]heptan-2-one,6-methyl -3-(1-methylethyl) present in *Cassia angustifolia* with RT = 7.750 using GC-MS analysis.

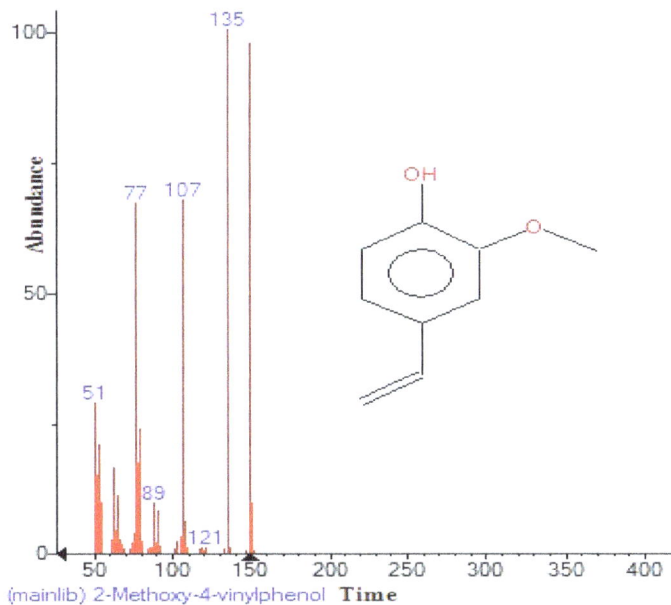

Figure 9. Structure of 2-Methoxy-4-vinylphenol present in *Cassia angustifolia* with RT= 7.933 using GC-MS analysis.

Conclusion

From the results obtained in this study, it could be concluded that *C. angustifolia* possesses remarkable antimicrobial activity which is mainly due to 2-Propyl-tetrahydropyran-3-ol, 1,2,2-Trimethylcyclopentane-1,3-dicarboxylic acid and Diisooctyl phthalate. According to these findings, it could be said that the methanol extract act as antifungal agent.

Conflict of Interests

The authors have not declared any conflict of interests.

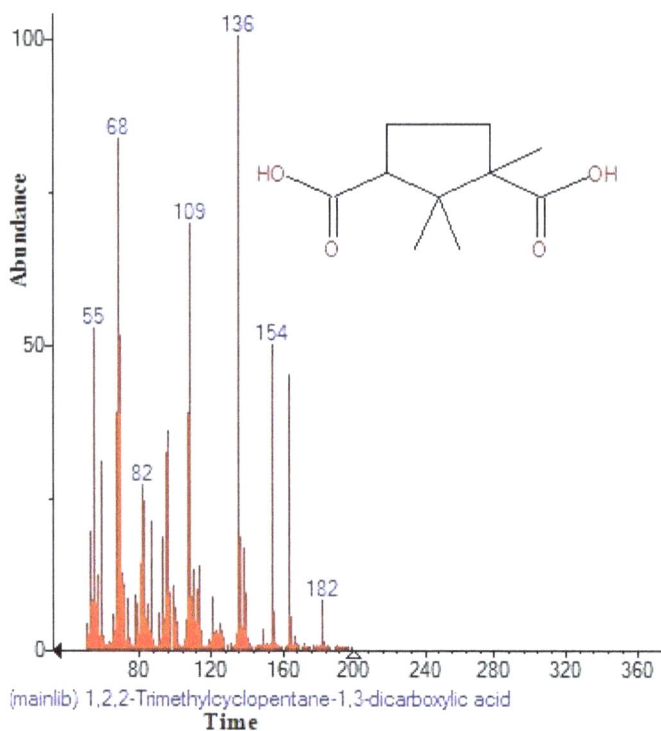

Figure 10. Structure of 1,2,2-Trimethylcyclopentane-1,3-dicarboxylic acid present in *Cassia angustifolia* with RT= 8.431 using GC-MS analysis.

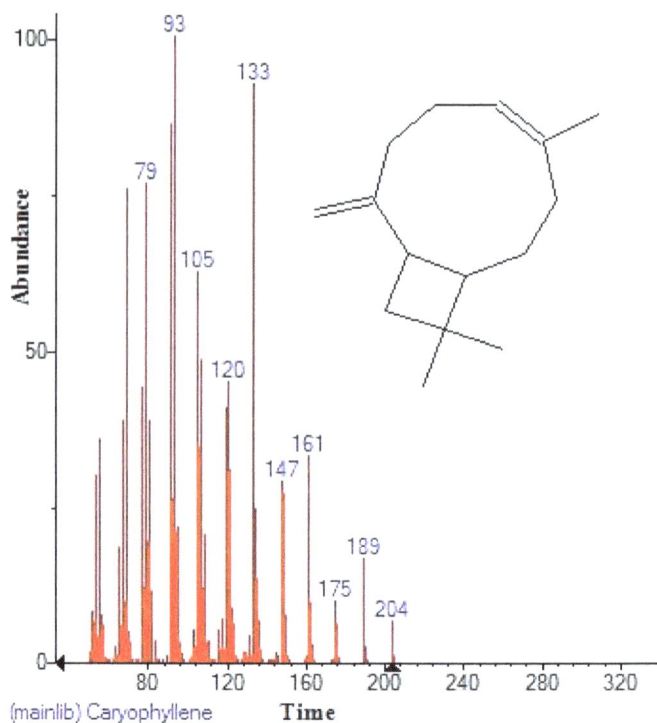

Figure 12. Structure of Caryophyllene present in *Cassia angustifolia* with RT= 9.301 using GC-MS analysis.

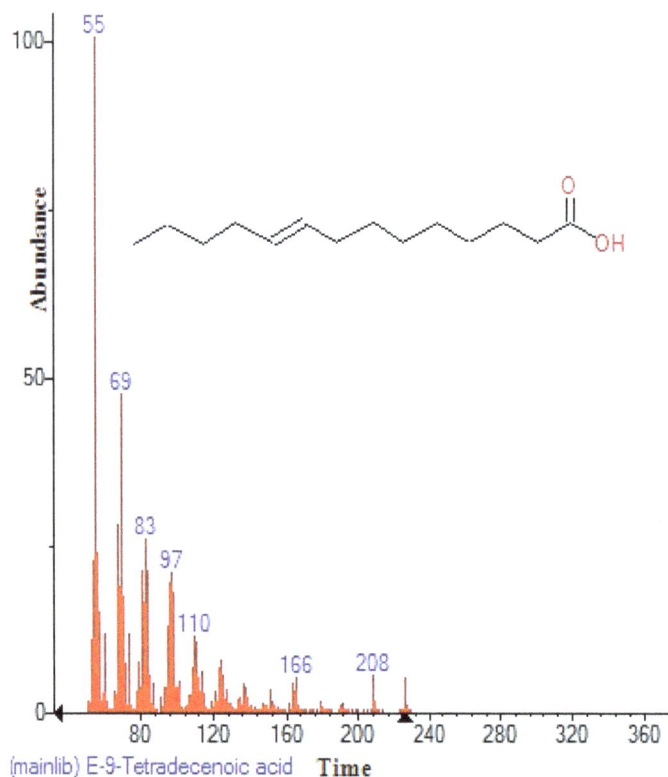

Figure 11. Structure of E-9-Tetradecenoic acid present in *Cassia angustifolia* with RT= 8.746 using GC-MS analysis.

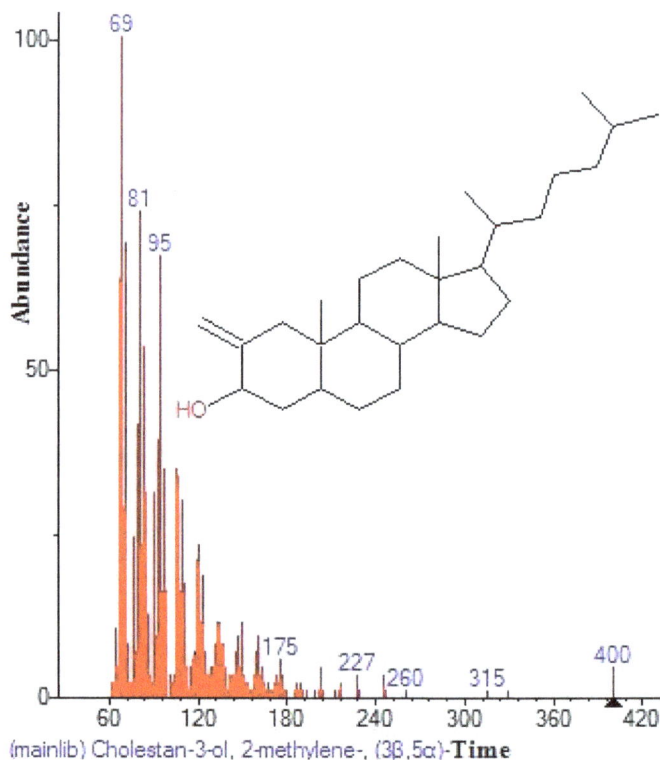

Figure 13. Structure of Cholestan-3-ol,2-methylene-,(3ß,5α)- present in *Cassia angustifolia* with RT= 9.616 using GC-MS analysis.

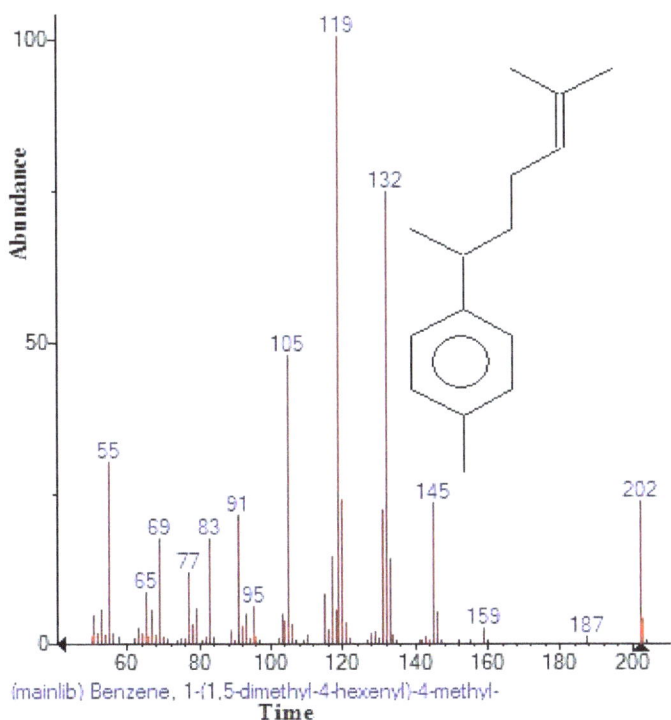

Figure 14. Structure of Benzene , 1-(1,5-dimethyl-4-hexenyl)-4-methyl present in *Cassia angustifolia* with RT= 10.010 using GC-MS analysis.

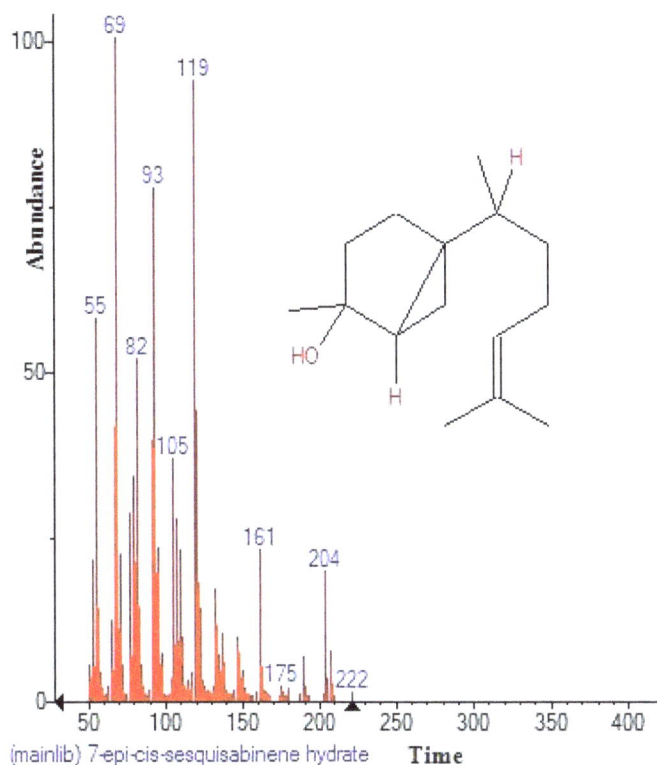

Figure 16. Structure of 7-epi-cis-sesquisabinene hydrate present in *Cassia angustifolia* with RT = 10.274 using GC-MS analysis.

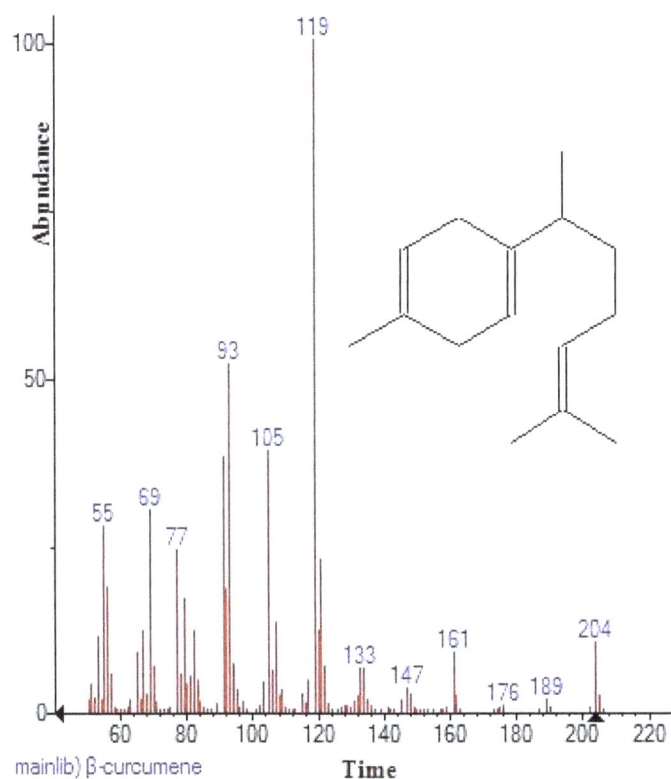

Figure 15. Structure of ß-curcumene present in *Cassia angustifolia* with RT= 10.165 using GC-MS analysis.

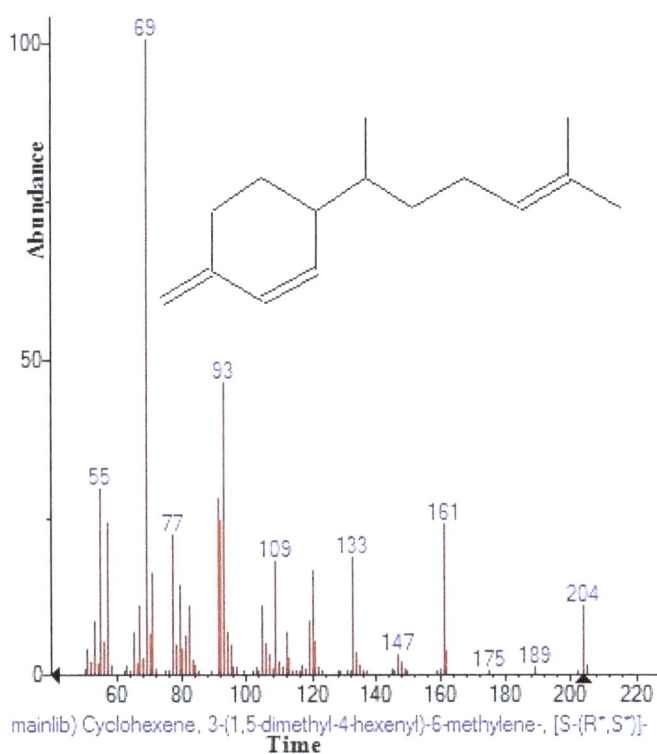

Figure 17. Structure of Cyclohexene ,3-(1,5-dimethyl-4-hexenyl)-6-methylene-,[S-(R*,S*)] present in *Cassia angustifolia* with RT= 10.508 using GC-MS analysis.

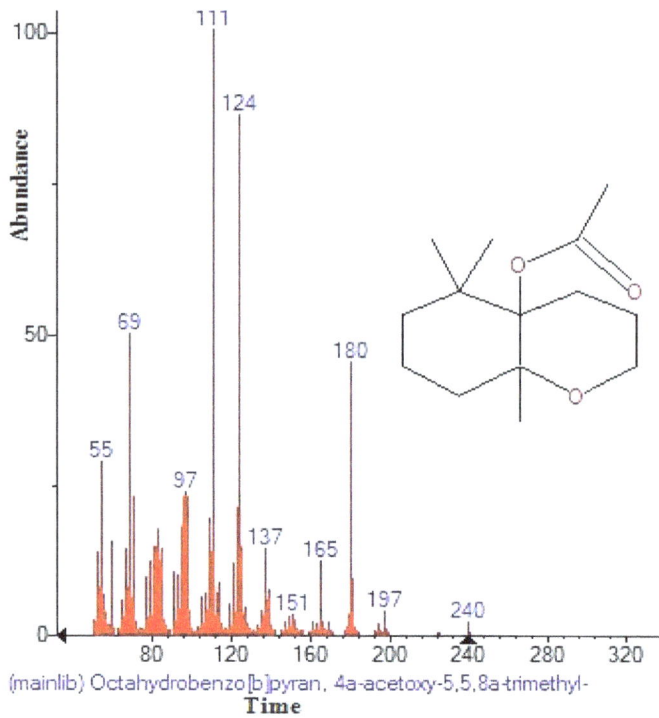

(mainlib) Octahydrobenzo[b]pyran, 4a-acetoxy-5,5,8a-trimethyl-

Figure 18. Structure of Octahydrobenzo[b]pyran,4a-acetoxy-5,5,8a,-trimethyl present in *Cassia angustifolia* with RT= 10.771 using GC-MS analysis.

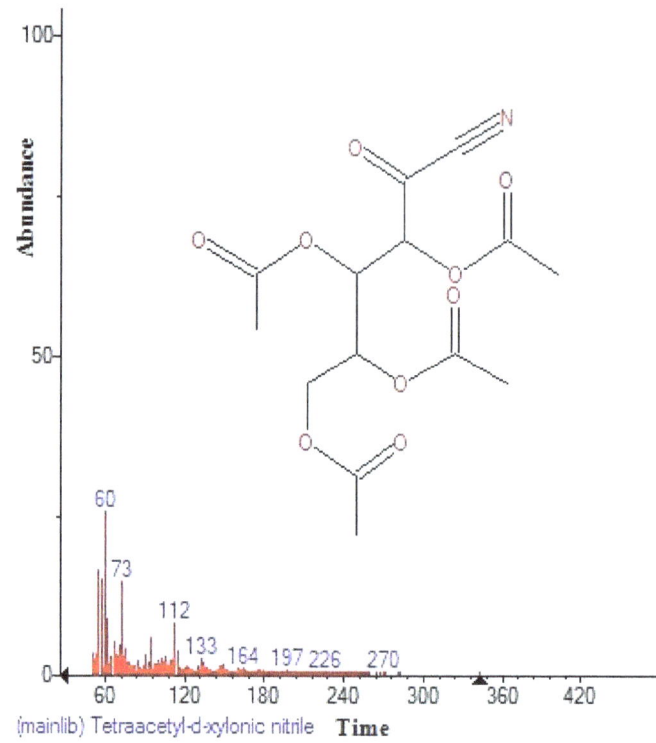

(mainlib) Tetraacetyl-d-xylonic nitrile

Figure 20. Structure of Tetraacetyl-d-xylonic nitrile present in *Cassia angustifolia* with RT= 11.012 using GC-MS analysis.

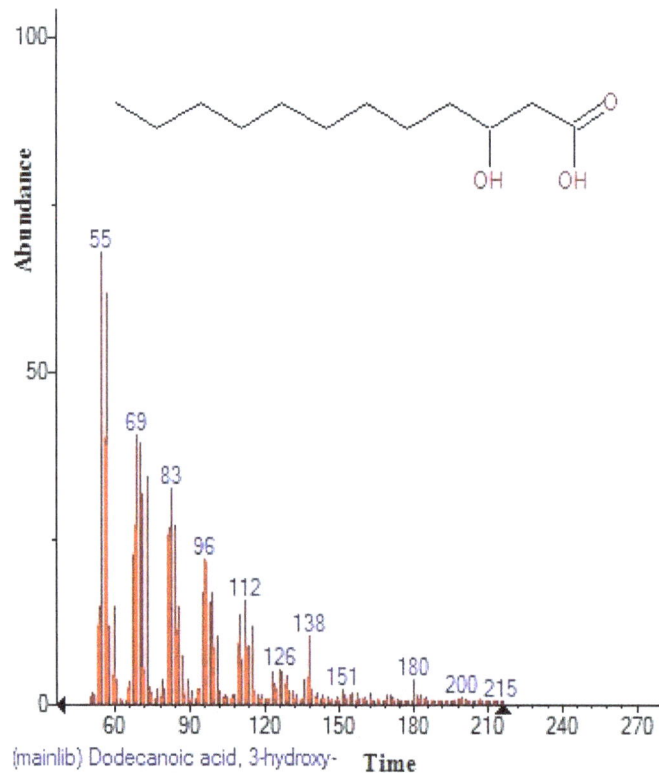

(mainlib) Dodecanoic acid, 3-hydroxy-

Figure 19. Structure of Dodecanoic acid , 3-hydroxy present in *Cassia angustifolia* with RT= 11.218 using GC-MS analysis.

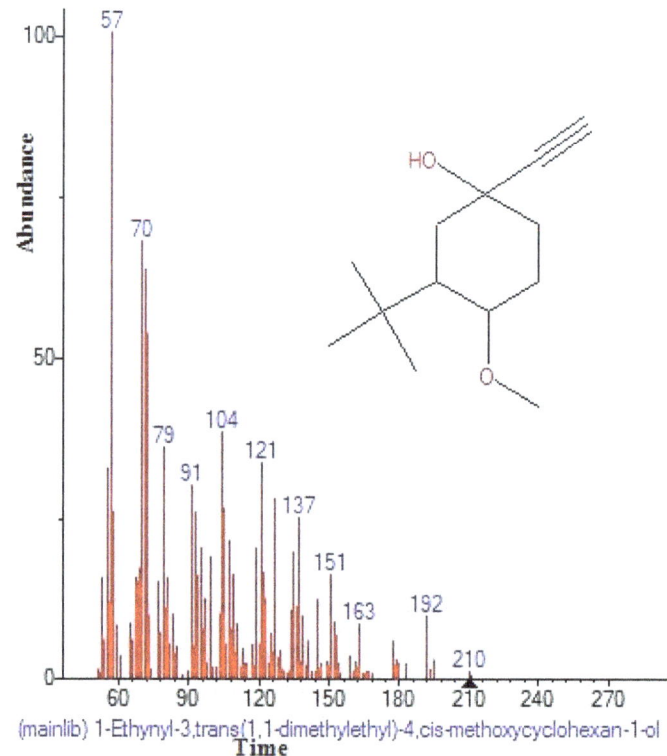

(mainlib) 1-Ethynyl-3,trans(1,1-dimethylethyl)-4,cis-methoxycyclohexan-1-ol

Figure 21. Structure of 1-Ethenyl 3,trans(1,1-dimethylethyl)-4,cis-methoxycyclohexan-1-ol present in *Cassia angustifolia* with RT= 11.246 using GC-MS analysis.

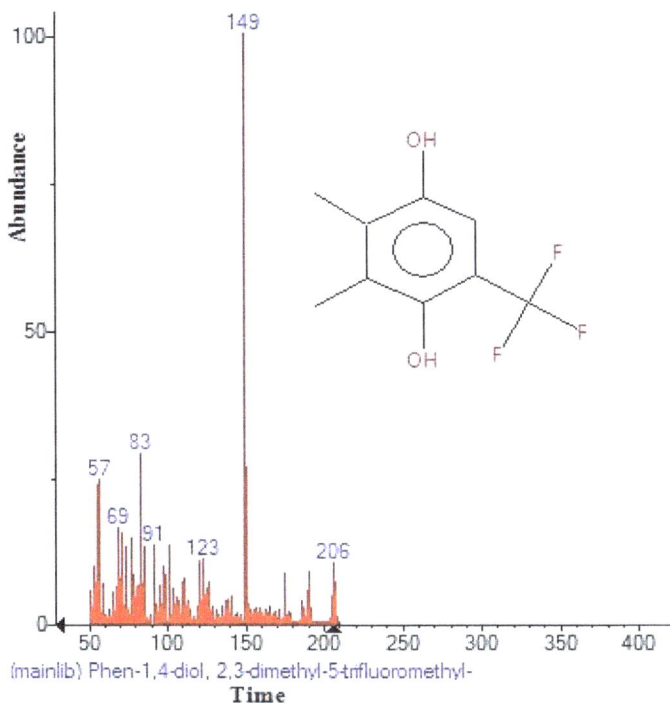

Figure 22. Structure of Phen-1,4-diol,2,3-dimethyl-5-trifluoromethyl present in *Cassia angustifolia* with RT= 11.378 using GC-MS analysis.

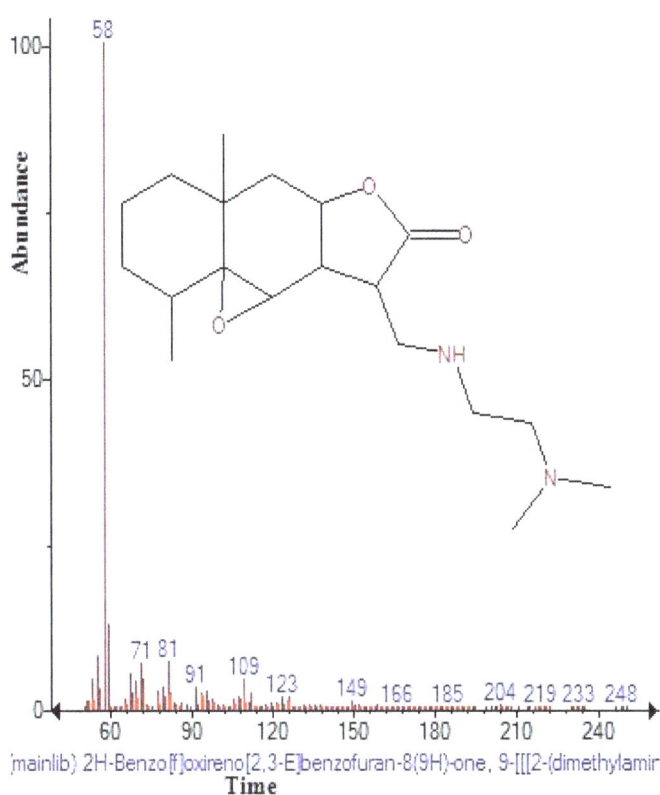

Figure 24. Structure of 2H-Benzo[f]oxireno[2,3-E]benzofuran-8(9H)-one,9-[[[2-(dimethylamin present in *Cassia angustifolia* with RT= 12.877 using GC-MS analysis.

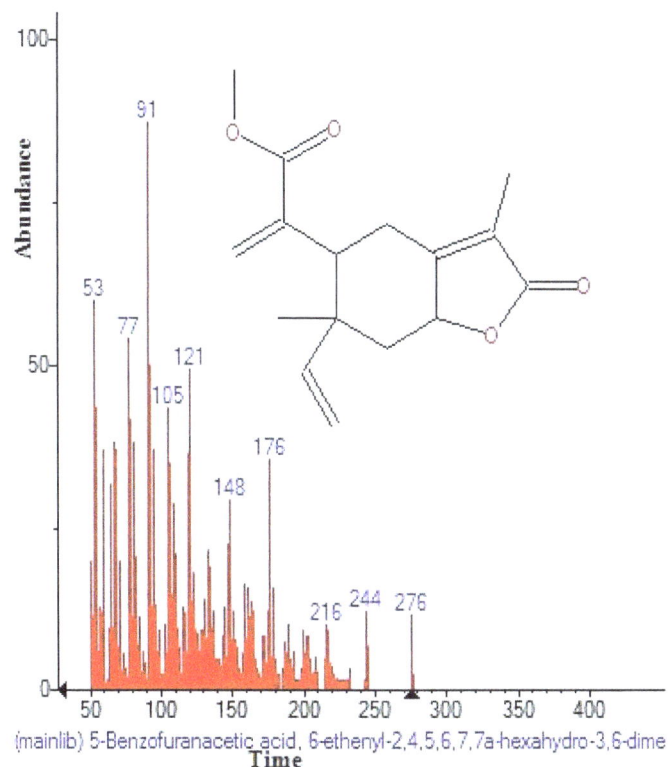

Figure 23. Structure of 5-Benzofuranacetic acid,6-ethenyl - 2,4,5,6,7,7a-hexahydro-3,6-dime present in *Cassia angustifolia* with RT= 12.036 using GC-MS analysis.

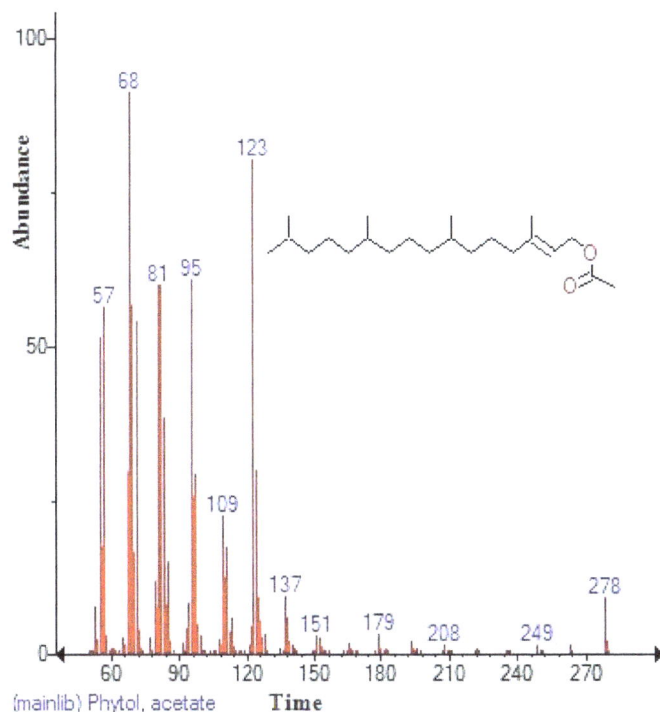

Figure 25. Structure of Phytol, acetate present in *Cassia angustifolia* with RT= 13.953 using GC-MS analysis.

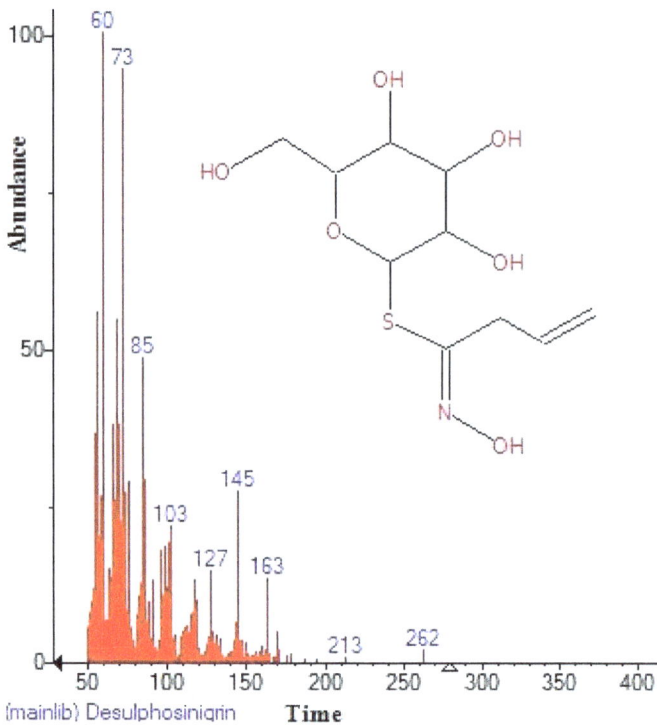

Figure 26. Structure of Desulphosiniqrin present in *Cassia angustifolia* with RT= 14.399 using GC-MS analysis.

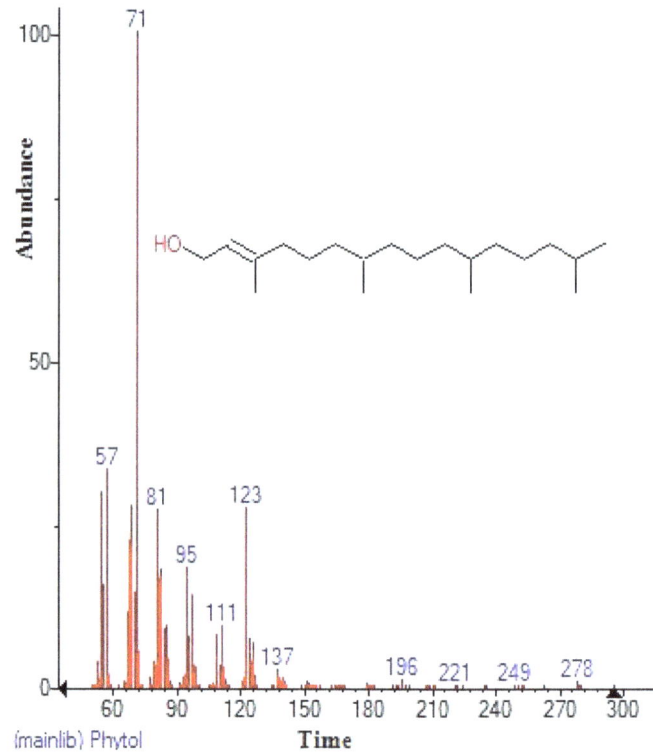

Figure 28. Structure of Phytol present in *Cassia angustifolia* with RT= 16.665 using GC-MS analysis.

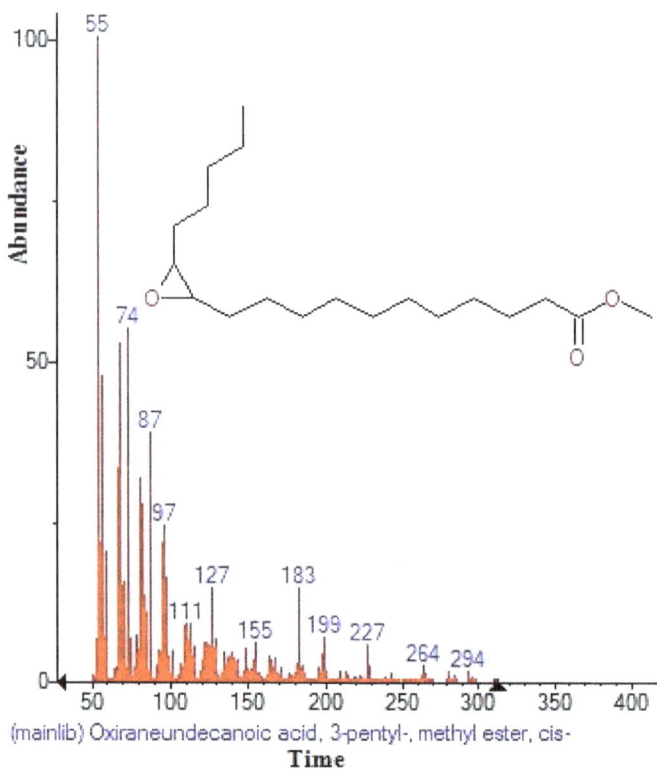

Figure 27. Structure of Oxiraneundecanoic acid ,3-pentyl-,methyl ester , cis present in *Cassia angustifolia* with RT= 16.482 using GC-MS analysis.

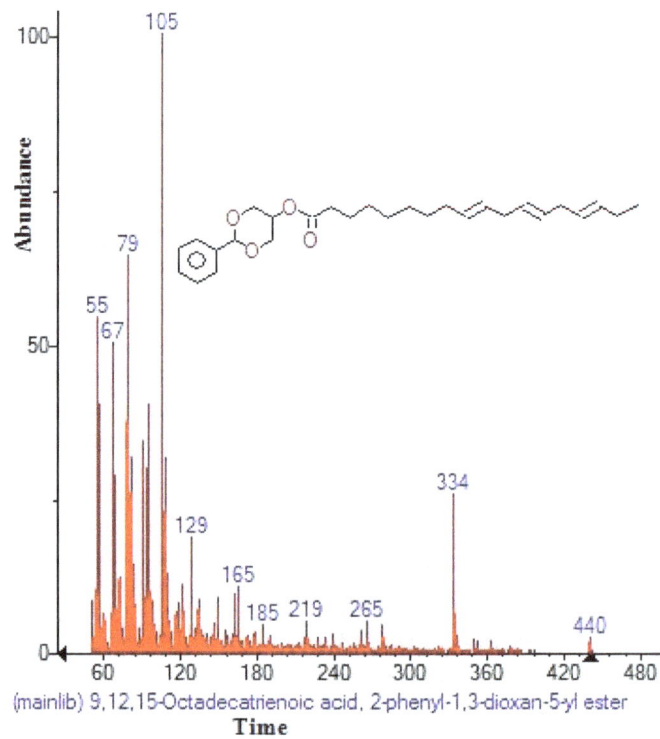

Figure 29. Structure of 9,12,15-Octadecatrienoic acid , 2-phenyl 1,3-dioxan-5-yl ester present in *Cassia angustifolia* with RT= 18.29 using GC-MS analysis.

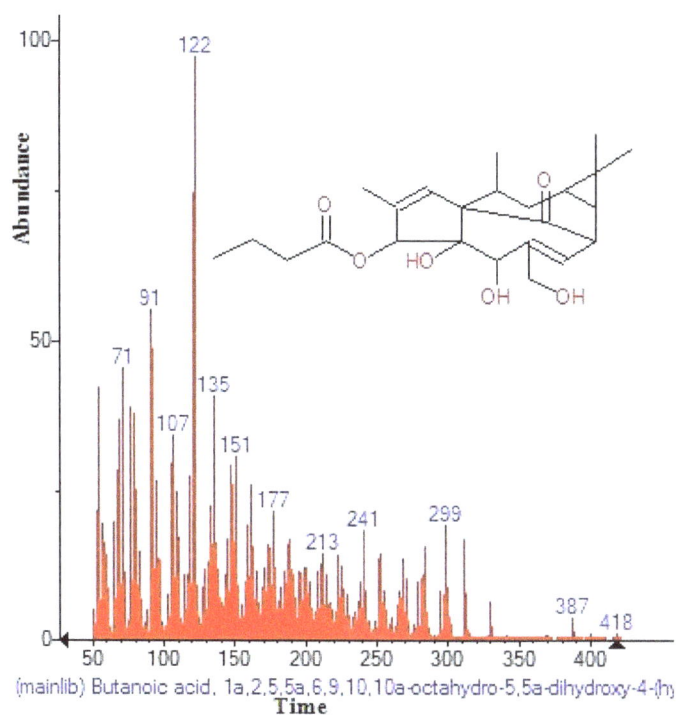

(mainlib) Butanoic acid, 1a,2,5,5a,6,9,10,10a-octahydro-5,5a-dihydroxy-4-(h)

Figure 30. Structure of Butanoic acid, 1a,2,5,5a,6,9,10,10a-octahydro-5,5adihydroxy-4-(h) present in *Cassia angustifolia* with RT= 18.874 using GC-MS analysis.

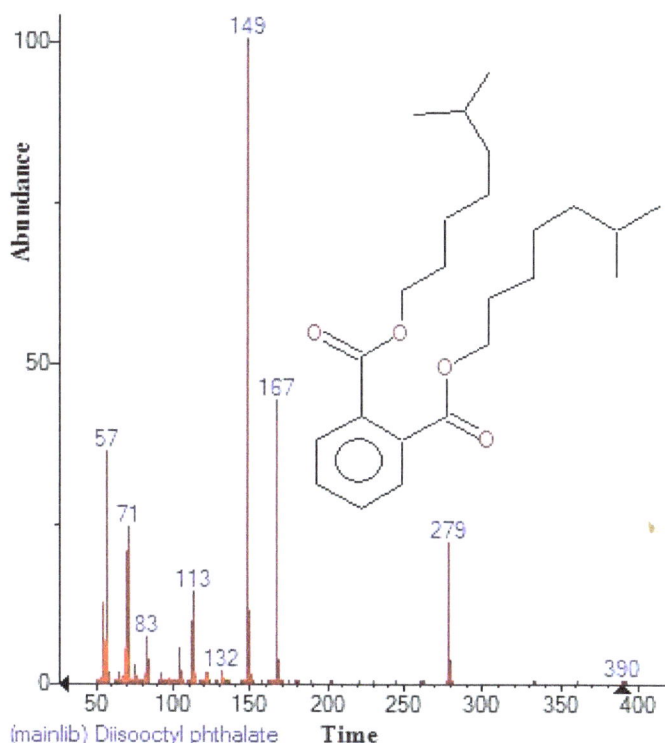

(mainlib) Diisooctyl phthalate

Figure 32. Structure of Diisooctyl phthalate present in *Cassia angustifolia* with RT= 20.373 using GC-MS analysis.

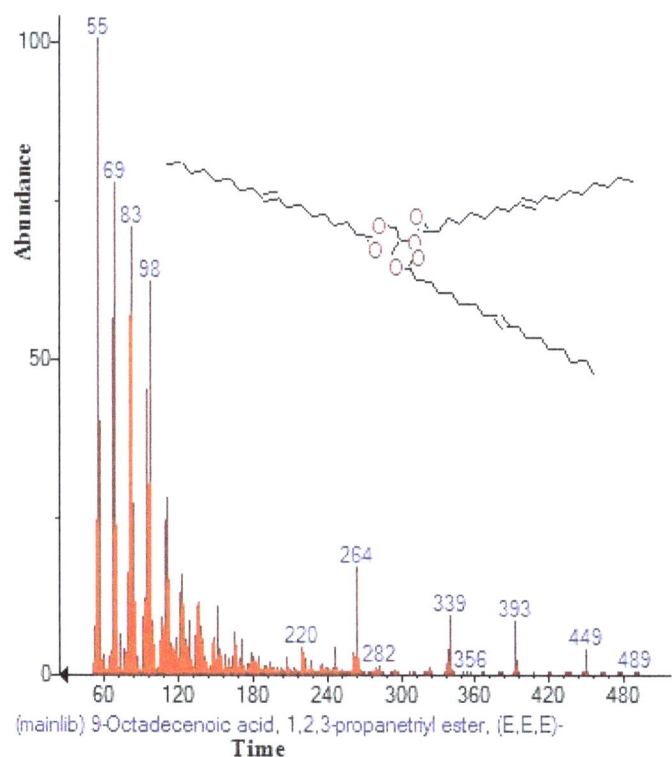

(mainlib) 9-Octadecenoic acid, 1,2,3-propanetriyl ester, (E,E,E)-

Figure 31. Structure of 9-Octadecenoic acid , 1,2,3-propanetriyl ester , (E,E,E) present in *Cassia angustifolia* with RT= 19.846 using GC-MS analysis.

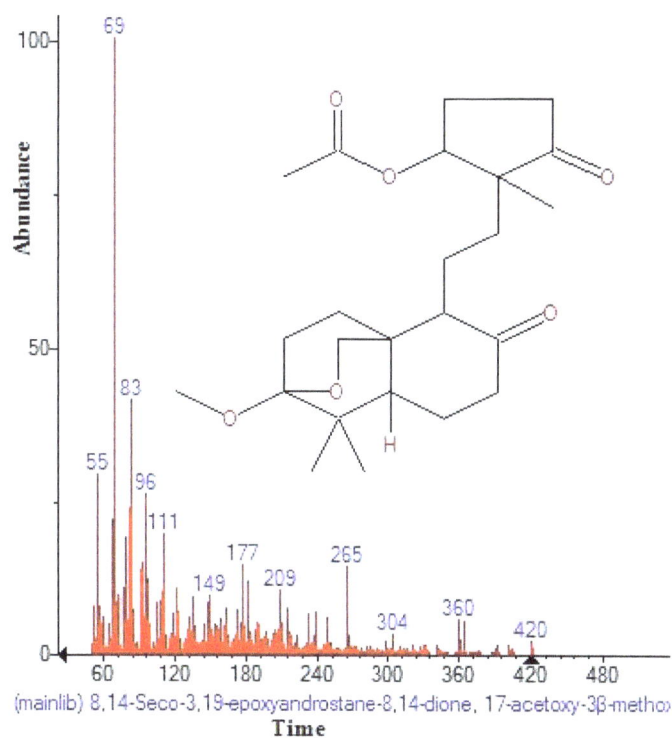

(mainlib) 8,14-Seco-3,19-epoxyandrostane-8,14-dione, 17-acetoxy-3β-metho>

Figure 33. Structure of 8,14-Seco -3,19-epoxyandrostane-8,14-dione,17-acetoxy-3ß-methoxy present in *Cassia angustifolia* with RT= 21.449 using GC-MS analysis.

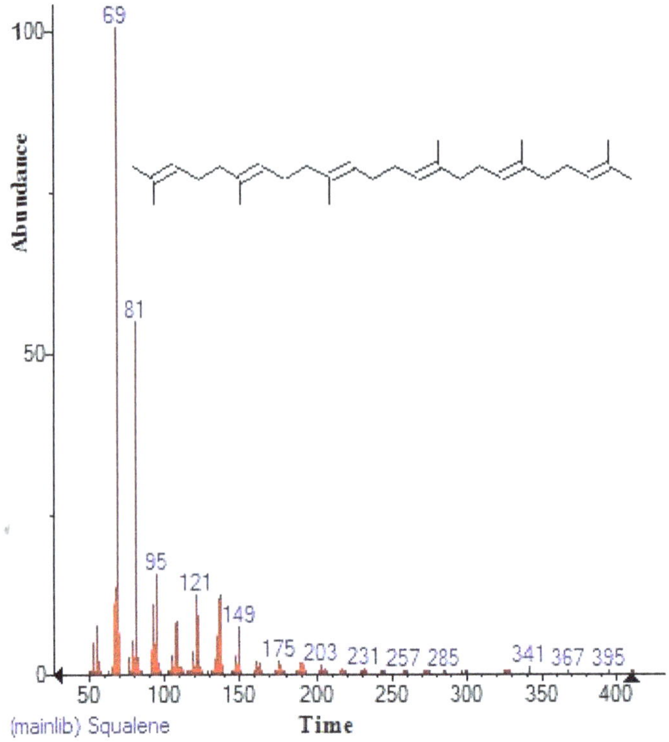

Figure 34. Structure of Squalene present in *Cassia angustifolia* with RT= 22.604 using GC-MS analysis.

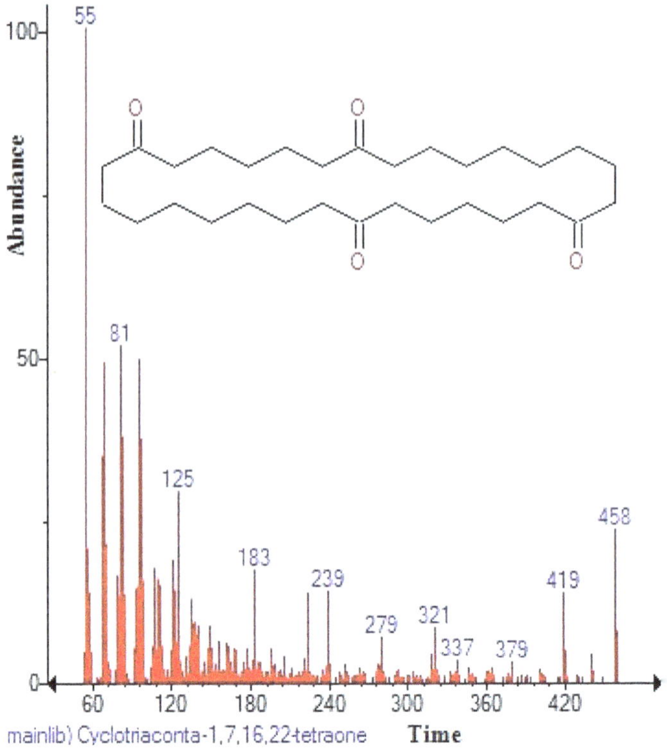

Figure 36. Structure of Cyclotriaconta-1,7,16,22,-tetraone present in *Cassia angustifolia* with RT= 23.159 using GC-MS analysis.

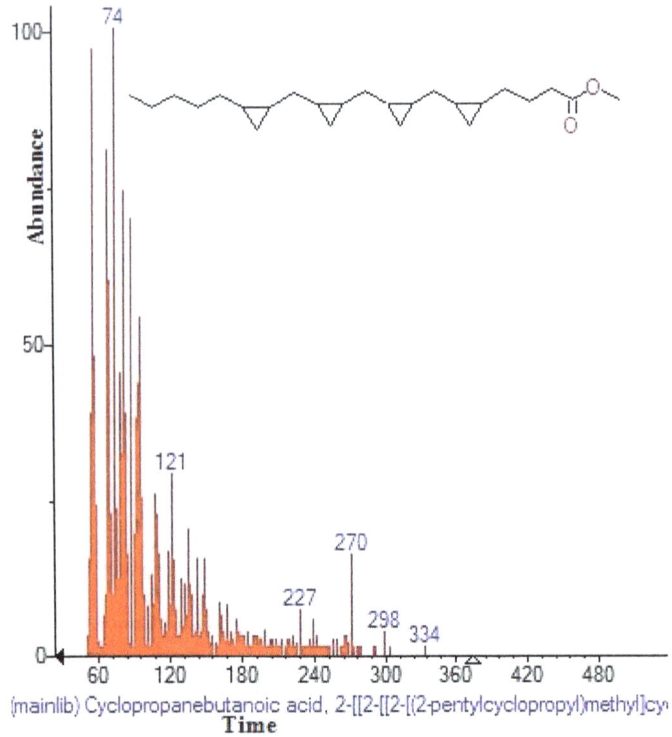

Figure 35. Structure of Cyclopropanebutanoic acid, 2-[[2-[[2-[(2-pentylcyclopropyl)methyl]cyclo present in *Cassia angustifolia* with RT= 22.845 using GC-MS analysis.

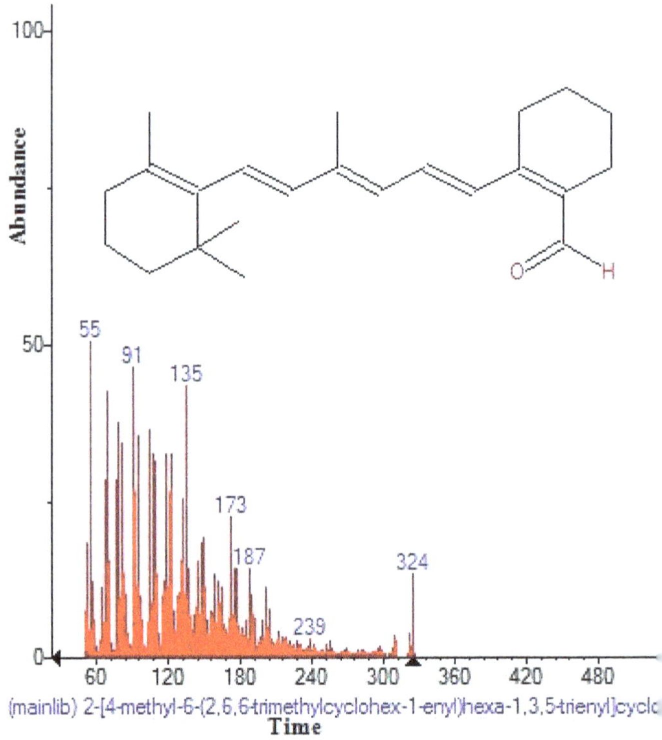

Figure 37. Structure of 2-[4-methyl-6-(2,6,6-trimethylcyclohex-1-enyl)hexa-1,3,5-trienyl]cyclo present in *Cassia angustifolia* with RT= 23.451using GC-MS analysis.

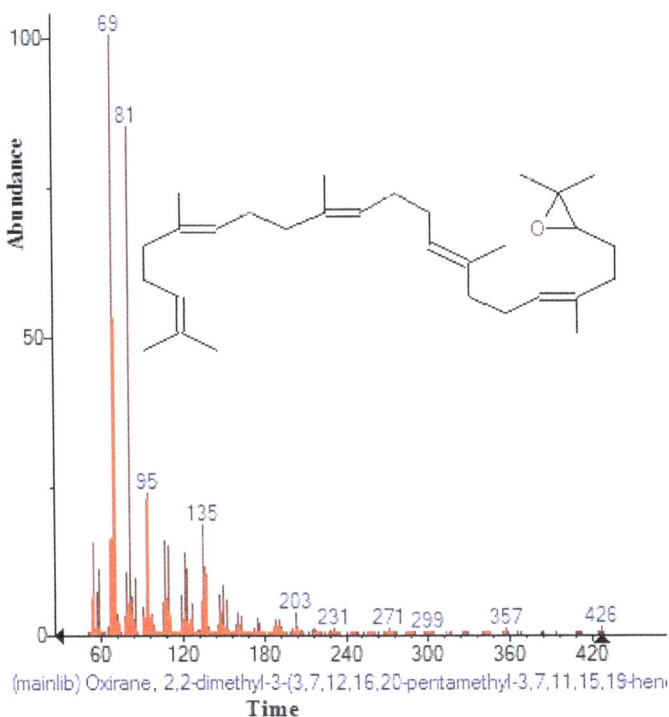

Figure 38. Structure of Oxirane ,2,2-dimethyl-3-(3,7,12,16,20-pentamethyl-3,7,11,15,19,-hen present in *Cassia angustifolia* with RT= 23.657 using GC-MS analysis.

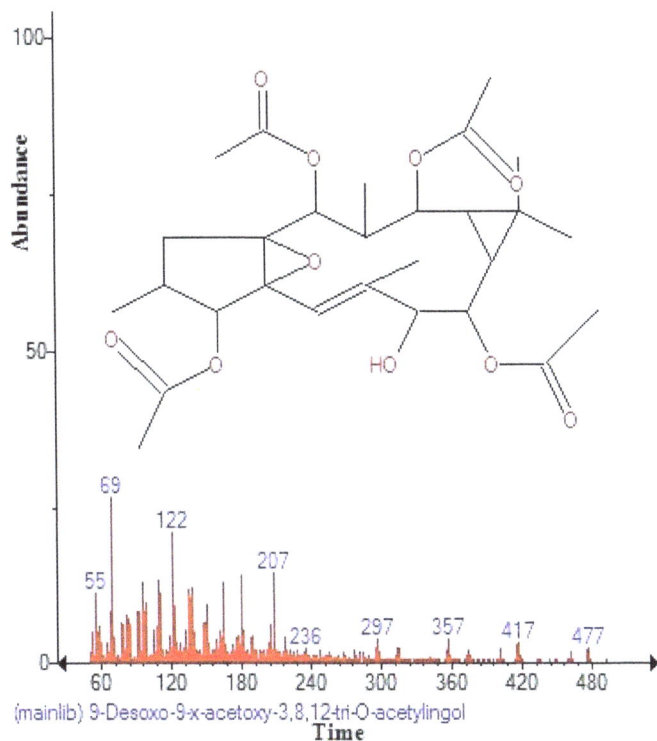

Figure 40. Structure of 9-Desoxo-9-x-acetoxy-3,8,12-tri-O-acetylingol present in *Cassia angustifolia* with RT= 25.025 using GC-MS analysis.

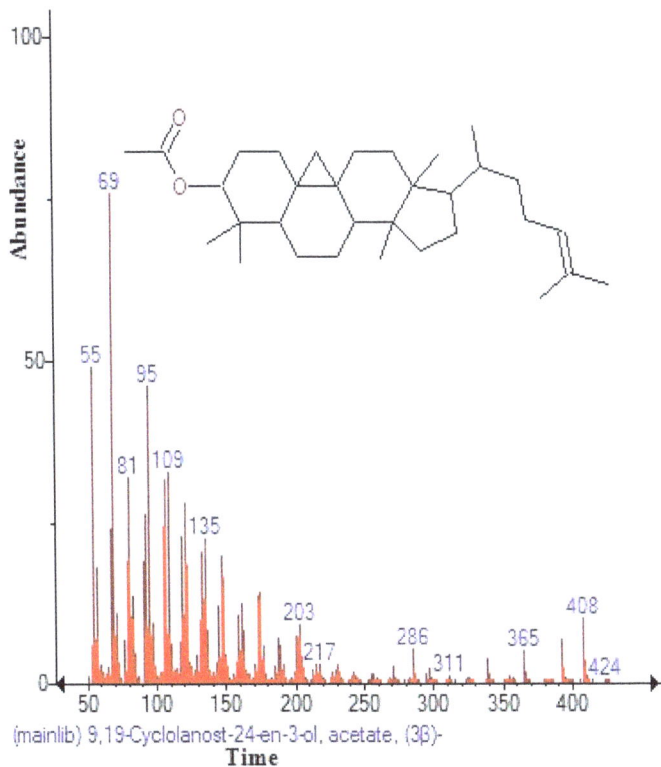

Figure 39. Structure of 9,19-Cyclolanost-24-en-3-ol,acetate , (3ß) present in *Cassia angustifolia* with RT= 23.686 using GC-MS analysis.

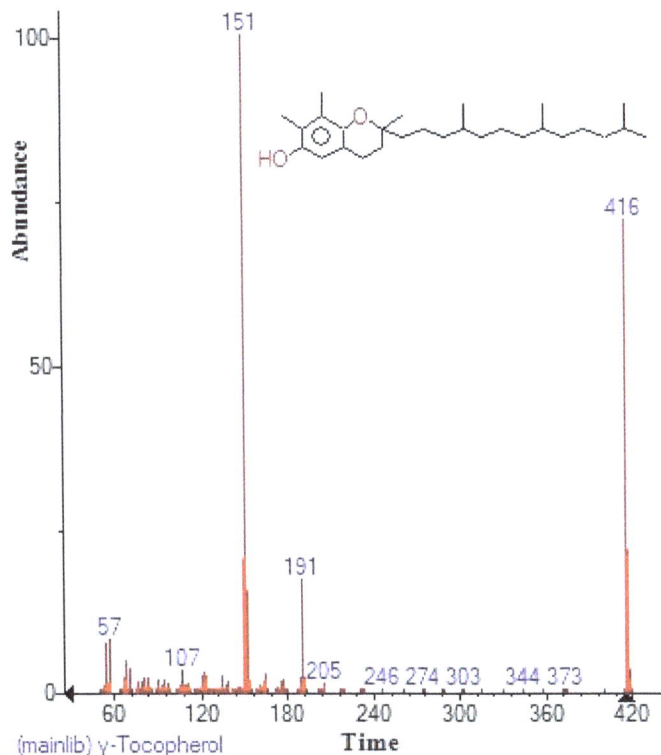

Figure 41. Structure of y-Tocopherol present in *Cassia angustifolia* with RT= 25.236 using GC-MS analysis.

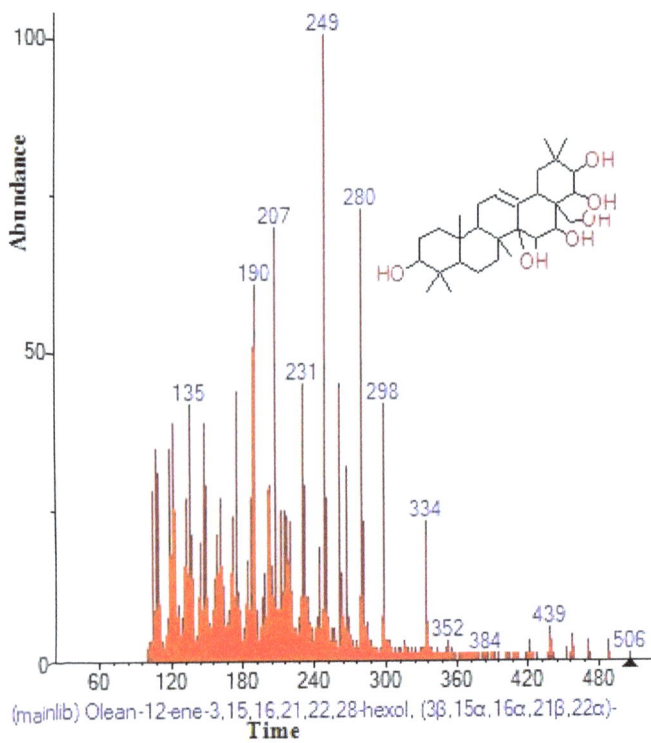

Figure 42. Structure of Olean-12-ene-3,15,16,21,22,28-hexol,(3ß,15α,16α,21ß,22α) present in *Cassia angustifolia* with RT= 25.683 using GC-MS analysis.

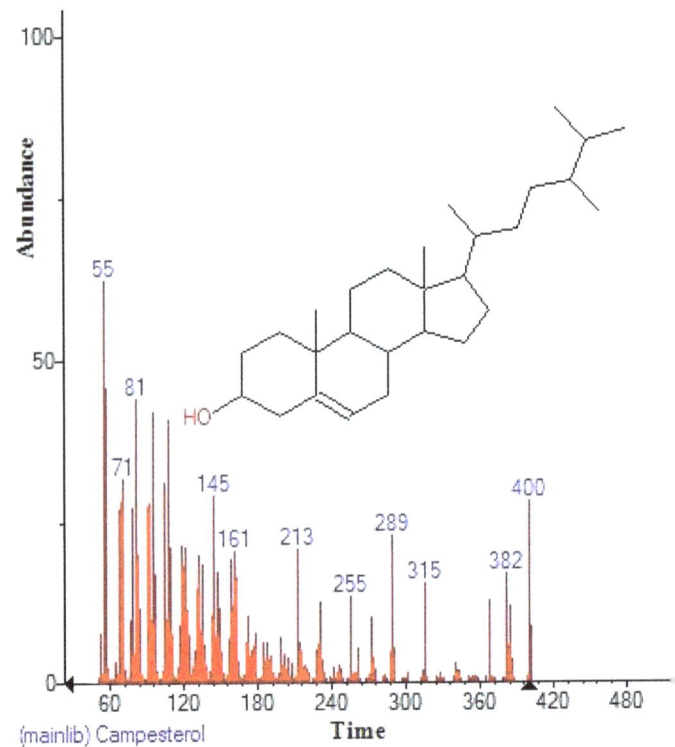

Figure 44. Structure of Campesterol present in *Cassia angustifolia* with RT= 28.315 using GC-MS analysis.

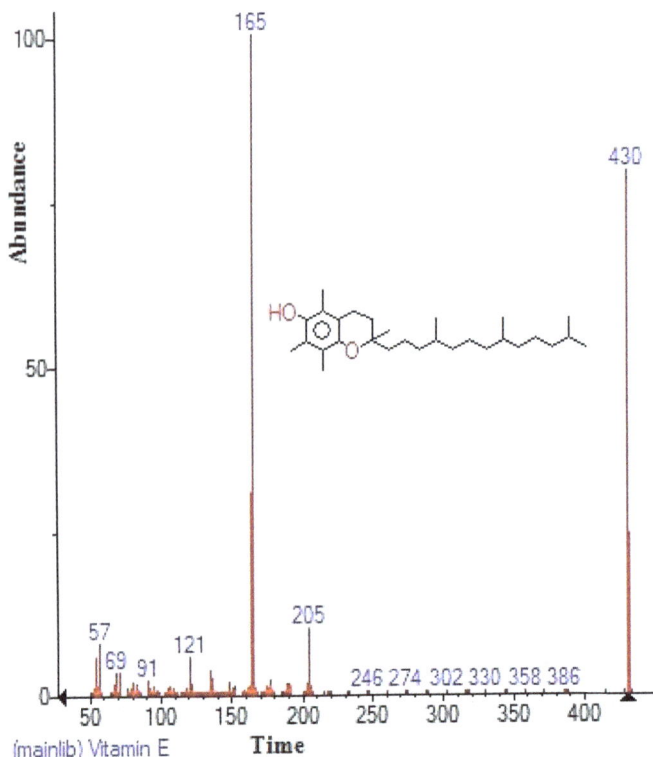

Figure 43. Structure of Vitamin E present in *Cassia angustifolia* with RT= 26.581 using GC-MS analysis.

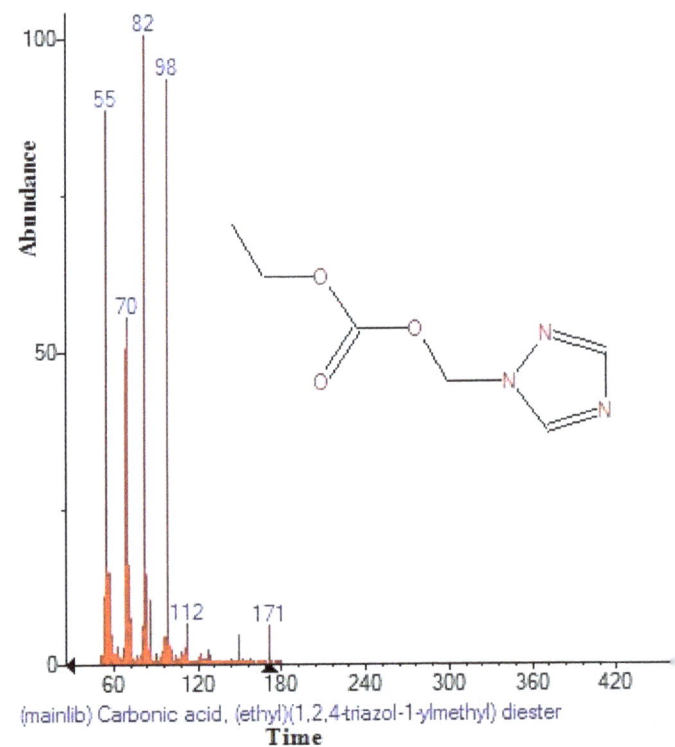

Figure 45. Structure of Carbonic acid, (ethyl)(1,2,4-triazol-1-ylmethyl)diester present in *Cassia angustifolia* with RT= 3.224 using GC-MS analysis.

ACKNOWLEDGEMENT

The authors thank Dr. Abdul-Kareem Al-Bermani, Lecturer, Department of Biology, for valuable suggestions and encouragement.

REFERENCES

Altameme HJ, Hameed IH, Idan SA, Hadi MY (2015a). Biochemical analysis of *Origanum vulgare* seeds by Fourier-transform infrared (FTIR) spectroscopy and gas chromatography-mass spectrometry (GCMS). J. Pharmacogn. Phytother. 7(9):221-237.

Altameme HJ, Hameed IH, Kareem MA (2015b). Analysis of alkaloid phytochemical compounds in the ethanolic extract of *Datura stramonium* and evaluation of antimicrobial activity. Afr. J. Biotechnol. 14(19):1668-1674.

Bako SP, Bakfur MJ, John I, Bala EI (2005). Ethnomedicinal and Phytochemical profile of some savanna plant species in Nigeria. Int. J. Bot. 1(2):147-150.

Bansal S, Malwal M, Sarin R (2010). Antibacterial efficacy of some plants used in folkloric medicines in arid zone. J. Pharm. Res. 3(11):2640-2642.

Basgel S, Erdemoglu SB (2006). Determination of mineral and trace elements in some medicinal herbs and their infusions consumed in Turkey. Sci. Total Environ. 359:82-89.

Bournemouth PR (1992). British Herbal Compendium, Volume 1, BHMA, Bournemouth.

Chahal JK, Sarin R, Malwal M (2010). Efficacy of *Clerodendrum inerme* L. (Garden quinine) against some human pathogenic strains. Int. J. Pharm. Biol. Sci. 1(4):219-223.

Ernst E (1998). Harmless herbs: A review of the recent literature. Am. J. Med. 104(2):170-178.

Gupta RK (2010). Medicinal and Aromatic plants, 1st ed. CBS Publishers & Distributors, India. pp. 116-117.

Hameed IH, Hussein HJ, Kareem MA, Hamad NS (2015a). Identification of five newly described bioactive chemical compounds in methanolic extract of *Mentha viridis* by using gas chromatography-mass spectrometry (GC-MS). J. Pharmacogn. Phytother. 7(7):107-125.

Hameed IH, Ibraheam IA, Kadhim HJ (2015b). Gas chromatography mass spectrum and fourier-transform infrared spectroscopy analysis of methanolic extract of *Rosmarinus oficinalis* leaves. J. Pharmacogn. Phytother. 7(6):90-106.

Hameed IH, Jasim H, Kareem MA, Hussein AO (2015c). Alkaloid constitution of Nerium oleander using gas chromatography-mass spectroscopy (GC-MS). J. Med. Plants Res. 9(9):326-334.

Hameed IH, Hamza LF, Kamal SA (2015d). Analysis of bioactive chemical compounds of *Aspergillus niger* by using gas chromatography-mass spectrometry and Fourier-transform infrared spectroscopy. J. Pharmacogn. Phytother. 7(8):132-163.

Hamza LF, Kamal SA, Hameed IH (2015). Determination of metabolites products by *Penicillium expansum* and evaluating antimicrobial activity. J. PharmacogN. Phytother. 7(9):194-220.

Hoffmann D (1990). The new holistic herbal: A herbal celebrating the wholeness of life. Element Books.

Hussein AO, Hameed IH, Jasim H, Kareem MA (2015). Determination of alkaloid compounds of *Ricinus communis* by using gas chromatography-mass spectroscopy (GC-MS). J. Med. Plants Res. 9(10):349-359.

Imad H, Mohammed A, Aamera J (2014a). Genetic variation and DNA markers in forensic analysis. Afr. J. Biotechnol. 13(31):3122-3136.

Imad H, Mohammed A, Cheah Y, Aamera J (2014b). Genetic variation of twenty autosomal STR loci and evaluate the importance of these loci for forensic genetic purposes. Afr. J. Biotechnol. 13:1-9.

Imad H, Muhanned A, Aamera J, Cheah Y (2014c). Analysis of eleven Y-chromosomal STR markers in middle and south of Iraq. Afr. J. Biotechnol. 13(38):3860-3871.

Jasim H, Hussein AO, Hameed IH, Kareem MA (2015). Characterization of alkaloid constitution and evaluation of antimicrobial activity of *Solanum nigrum* using gas chromatography mass spectrometry (GC-MS). J. Pharmacogn. Phytother. 7(4):56-72.

Kareem MA, Hussein AO, Hameed IH (2015). Y-chromosome short tandem repeat, typing technology, locus information and allele frequency in different population: A review. Afr. J. Biotechnol. 14(27):2175-2178.

Kinjo J, Ikeda T, Watanabe K, Nohara T (1994). An anthraquinone glycoside from *Cassia angustifolia* leaves. Phytochemistry 37(6):1685-1687.

Malwal M, Sarin R (2011). Antimicrobial efficacy of Murray koenigii (Linn.) Spreng root extract. Indian J. Nat. Prod. Res. 2(1):48-51.

Mills SY (1993). The Essential Book of Herbal Medicine, Penguin, London (First published in 1991 as Out of the Earth, Arkana.

Mohammed A, Imad H (2013). Autosomal STR: From locus information to next generation sequencing technology. Res. J. Biotechnol. 8(10):92-105.

Sarin R (2005). Useful metabolites from plant tissue culture. Biotechnology 4(2):79-83.

Seth R, Sarin R (2010). Analysis of the phytochemical content and antimicrobial activity of *J. gossypifolia* L. Arch. Appl. Sci. Res. 2(5):285-291.

Sofowora EA (1982). The State of Medicinal Plants' Research in Nigeria. Ibadan University Press, Nigeria. P 404.

Spiller H, Winter M, Weber J, Krenzelok E, Anderson D, Ryan M (2003). Skin breakdown and blisters from senna-containing laxatives in young children. Ann. Pharmacother. 37(5):636-639.

Vanderperren B, Rizzo M, Angenot L, Haufroid V, Jadoul M, Hantson P (2005). Acute liver failure with renal impairment related to the abuse of senna anthraquinone glycosides. Ann. Pharmacother. 39(7-8):1353-1357.

Permissions

All chapters in this book were first published in JPP, by Academic Journals; hereby published with permission under the Creative Commons Attribution License or equivalent. Every chapter published in this book has been scrutinized by our experts. Their significance has been extensively debated. The topics covered herein carry significant findings which will fuel the growth of the discipline. They may even be implemented as practical applications or may be referred to as a beginning point for another development.

The contributors of this book come from diverse backgrounds, making this book a truly international effort. This book will bring forth new frontiers with its revolutionizing research information and detailed analysis of the nascent developments around the world.

We would like to thank all the contributing authors for lending their expertise to make the book truly unique. They have played a crucial role in the development of this book. Without their invaluable contributions this book wouldn't have been possible. They have made vital efforts to compile up to date information on the varied aspects of this subject to make this book a valuable addition to the collection of many professionals and students.

This book was conceptualized with the vision of imparting up-to-date information and advanced data in this field. To ensure the same, a matchless editorial board was set up. Every individual on the board went through rigorous rounds of assessment to prove their worth. After which they invested a large part of their time researching and compiling the most relevant data for our readers.

The editorial board has been involved in producing this book since its inception. They have spent rigorous hours researching and exploring the diverse topics which have resulted in the successful publishing of this book. They have passed on their knowledge of decades through this book. To expedite this challenging task, the publisher supported the team at every step. A small team of assistant editors was also appointed to further simplify the editing procedure and attain best results for the readers.

Apart from the editorial board, the designing team has also invested a significant amount of their time in understanding the subject and creating the most relevant covers. They scrutinized every image to scout for the most suitable representation of the subject and create an appropriate cover for the book.

The publishing team has been an ardent support to the editorial, designing and production team. Their endless efforts to recruit the best for this project, has resulted in the accomplishment of this book. They are a veteran in the field of academics and their pool of knowledge is as vast as their experience in printing. Their expertise and guidance has proved useful at every step. Their uncompromising quality standards have made this book an exceptional effort. Their encouragement from time to time has been an inspiration for everyone.

The publisher and the editorial board hope that this book will prove to be a valuable piece of knowledge for researchers, students, practitioners and scholars across the globe.

List of Contributors

Idayat Titilayo Gbadamosi
Department of Botany, University of Ibadan, Nigeria

C. N. Fokunang and E. Tembe-Fokunang
Department of Pharmacotoxicology and Pharmacokinetics, Faculty of Medicine and Biomedical Sciences, University of Yaoundé I, Yaoundé Cameroon

F. K. Mushagalusa
Department of Pharmacy, Faculty of Medicine and Pharmacy, Official University of Bukavu, Bukavu, Democratic Republic of Congo

J. Ngoupayo, B. Ngameni and B. T. Ngadjui
Department of Pharmacognosy and Pharmaceutical chemistry, University of Bamenda, Cameroon

L. N. Njinkio and F. A. Kechia
Department of Medical Laboratory Sciences, University of Bamenda, Cameroon

B. Atogho-Tiedeu
Department of Biochemistry, Faculty of Sciences; University of Yaounde I, Yaounde, Cameroon

J. N. Kadima and W. F. Mbacham
Department of Pharmacology, School of Medicine and Health Sciences, University of Rwanda, Rwanda

Abdelkrim Berroukche, Abdelkrim Attaoui and Mustafa Loth
Laboratory of BioToxicology, Pharmacognosy and Biological Recycling of Plants Biology Department, Faculty of Sciences, Moulay Tahar University, Saida 20000, Algeria

Iwara Arikpo Iwara, Godwin Oju Igile, Friday Effiong Uboh, Kelvin Ngwu Elot and Mbeh Ubana Eteng
Department of Biochemistry, Faculty of Basic Medical Sciences, University of Calabar, P. M. B. 1115, Calabar, Nigeria

Riham O. Bakr
Department of Pharmacognosy, Faculty of Pharmacy, MSA University, Giza 11787, Egypt

Shaza A. Mohamed
Department of Pharmacognosy, Faculty of Pharmacy, Al-Azhar University (Girls), Cairo, Egypt

Nermien E. Waly
Department of Physiology, Faculty of Medicine, Helwan University, Helwan 11795, Egypt

Hussein J. Hussein and Imad Hadi Hameed
Department of Biology, Babylon University, Iraq

Mohammed Yahya Hadi
College of Biotechnology, Al-Qasim Green University, Iraq

M. Laadim, M. L. Ouahidi, L. Zidane, A. El Hessni, A. Ouichou and A. Mesfioui
Laboratory of Genetics, Neuroendocrinology and Biotechnology, Department of Biology, Faculty of Sciences, Ibn Tofail University, Kenitra, Morocco

Sneeha Veerakumar and Safreen Shaikh Dawood Amanulla
Department of Biotechnology, Periyar Maniammai University, Vallam, Thanjavur-613 403, India

Kumaresan Ramanathan
Department of Biotechnology, Periyar Maniammai University, Vallam, Thanjavur-613 403, India
Department of Biochemistry, Institute of Biomedical Sciences, College of Health Sciences, Mekelle University (Ayder Campus), Mekelle, Ethiopia

Abdullah-Al-Ragib and Md. Tanvir Hossain
Department of Applied Chemistry and Chemical Engineering, Noakhali Science and Technology University, Sonapur, Noakhali-3814, Bangladesh

Javed Hossain
Department of Pharmacy, International Islamic University Chittagong, Chittagong-4314, Bangladesh

Md. Jakaria
Department of Pharmacy, International Islamic University Chittagong, Chittagong-4314, Bangladesh
Department of Pharmacy, Southern University Bangladesh, Chittagong-4000, Bangladesh

Amel M. Kamal, Mohamed I. S. Abdelhady, Heba Tawfeek and Eman G. Haggag
Department of Pharmacognosy, Faculty of Pharmacy, Helwan University, Cairo 11795, Egypt

Maha G. Haggag
Department of Microbiology, Research Institute of Ophthalmology, Giza, Egypt

Ghaidaa Jihadi Mohammed
College of Science, Al-Qadisia University, Iraq

Imad Hadi Hameed
Department of Biology, Babylon University, Iraq

Mohanad Jawad Kadhim
Department of Genetic Engineering, Al-Qasim Green University, Iraq

Azhar Abdulameer Sosa
College of Education for Women, Al-Qadisyia University, Iraq

Imad Hadi Hameed
College of Nursing, Babylon University, Iraq

Mojirayo Rebecca Ibukunoluwa
Department of Biology, Adeyemi College of Education, Ondo State, Nigeria

Kanokwan Kiattisin, Thananya Nantarat and Pimporn Leelapornpisid
Department of Pharmaceutical Sciences, Faculty of Pharmacy, Chiang Mai University, Suthep Road, Chiang Mai, Thailand

Celestine Uzoma Aguoru, Christopher Gbokaiji Bashayi and Innocent Okonkwo Ogbonna
Department of Biological Sciences, University of Agriculture, Makurdi, Benue State, Nigeria

Sameer H. Qari
Biology Department, Aljamom University College, Umm Al-Qura University Saudi Arabia

José Luis Martínez-Rodríguez, Claudia Araceli Reyes-Estrada and Rosalinda Gutiérrez- Hernández
Doctorado en Ciencias en la Especialidad en Farmacología Médica y Molecular de la Unidad Académica de Medicina Humana y Ciencias de la Salud de la Universidad Autónoma de Zacatecas. Campus Siglo XXI, Kilómetro 6, Ejido la Escondida, CP 98160. Zacatecas, Zac. México

Jesús Adrián López
Laboratorio de microRNAs de la Unidad Académica de Ciencias Biológicas de la Universidad Autónoma de Zacatecas. Av. Preparatoria S/N, Hidraulica, CP 98068 Zacatecas, Zac. México

Shihab Uddin
Department of Biochemistry and Molecular Biology, Jahangirnagar University, Savar, Bangladesh

Md. Mahmodul Islam
Department of Pharmacy, Dhaka International University, Banani, Dhaka, Bangladesh

Md. Mynul Hassan
Dept of Biotechnology and Genetic Engineering, Khulna University, Khulna, Bangladesh

Amrita Bhowmik
Department of Applied Laboratory Sciences, Bangladesh University of Health Sciences, Dhaka, Bangladesh

Begum Rokeya
Department of Pharmacology, Bangladesh University of Health Sciences, Dhaka, Bangladesh

Ali Hussein Al-Marzoqi and Imad Hadi Hameed
Department of Biology, Babylon University, Hilla City, Iraq

Mohammed Yahya Hadi
College of Biotechnology, Al-Qasim Green University, Iraq

Index